YO-BTA-217

ANNUAL EDITIONS

Health 10/11

Thirty-First Edition

EDITOR

Eileen L. Daniel
SUNY at Brockport

Eileen Daniel, a registered dietitian and licensed nutritionist, is a Professor in the Department of Health Science and Associate Dean of Professions at the State University of New York at Brockport. She received a BS in Nutrition and Dietetics from the Rochester Institute of Technology in 1977, an MS in Community Health Education from SUNY at Brockport in 1987, and a PhD in Health Education from the University of Oregon in 1986. A member of the American Dietetics Association and other professional and community organizations, Dr. Daniel has published more than 40 journal articles on issues of health, nutrition, and health education. She is also the editor of *Taking Sides: Clashing Views on Controversial Issues in Health and Society,* ninth edition, (McGraw-Hill/ Contemporary Learning Series, 2010).

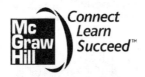

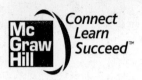

Connect
Learn
Succeed™

ANNUAL EDITIONS: HEALTH, THIRTY-FIRST EDITION

Published by McGraw-Hill, a business unit of The McGraw-Hill Companies, Inc., 1221 Avenue of the Americas, New York, NY 10020. Copyright © 2010 by The McGraw-Hill Companies, Inc. All rights reserved. Previous edition(s) 1978–2009. No part of this publication may be reproduced or distributed in any form or by any means, or stored in a database or retrieval system, without the prior written consent of The McGraw-Hill Companies, Inc., including, but not limited to, in any network or other electronic storage or transmission, or broadcast for distance learning.

Some ancillaries, including electronic and print components, may not be available to customers outside the United States.

Annual Editions® is a registered trademark of the McGraw-Hill Companies, Inc.

Annual Editions is published by the **Contemporary Learning Series** group within the McGraw-Hill Higher Education division.

1 2 3 4 5 6 7 8 9 0 QPD/QPD 0 9

ISBN 978–0–07–812783–0
MHID 0–07–812783–1
ISSN 0278–4653

Managing Editor: *Larry Loeppke*
Senior Managing Editor: *Faye Schilling*
Developmental Editor: *Debra Henricks*
Editorial Coordinator: *Mary Foust*
Editorial Assistant: *Cindy Hedley*
Production Service Assistant: *Rita Hingtgen*
Permissions Coordinator: *Lenny J. Behnke*
Senior Marketing Manager: *Julie Keck*
Senior Marketing Communications Specialist: *Mary Klein*
Marketing Coordinator: *Alice Link*
Project Manager: *Joyce Watters*
Design Specialist: *Tara McDermott*
Senior Production Supervisor: *Laura Fuller*
Cover Graphics: *Kristine Jubeck*

Compositor: Laserwords Private Limited
Cover Image: © Digital Vision Ltd. (inset); © Design Pics/Punchstock (background)

Library in Congress Cataloging-in-Publication Data
Main entry under title: Annual Editions: Health. 2010/2011.
 1. Health—Periodicals. I. Daniel, Eileen L., *comp.* II. Title: Health.
658'.05

www.mhhe.com

Editors/Academic Advisory Board

Members of the Academic Advisory Board are instrumental in the final selection of articles for each edition of ANNUAL EDITIONS. Their review of articles for content, level, and appropriateness provides critical direction to the editors and staff. We think that you will find their careful consideration well reflected in this volume.

ANNUAL EDITIONS: Health 10/11
31st Edition

EDITOR

Eileen L. Daniel
SUNY at Brockport

ACADEMIC ADVISORY BOARD MEMBERS

Harry Barney
Clemens College

David Birch
Southern Illinois University at Carbondale

F. Stephen Bridges
University of West Florida

Jeff Burnett
Fort Hays State University

Evia L. Davis
Langston University

Diane Dettmore
Fairleigh Dickinson University

Jonathan Deutsch
Kingsborough Community College

Brad Engeldinger
Sierra College

William English
Clarion University of Pennsylvania

Kelly Evans
Brigham Young University—Idaho

Julie Feeny
Illinois Central College

Lisa K. Fender-Scarr
University of Akron

Bernard Frye
University of Texas at Arlington

Zaje A.T. Harrell
Michigan State University

Nicholas K. Iammarino
Rice University

Allen Jackson
Chadron State College

John Janowiak
Appalachian State University

Barry Johnson
Forsyth Technical Community College

John Judkins
University of Phoenix

Manjit Kaur
East Los Angeles College

Julie Leonard
Ohio State University—Marion

Gary Liguori
North Dakota State University

Willis McAleese
Idaho State University

M.J. McMahon
Northern Arizona University

Danny Mielke
Eastern Oregon University

Laura M. Miller
Edinboro University

Scott J. Modell
California State University—Sacramento

Linda Mukina Felker
Edinboro University

Judy Peel
North Carolina State University

John A. Perrotto
Nassau Community College

Glen J. Peterson
Lakewood Community College

Susan K. (Skip) Pollock
Mesa Community College

Thomas G. Porrazzo
Alvernia College

Joshua Searcy
Central State University

Loren Toussaint
Luther College

Alex Waigandt
University of Missouri—Columbia

Kenneth Wolf
Anne Arundel Community College

Deborah A. Wuest
Ithaca College

Elizabeth Zicha
Muskingum College

Lana Zinger
Queensborough Community College

Preface

In publishing ANNUAL EDITIONS we recognize the enormous role played by the magazines, newspapers, and journals of the public press in providing current, first-rate educational information in a broad spectrum of interest areas. Many of these articles are appropriate for students, researchers, and professionals seeking accurate, current material to help bridge the gap between principles and theories and the real world. These articles, however, become more useful for study when those of lasting value are carefully collected, organized, indexed, and reproduced in a low-cost format, which provides easy and permanent access when the material is needed. That is the role played by ANNUAL EDITIONS.

America is in the midst of a revolution that is changing the way millions of Americans view their health. Traditionally, most people delegated responsibility for their health to their physicians and hoped that medical science would be able to cure whatever ailed them. This approach to health care emphasized the role of medical technology and funneled billions of dollars into medical research. The net result of all this spending is the most technically advanced and expensive health care system in the world. In an attempt to rein in health care costs, the health care delivery system moved from privatized health care coverage to what is termed "managed care."

While managed care has turned the tide regarding the rising cost of health care, it has done so by limiting reimbursement for many cutting edge technologies. Unfortunately, many people also feel that it has lowered the overall quality of care that is being given. Perhaps the saving grace is that we live at a time in which chronic illnesses, rather than acute illnesses, are our number one health threat, and many of these illnesses can be prevented or controlled by our lifestyle choices. The net result of these changes has prompted millions of individuals to assume more personal responsibility for safeguarding their own health. Evidence of this change in attitude can be seen in the growing interest in nutrition, physical fitness, dietary supplements, and stress management.

If we, as a nation, are to capitalize on this new health consciousness, we must devote more time and energy to educating Americans in the health sciences, so that they will be better able to make informed choices about their health. Health is a complex and dynamic subject, and it is practically impossible for anyone to stay abreast of all the current research findings. In the past, most of us have relied on books, newspapers, magazines, and television as our primary sources for medical/health information, but today, with the widespread use of personal computers connected to the World Wide Web, it is possible to access vast amounts of health information, any time of the day, without even leaving one's home. Unfortunately, quantity and availability does not necessarily translate into quality, and this is particularly true in the area of medical/health information. Just as the Internet is a great source for reliable timely information, it is also a vehicle for the dissemination of misleading and fraudulent information.

Currently, there are no standards or regulations regarding the posting of health content on the Internet, and this has led to a plethora of misinformation and quackery in the medical/health arena. Given this vast amount of health information, our task as health educators is twofold: (1) To provide our students with the most up-to-date and accurate information available on major health issues of our time, and (2) to teach our students the skills that will enable them to sort out facts from fiction in order to become informed consumers. *Annual Editions: Health 10/11* was designed to aid this task. It offers a sampling of quality articles that represent the latest thinking on a variety of health issues, and it also serves as a tool for developing critical thinking skills.

The articles in this volume were carefully chosen on the basis of their quality and timeliness. Because this book is revised and updated annually, it contains information that is not generally available in any standard textbook. As such, it serves as a valuable resource for both teachers and students. This edition of *Annual Editions: Health* has been updated to reflect the latest thinking on a variety of contemporary health issues. We hope that you find this edition to be a helpful learning tool filled with information and the presentation user-friendly. The 10 topical areas presented in this edition mirror those that are normally covered in introductory health courses: Promoting Healthy Behavior Change, Stress and Mental Health, Nutritional Health, Exercise and Weight Management, Drugs and Health, Sexuality and Relationships, Preventing and Fighting Disease, Health Care and the Health Care System, Consumer Health, and Contemporary Health Hazards. Because of the interdependence of the various elements that constitute health, the articles selected were written by authors with diverse educational backgrounds and expertise including: naturalists, environmentalists, psychologists, economists, sociologists, nutritionists, consumer advocates, and traditional health practitioners.

Annual Editions: Health 10/11 was designed to be one of the most useful and up-to-date publications currently available in the area of health. Please let us know what you think of it by filling out and returning the postage paid *article rating form* on the last page of this book. Any anthology can be improved. This one will be—annually.

Elieen L. Daniel
Editor

Contents

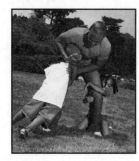

UNIT 1
Promoting Healthy Behavior Change

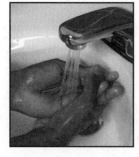

UNIT 2
Stress and Mental Health

The concepts in bold italics are developed in the article. For further expansion, please refer to the Topic Guide.

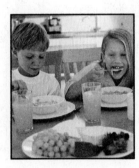

UNIT 3
Nutritional Health

The concepts in bold italics are developed in the article. For further expansion, please refer to the Topic Guide.

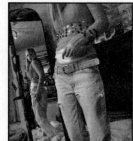

UNIT 4
Exercise and Weight Management

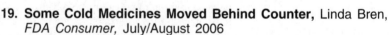

UNIT 5
Drugs and Health

The concepts in bold italics are developed in the article. For further expansion, please refer to the Topic Guide.

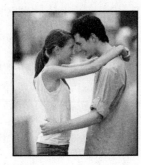

UNIT 6
Sexuality and Relationships

The concepts in bold italics are developed in the article. For further expansion, please refer to the Topic Guide.

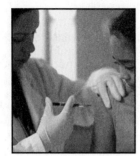

UNIT 7
Preventing and Fighting Disease

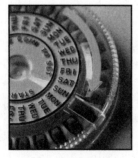

UNIT 8
Health Care and the Health Care System

The concepts in bold italics are developed in the article. For further expansion, please refer to the Topic Guide.

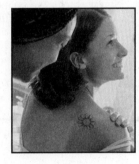

UNIT 9
Consumer Health

The concepts in bold italics are developed in the article. For further expansion, please refer to the Topic Guide.

UNIT 10
Contemporary Health Hazards

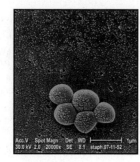

The concepts in bold italics are developed in the article. For further expansion, please refer to the Topic Guide.

The concepts in bold italics are developed in the article. For further expansion, please refer to the Topic Guide.

Correlation Guide

The *Annual Editions* series provides students with convenient, inexpensive access to current, carefully selected articles from the public press. **Annual Editions: Health 10/11** is an easy-to-use reader that presents articles on important topics such as *consumer health, exercise, nutrition,* and many more. For more information on *Annual Editions* and other *McGraw-Hill Contemporary Learning Series* titles, visit www.mhhe.com/cls.

This convenient guide matches the units in **Annual Editions: Health 10/11** with the corresponding chapters in three of our best-selling McGraw-Hill Health textbooks by Hahn et al., Payne et al., and Insel/Roth.

Annual Editions: Health 10/11	Focus on Health, 10/e by Hahn et al.	Understanding Your Health, 11/e by Payne et al.	Core Concepts in Health, 11/e by Insel/Roth
Unit 1: Promoting Healthy Behavior Change	**Chapter 1:** Shaping Your Health	**Chapter 1:** Shaping Your Health	**Chapter 1:** Taking Charge of Your Health
Unit 2: Stress and Mental Health	**Chapter 2:** Achieving Psychological Health **Chapter 3:** Managing Stress	**Chapter 2:** Achieving Psychological Health **Chapter 3:** Managing Stress	**Chapter 2:** Stress: The Constant Challenge **Chapter 3:** Psychological Health
Unit 3: Nutritional Health	**Chapter 5:** Understanding Nutrition and Your Diet	**Chapter 5:** Understanding Nutrition and Your Diet	**Chapter 12:** Nutrition Basics
Unit 4: Exercise and Weight Management	**Chapter 4:** Becoming Physically Fit **Chapter 6:** Maintaining a Healthy Weight	**Chapter 4:** Becoming Physically Fit **Chapter 6:** Maintaining a Healthy Weight	**Chapter 13:** Exercise for Health and Fitness **Chapter 14:** Weight Management
Unit 5: Drugs and Health	**Chapter 7:** Making Decisions About Drug and Alcohol Use **Chapter 8:** Rejecting Tobacco Use	**Chapter 7:** Making Decisions About Drug Use **Chapter 8:** Taking Control of Alcohol Use **Chapter 9:** Rejecting Tobacco Use	**Chapter 9:** The Use and Abuse of Psychoactive Drugs **Chapter 10:** The Responsible Use of Alcohol **Chapter 11:** Toward a Tobacco-Free Society
Unit 6: Sexuality and Relationships	**Chapter 12:** Understanding Sexuality **Chapter 13:** Managing Your Fertility	**Chapter 14:** Exploring the Origins of Sexuality **Chapter 15:** Understanding Sexual Behavior and Relationships **Chapter 16:** Managing Your Fertility **Chapter 17:** Becoming a Parent	**Chapter 4:** Intimate Relationships and Communication **Chapter 5:** Sex and Your Body **Chapter 8:** Pregnancy and Childbirth
Unit 7: Preventing and Fighting Disease	**Chapter 9:** Reducing Your Risk of Cardiovascular Disease **Chapter 10:** Living with Cancer and Chronic Conditions **Chapter 11:** Preventing Infectious Diseases	**Chapter 10:** Enhancing Your Cardiovascular Health **Chapter 11:** Living with Cancer **Chapter 12:** Managing Chronic Conditions **Chapter 13:** Preventing Infectious Diseases	**Chapter 15:** Cardiovascular Health **Chapter 16:** Cancer **Chapter 17:** Immunity and Infection **Chapter 18:** Sexually Transmitted Diseases
Unit 8: Health Care and the Health Care System	**Chapter 14:** Becoming an Informed Health Care Consumer	**Chapter 18:** Becoming an Informed Health Care Consumer	**Chapter 20:** Conventional and Complementary Medicine
Unit 9: Consumer Health	**Chapter 15:** Protecting Your Safety	**Chapter 19:** Protecting Your Safety	**Chapter 21:** Personal Safety
Unit 10: Contemporary Health Hazards	**Chapter 16:** The Environment and Your Health	**Chapter 20:** The Environment and Your Health	**Chapter 19:** Environmental Health

Topic Guide

This topic guide suggests how the selections in this book relate to the subjects covered in your course. You may want to use the topics listed on these pages to search the web more easily.

On the following pages a number of websites have been gathered specifically for this book. They are arranged to reflect the units of this Annual Editions reader. You can link to these sites by going to *http://www.mhcls.com*.

All the articles that relate to each topic are listed below the bold-faced term.

Internet References

The following Internet sites have been selected to support the articles found in this reader. These sites were available at the time of publication. However, because websites often change their structure and content, the information listed may no longer be available. We invite you to visit http://www.mhcls.com for easy access to these sites.

Annual Editions: Health 10/11

General Sources

National Institute on Aging (NIA)
http://www.nia.nih.gov/

The NIA, one of the institutes of the U.S. National Institutes of Health, presents this home page to lead you to a variety of resources on health and lifestyle issues on aging.

U.S. Department of Agriculture (USDA)/Food and Nutrition Information Center (FNIC)
http://www.nal.usda.gov/fnic/

Use this site to find nutrition information provided by various USDA agencies, to find links to food and nutrition resources on the Internet, and to access FNIC publications and databases.

U.S. Department of Health and Human Services
http://www.os.dhhs.gov

This site has extensive links to information on such topics as the health benefits of exercise, weight control, and prudent lifestyle choices.

U.S. National Institutes of Health (NIH)
http://www.nih.gov

Consult this site for links to extensive health information and scientific resources. Comprising 24 separate institutes, centers, and divisions, the NIH is one of eight health agencies of the Public Health Service, which, in turn, is part of the U.S. Department of Health and Human Services.

U.S. National Library of Medicine
http://www.nlm.nih.gov

This huge site permits a search of a number of databases and electronic information sources such as MEDLINE. You can learn about research projects and programs and peruse the national network of medical libraries here.

World Health Organization
http://www.who.int/en

This home page of the World Health Organization will provide links to a wealth of statistical and analytical information about health around the world.

UNIT 1: Promoting Healthy Behavior Change

Columbia University's Go Ask Alice!
http://www.goaskalice.columbia.edu/index.html

This interactive site provides discussion and insight into a number of personal issues of interest to college-age people and often those younger and older. Many questions about physical and emotional health and well-being are answered.

The Society of Behavioral Medicine
http://www.sbm.org/

This site provides listings of major, general health institutes and organizations as well as discipline-specific links and resources in medicine, psychology, and public health.

UNIT 2: Stress and Mental Health

The American Institute of Stress
http://www.stress.org

This site provides comprehensive information on stress: its dangers, the beliefs that build helpful techniques for overcoming stress, and so on. This easy-to-navigate site has good links to information on anxiety and related topics.

National Mental Health Association (NMHA)
http://www.nmha.org/index.html

The NMHA is a citizen volunteer advocacy organization that works to improve the mental health of all individuals. The site provides access to guidelines that individuals can use to reduce stress and improve their lives in small, yet tangible, ways.

Self-Help Magazine
http://www.selfhelpmagazine.com/index.html

Reach lots of links to self-help resources on the Net at this site, including resources on stress, anxiety, fears, and more.

UNIT 3: Nutritional Health

The American Dietetic Association
http://www.eatright.org

This organization, along with its National Center of Nutrition and Dietetics, promotes optimal nutrition, health, and well-being. This easy-to-navigate site presents FAQs about nutrition and dieting, nutrition resources, and career and member information.

Center for Science in the Public Interest (CSPI)
http://www.cspinet.org/

CSPI is a nonprofit education and advocacy organization that focuses on improving the safety and nutritional quality of our food supply and on reducing the health problems caused by alcohol. This agency also evaluates the nutritional composition of fast foods, movie popcorn, and chain restaurants. There are also good links to related sites.

Food and Nutrition Information Center
http://www.nalusda.gov/fnic/index.html

This is an official Agriculture Network Information Center website. The FNIC is one of several information centers at the National Agriculture Library, the Agricultural Research Service, and the U.S. Department of Agriculture. The website has information on nutrition-related publications, an index of food and nutrition related Internet resources, and an on-line catalog of materials.

UNIT 4: Exercise and Weight Management

American Society of Exercise Physiologists (ASEP)
http://www.asep.org

Internet References

The ASEP is devoted to promoting people's health and physical fitness. This extensive site provides links to publications related to exercise and career opportunities in exercise physiology.

Cyberdiet
http://www.cyberdiet.com/reg/index.html

This site, maintained by a registered dietician, offers CyberDiet's interactive nutritional profile, food facts, menus and meal plans, and exercise and food-related sites.

Shape Up America!
http://www.shapeup.org

At the Shape Up America! website you will find the latest information about safe weight management, healthy eating, and physical fitness.

UNIT 5: Drugs and Health

Food and Drug Administration (FDA)
http://www.fda.gov/

This site includes FDA news, information on drugs, and drug toxicology facts.

National Institute on Drug Abuse (NIDA)
http://www.nida.nih.gov/

Use this site index for access to NIDA publications and communications, information on drugs of abuse, and links to other related websites.

UNIT 6: Sexuality and Relationships

Planned Parenthood
http://www.plannedparenthood.org/

This home page provides links to information on contraceptives (including outercourse and abstinence) and to discussions of other topics related to sexual health.

Sexuality Information and Education Council of the United States (SIECUS)
http://www.siecus.org/

SIECUS is a nonprofit, private advocacy group that affirms that sexuality is a natural and healthy part of living. This home page offers publications, what's new, descriptions of programs, and a listing of international sexuality education initiatives.

UNIT 7: Preventing and Fighting Disease

American Cancer Society
http://www.cancer.org

Open this site and its various links to learn the concerns and lifestyle advice of the American Cancer Society. It provides information on tobacco and alternative cancer therapies.

American Diabetes Association Home Page
http://www.diabetes.org

This site offers information on diabetes including treatment, diet, and insulin therapy.

American Heart Association
http://www.amhrt.org

This award-winning, comprehensive site of the American Heart Association offers information on heart disease, prevention, patient facts, eating plans, what's new, nutrition, smoking cessation, and FAQs.

National Institute of Allergy and Infectious Diseases (NIAID)
http://www3.niaid.nih.gov/

Open this site and its various links to learn the concerns and lifestyle advice of the National Institute of Allergy and Infectious Diseases.

UNIT 8: Health Care and the Health Care System

American Medical Association (AMA)
http://www.ama-assn.org

The AMA offers this site to find up-to-date medical information, peer-review resources, discussions of such topics as HIV/AIDS and women's health, examination of issues related to managed care, and important publications.

MedScape: The Online Resource for Better Patient Care
http://www.medscape.com

For health professionals and interested consumers, this site offers peer-reviewed articles, self-assessment features, medical news, and annotated links to Internet resources. It also contains the Morbidity & Mortality Weekly Report, which is a publication of the Centers for Disease Control and Prevention.

UNIT 9: Consumer Health

FDA Consumer Magazine
http://www.fda.gov/fdac

This site offers articles and information that appears in the FDA Consumer Magazine.

Global Vaccine Awareness League
http://www.gval.com

This site addresses side effects related to vaccination. Its many links are geared to provide copious information.

UNIT 10: Contemporary Health Hazards

Centers for Disease Control: Flu
http://www.cdc.gov/flu

This CDC site provides updates, information, key facts, questions and answers, and ways to prevent influenza (the flu). Updated regularly during the flu season.

Food and Drug Administration Mad Cow Disease Page
http://www.fda.gov/oc/opacom/hottopics/bse.html

This Food and Drug Administration page includes information, articles, and updates about Bovine Spongiform Encephalopathy (BSE) also known as "Mad Cow Disease."

Environmental Protection Agency
http://www.epa.gov

Use this site to find environmental health information provided by various EPA agencies.

UNIT 1

Promoting Healthy Behavior Change

Unit Selections

Key Points to Consider

- Why do you think people continue to engage in behaviors that affect their health even when they know about the ill effects of these behaviors? Do you engage in any behavior that you know will have negative impact on health? If so, why?

- What are the negative behaviors practiced by college students that contribute to academic difficulties?

- What is the relationship between health behaviors and sexuality?

- What factors contribute to a successful lifestyle change?

- What are the personal health behaviors that you would like to improve? What prevents you from making these changes?

- How can you overcome these obstacles?

- What are the social and economic issues that have an impact on health behaviors?

- What are the five domains linked to better health?

Student Website

www.mhcls.com

Internet References

Columbia University's Go Ask Alice!
   http://www.goaskalice.columbia.edu/index.html

The Society of Behavioral Medicine
   http://www.sbm.org/

"Those of us who protect our health daily and those of us who put our health in constant jeopardy have exactly the same mortality: 100 percent. The difference, of course, is the timing." This quotation from Elizabeth M. Whelan, ScD, MPH, reminds us that we must all face the fact that we are going to die sometime. The question that is decided by our behavior is when and, to a certain extent, how. This book, and especially this unit, is designed to assist students to develop the cognitive skills and knowledge that, when put to use, help make the moment of our death come after the greatest number of years possible, and to maintain our health as long as possible. While we cannot control many of the things that happen to us, we must all strive to accept personal responsibility for, and make informed decisions about, things that we can control. This is no minor task, but it is one in which the potential reward is life itself. Perhaps the best way to start this process is by educating ourselves on the relative risks associated with the various behaviors and lifestyle choices we make. To minimize on all the risks to life and health would be to significantly limit the quality of our lives, and while this might be a choice that some would make, it certainly is not the goal of health education. A more logical approach to risk reduction would be to educate the public on the relative risks associated with various behaviors and lifestyle choices, so that they are capable of making informed decisions. While it may seem obvious that certain behaviors, such as smoking, entail a high level of risk, the significance of others such as toxic waste sites and food additives are frequently blown out of proportion to the actual risks involved. The net result of this type of distortion is that many Americans tend to minimize the dangers of known hazards such as tobacco and alcohol, and focus attention, instead, on potentially minor health hazards over which they have little or no control.

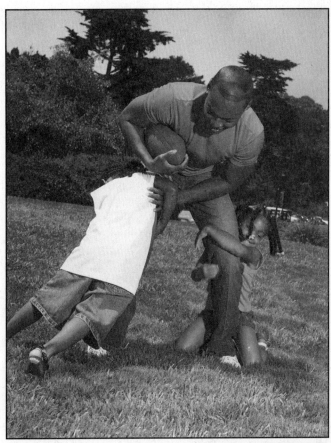

© Tanya Constantine/Getty Images

Educating the public on the relative risk of various health behaviors is only part of the job that health educators must tackle in order to assist individuals in making informed choices regarding their health. They must also teach the skills that will enable people to evaluate the validity and significance of new information as it becomes available. Just how important informed decision making is in our daily lives is evidenced by the numerous health-related media announcements and articles that fill our newspapers, magazines, and television broadcasts. Rather than informing and enlightening the public on significant new medical discoveries, many of these announcements do little more than add to the level of confusion or exaggerate or sensationalize health issues. Tara Parker-Pope joins two relevant issues for many people—their health and the health of the economy. She points out that when times are bad people's health habits tend to improve. Steven A. Schroeder addresses these issues in "We Can Do Better—Improving the Health of the American People."

Let's assume for a minute that the scientific community is in general agreement that certain behaviors clearly promote our health while others damage our health. Given this information, are you likely to make adjustments to your lifestyle to comply with the findings? Logic would suggest that of course you would, but experience has taught us that information alone isn't enough to bring about behavioral change in many people. Why is it that so many people continue to make bad choices regarding their health behaviors when they are fully aware of the risks involved? We can take vows to try and undo or minimize the negative health behaviors of our past. While strategies such as these may work for those who feel they are at risk, how do we help those who do not feel that they are at risk, or those who feel that it is too late in their lives for the changes to matter? In "The Perils of Higher Education," the author maintains that while college is a place to learn and grow, for many students it becomes four years of bad diet, too little sleep, and too much alcohol. These negative health behaviors affect not only the students' health, but their grades too.

1

Are Bad Times Healthy?

Tara Parker-Pope

M ost people are worried about the health of the economy. But does the economy also affect your health?

It does, but not always in ways you might expect. The data on how an economic downturn influences an individual's health are surprisingly mixed.

It's clear that long-term economic gains lead to improvements in a population's overall health, in developing and industrialized societies alike.

But whether the current economic slump will take a toll on your own health depends, in part, on your health habits when times are good. And economic studies suggest that people tend not to take care of themselves in boom times—drinking too much (especially before driving), dining on fat-laden restaurant meals and skipping exercise and doctors' appointments because of work-related time commitments.

"The value of time is higher during good economic times," said Grant Miller, an assistant professor of medicine at Stanford. "So people work more and do less of the things that are good for them, like cooking at home and exercising; and people experience more stress due to the rigors of hard work during booms."

1936 In hard times, as in the Great Depression, laborers have more time to care for their children.

Similar patterns have been seen in some developing nations. Dr. Miller, who is studying the effects of fluctuating coffee prices on health in Colombia, says that even though falling prices are bad for the economy, they appear to improve health and mortality rates. When prices are low, laborers have more time to care for their children.

"When coffee prices suddenly rise, people work harder on their coffee plots and spend less time doing things around the home, including things that are good for their children," he said. "Because the things that matter most for infant and child health in rural Colombia aren't expensive, but require a substantial amount of time—such as breast-feeding, bringing clean water

from far away, taking your child to a distant health clinic for free vaccinations—infant and child mortality rates rise."

In this country, a similar effect appeared in the Dust Bowl during the Great Depression, according to a 2007 paper by Dr. Miller and colleagues in The Proceedings of the National Academy of Sciences.

The data seem to contradict research in the 1970s suggesting that in hard times there are more deaths from heart disease, cirrhosis, suicide and homicide, as well as more admissions to mental hospitals. But those findings have not been replicated, and several economists have pointed out flaws in the research.

In May 2000, the *Quarterly Journal of Economics* published a surprising paper called "Are Recessions Good for Your Health?" by Christopher J. Ruhm, professor of economics at the University of North Carolina, Greensboro, based on an analysis measuring death rates and health behavior against economic shifts and jobless rates from 1972 to 1991.

Dr. Ruhm found that death rates declined sharply in the 1974 and 1982 recessions, and increased in the economic recovery of the 1980s. An increase of one percentage point in state unemployment rates correlated with a 0.5 percentage point decline in the death rate—or about 5 fewer deaths per 100,000 people. Over all, the death rate fell by more than 8 percent in the 20-year period of mostly economic decline, led by drops in heart disease and car crashes.

The economic downturn did appear to take a toll on factors having less to do with prevention and more to do with mental well-being and access to health care. For instance, cancer deaths rose 23 percent, and deaths from flu and pneumonia increased slightly. Suicides rose 2 percent, homicides 12 percent.

The issue that may matter most in an economic crisis is not related to jobs or income, but whether the slump widens the gap between rich and poor, and whether there is an adequate health safety net available to those who have lost their jobs and insurance.

1999 In Japan, people who lost jobs and insurance were likely to be in poorer health than those who didn't.

During a decade of economic recession in Japan that began in the 1990s, people who were unemployed were twice as likely to be in poor health than those with secure jobs. During Peru's severe economic crisis in the 1980s, infant mortality jumped 2.5 percentage points—about 17,000 more children died as public health spending and social programs collapsed.

In August, researchers from the Free University of Amsterdam looked at health studies of twins in Denmark. They found that individuals born in a recession were at higher risk for heart problems later in life and lived, on average, 15 months less than those born under better conditions.

Gerard J. van den Berg, an economics professor who was a co-author of the study, said babies in poor households suffered the most in a recession, because their families lacked access to good health care. Poor economic conditions can also cause stress that may interfere with parent bonding and childhood development, he said.

He noted that other studies had found that recessions can benefit babies by giving their parents more time at home.

"This scenario may be relevant for well-to-do families where one of the parents loses a job and the other still brings in enough money," he said. "But in a crisis where the family may have to incur huge housing-cost losses and the household income is insufficient for adequate nutrition and health care, the adverse effects of being born in a recession seem much more relevant."

2008 The rising cost of prepared foods in the United States is forcing people to cook from scratch.

In this country, there are already signs of the economy's effect on health. In May, the market research firm Information Resources reported that 53 percent of consumers said they were cooking from scratch more than they did just six months before—in part, no doubt, because of the rising cost of prepared foods. At the same time, health insurance costs are rising. With premiums and co-payments, the average employee with insurance pays nearly one-third of medical costs—about twice as much as four years ago, according to Paul H. Keckley, executive director of the Deloitte Center for Health Solutions.

In the United States, which unlike other industrialized nations lacks a national health plan, the looming recession may take a greater toll. About 46 million Americans lack health insurance, Dr. Keckley says, and even among the 179 million who have it, an estimated 1 in 7 would be bankrupted by a single health crisis.

The economic downturn "is not good news for the health care industry," he said. "There may be slivers of positive, but I view this as sobering."

From *The New York Times*, October 7, 2008. Copyright © 2008 by The New York Times Company. Reprinted by permission via PARS International.

The Perils of Higher Education

Can't remember the difference between declensions and derivatives? Blame college. The undergrad life is a blast, but it may lead you to forget everything you learn.

STEVEN KOTLER

We go to college to learn, to soak up a dazzling array of information intended to prepare us for adult life. But college is not simply a data dump; it is also the end of parental supervision. For many students, that translates into four years of late nights, pizza banquets and boozy week ends that start on Wednesday. And while we know that bad habits are detrimental to cognition in general—think drunk driving—new studies show that the undergrad urges to eat, drink and be merry have devastating effects on learning and memory. It turns out that the exact place we go to get an education may in fact be one of the worst possible environments in which to retain anything we've learned.

Dude, I Haven't Slept in Three Days!

Normal human beings spend one-third of their lives asleep, but today's college students aren't normal. A recent survey of undergraduates and medical students at Stanford University found 80 percent of them qualified as sleep-deprived, and a poll taken by the National Sleep Foundation found that most young adults get only 6.8 hours a night.

All-night cramfests may seem to be the only option when the end of the semester looms, but in fact getting sleep—and a full dose of it—might be a better way to ace exams. Sleep is crucial to declarative memory, the hard, factual kind that helps us remember which year World War I began, or what room the French Lit class is in. It's also essential for procedural memory, the "know-how" memory we use when learning to drive a car or write a five-paragraph essay. "Practice makes perfect," says Harvard Medical School psychologist Matt Walker, "but having a night's rest after practicing might make you even better."

Walker taught 100 people to bang out a series of nonsense sequences on a keyboard—a standard procedural memory task. When asked to replay the sequence 12 hours later, they hadn't improved. But when one group of subjects was allowed to sleep overnight before being retested, their speed and accuracy improved by 20 to 30 percent. "It was bizarre," says Walker. "We were seeing people's skills improve just by sleeping."

For procedural memory, the deep slow-wave stages of sleep were the most important for improvement—particularly during the last two hours of the night. Declarative memory, by contrast, gets processed during the slow-wave stages that come in the first two hours of sleep. "This means that memory requires a full eight hours of sleep," says Walker. He also found that if someone goes without sleep for 24 hours after acquiring a new skill, a week later they will have lost it completely. So college students who pull all-nighters during exam week might do fine on their tests but may not remember any of the material by next semester.

Walker believes that the common practice of back-loading semesters with a blizzard of papers and exams needs a rethink. "Educators are just encouraging sleeplessness," says Walker. "This is just not an effective way to force information into the brain."

Who's up for Pizza?

Walk into any college cafeteria and you'll find a smorgasbord of French fries, greasy pizza, burgers, potato chips and the like. On top of that, McDonald's, Burger King, Wendy's and other fast-food chains have been gobbling up campus real estate in recent years. With hectic schedules and skinny budgets, students find fast food an easy alternative. A recent Tufts University survey found that 50 percent of students eat too much fat, and 70 to 80 percent eat too much saturated fat.

But students who fuel their studies with fast food have something more serious than the "freshman 15" to worry about: They may literally be eating themselves stupid. Researchers have known since the late 1980s that bad eating habits contribute to the kind of cognitive decline found in diseases like Alzheimer's. Since then, they've been trying to find out exactly how a bad diet might be hard on the brain. Ann-Charlotte Granholm, director of the Center for Aging at the Medical University of South Carolina, has recently focused on trans fat, widely used in fast-food cooking because it extends the shelf life of foods. Trans fat is made by bubbling hydrogen through unsaturated fat, with copper or zinc added to speed the chemical reaction along. These metals are frequently found in the brains of people with Alzheimer's, which sparked Granholm's concern.

To investigate, she fed one group of rats a diet high in trans fat and compared them with another group fed a diet that was just as greasy but low in trans fat. Six weeks later, she tested the animals in a water maze, the rodent equivalent of a final exam in organic chemistry. "The trans-fat group made many more errors," says Granholm, especially when she used more difficult mazes.

When she examined the rats' brains, she found that trans-fat eaters had fewer proteins critical to healthy neurological function. She also saw inflammation in and around the hippocampus, the part of the brain responsible for learning and memory. "It was alarming," says Granholm. "These are the exact types of changes we normally see at the onset of Alzheimer's, but we saw them after six weeks," even though the rats were still young.

Students who fuel their studies with fast food have something serious to worry about: They may literally be eating themselves stupid.

Her work corresponds to a broader inquiry conducted by Veerendra Kumar Madala Halagaapa and Mark Mattson of the National Institute on Aging. The researchers fed four groups of mice different diets—normal, high-fat, high-sugar and high-fat/high-sugar. Each diet had the same caloric value, so that one group of mice wouldn't end up heavier. Four months later, the mice on the high-fat diets performed significantly worse than the other groups on a water maze test.

The researchers then exposed the animals to a neurotoxin that targets the hippocampus, to assess whether a high-fat diet made the mice less able to cope with brain damage. Back in the maze, all the animals performed worse than before, but the mice who had eaten the high-fat diets were most seriously compromised. "Based on our work," says Mattson, "we'd predict that people who eat high-fat diets and high-fat/high-sugar diets are not only damaging their ability to learn and remember new information, but also putting themselves at much greater risk for all sorts of neurodegenerative disorders like Alzheimer's."

Welcome to Margaritaville State University

It's widely recognized that heavy drinking doesn't exactly boost your intellect. But most people figure that their booze-induced foolishness wears off once the hangover is gone. Instead, it turns out that even limited stints of overindulgence may have long-term effects.

Less than 20 years ago, researchers began to realize that the adult brain wasn't just a static lump of cells. They found that stem cells in the brain are constantly churning out new neurons, particularly in the hippocampus. Alcoholism researchers, in turn, began to wonder if chronic alcoholics' memory problems had something to do with nerve cell birth and growth.

In 2000, Kimberly Nixon and Fulton Crews at the University of North Carolina's Bowles Center for Alcohol Studies subjected lab rats to four days of heavy alcohol intoxication. They gave the rats a week to shake off their hangovers, then tested them on and off during the next month in a water maze. "We didn't find anything at first," says Nixon. But on the 19th day, the rats who had been on the binge performed much worse. In 19 days, the cells born during the binge had grown to maturity—and clearly, the neurons born during the boozy period didn't work properly once they reached maturity. "[The timing] was almost too perfect," says Nixon.

While normal rats generated about 2,500 new brain cells in three weeks, the drinking rats produced only 1,400. A month later, the sober rats had lost about half of those new cells through normal die-off. But all of the new cells died in the brains of the binge drinkers. "This was startling," says Nixon. "It was the first time anyone had found that alcohol not only inhibits the birth of new cells but also inhibits the ones that survive." In further study, they found that a week's abstinence produced a twofold burst of neurogenesis, and a month off the sauce brought cognitive function back to normal.

What does this have to do with a weekend keg party? A number of recent studies show that college students consume far more alcohol than anyone previously suspected. Forty-four percent of today's collegiates drink enough to be classified as binge drinkers, according to a nationwide survey of 10,000 students done at Harvard University. The amount of alcohol consumed by Nixon's binging rats far exceeded intake at a typical keg party—but other research shows that the effects of alcohol work on a sliding scale. Students who follow a weekend of heavy drinking with a week of heavy studying might not forget everything they learn. They just may struggle come test time.

Can I Bum a Smoke?

If this ledger of campus menaces worries you, here's something you really won't like: Smoking cigarettes may actually have some cognitive benefits, thanks to the power of nicotine. The chemical improves mental focus, as scientists have known since the 1950s. Nicotine also aids concentration in people who have ADHD and may protect against Alzheimer's disease. Back in 2000, a nicotine-like drug under development by the pharmaceutical company Astra Arcus USA was shown to restore the ability to learn and remember in rats with brain lesions similar to those found in Alzheimer's patients. More recently Granholm, the scientist investigating trans fats and memory, found that nicotine enhances spatial memory in healthy rats. Other researchers have found that nicotine also boosts both emotional memory (the kind that helps us *not* put our hands back in the fire after we've been burned) and auditory memory.

There's a catch: Other studies show that nicotine encourages state-dependent learning. The idea is that if, for example, you study in blue sweats, it helps to take the exam in blue sweats. In other words, what you learn while smoking is best recalled while smoking. Since lighting up in an exam room might cause problems, cigarettes probably aren't the key to getting on the dean's list.

Nonetheless, while the number of cigarette smokers continues to drop nationwide, college students are still lighting up: As many as 30 percent smoke during their years of higher education. The smoking rate for young adults between the ages of 18 and 24 has actually risen in the past decade.

All this news makes you wonder how anyone's ever managed to get an education. Or what would happen to GPAs at a vegetarian university with a 10 P.M. curfew. But you might not need to go to such extremes. While Granholm agrees that the excesses of college can be "a perfect example of what you shouldn't do to yourself if you are trying to learn," she doesn't recommend abstinence. "Moderation," she counsels, "just like in everything else. Moderation is the key to collegiate success."

STEVEN KOTLER, based in Los Angeles, has written for *The New York Times Magazine, National Geographic, Details, Wired* and *Outside.*

From *Psychology Today*, Vol. 38, No. 2, March/April 2005, pp. 66, 68, 70. Copyright © 2005 by Sussex Publishers, LLC. Reprinted by permission.

We Can Do Better—Improving the Health of the American People

STEVEN A. SCHROEDER, MD

The United States spends more on health care than any other nation in the world, yet it ranks poorly on nearly every measure of health status. How can this be? What explains this apparent paradox?

The two-part answer is deceptively simple—first, the pathways to better health do not generally depend on better health care, and second, even in those instances in which health care is important, too many Americans do not receive it, receive it too late, or receive poor-quality care. In this lecture, I first summarize where the United States stands in international rankings of health status. Next, using the concept of determinants of premature death as a key measure of health status, I discuss pathways to improvement, emphasizing lessons learned from tobacco control and acknowledging the reality that better health (lower mortality and a higher level of functioning) cannot be achieved without paying greater attention to poor Americans. I conclude with speculations on why we have not focused on improving health in the United States and what it would take to make that happen.

Health Status of the American Public

Among the 30 developed nations that make up the Organization for Economic Cooperation and Development (OECD), the United States ranks near the bottom on most standard measures of health status (Table 1). [1-4] (One measure on which the United States does better is life expectancy from the age of 65 years, possibly reflecting the comprehensive health insurance provided for this segment of the population.) Among the 192 nations for which 2004 data are available, the United States ranks 46th in average life expectancy from birth and 42nd in infant mortality. [5,6] It is remarkable how complacent the public and the medical profession are in their acceptance of these unfavorable comparisons, especially in light of how carefully we track health-systems measures, such as the size of the budget for the National Institutes of Health, trends in national spending on health, and the number of Americans who lack health insurance. One reason for the complacency may be the rationalization that the United States is more ethnically heterogeneous than the

nations at the top of the rankings, such as Japan, Switzerland, and Iceland. It is true that within the United States there are large disparities in health status—by geographic area, race and ethnic group, and class. [7-9] But even when comparisons are limited to white Americans, our performance is dismal (Table 1). And even if the health status of white Americans matched that in the leading nations, it would still be incumbent on us to improve the health of the entire nation.

Pathways to Improving Population Health

Health is influenced by factors in five domains—genetics, social circumstances, environmental exposures, behavioral patterns, and health care (Fig. 1). [10,11] When it comes to reducing early deaths, medical care has a relatively minor role. Even if the entire U.S. population had access to excellent medical care—which it does not—only a small fraction of these deaths could be prevented. The single greatest opportunity to improve health and reduce premature deaths lies in personal behavior. In fact, behavioral causes account for nearly 40% of all deaths in the United States. [12] Although there has been disagreement over the actual number of deaths that can be attributed to obesity and physical inactivity combined, it is clear that this pair of factors and smoking are the top two behavioral causes of premature death (Fig. 2). [12]

Addressing Unhealthy Behavior

Clinicians and policymakers may question whether behavior is susceptible to change or whether attempts to change behavior lie outside the province of traditional medical care. [13] They may expect future successes to follow the pattern whereby immunization and antibiotics improved health in the 20th century. If the public's health is to improve, however, that improvement is more likely to come from behavioral change than from technological innovation. Experience demonstrates that it is in fact possible to change behavior, as illustrated by increased seat-belt use and decreased consumption of products high in saturated fat. The case of tobacco best demonstrates how rapidly positive behavioral change can occur.

Table 1 Health Status of the United States and Rank among the 29 Other OECD Member Countries

Health-Status Measure	United States	U.S. Rank in OECD	Top-Ranked Country in OECD*
Infant mortality (first year of life), 2001			
All races	6.8 deaths/1000 live births	25	Iceland (2.7 deaths/1000 live births)
Whites only	5.7 deaths/1000 live births	22	
Maternal mortality, 2001†			
All races	9.9 deaths/100,000 births	22	Switzerland (1.4 deaths/100,000 births)
Whites only	7.2 deaths/100,000 births	19	
Life expectancy from birth, 2003			
All women	80.1 yr	23	Japan (85.3 yr)
White women	80.5 yr	22	
All men	74.8 yr	22	Iceland (79.7 yr)
White men	75.3 yr	19	
Life expectancy from age 65, 2003‡			
All women	19.8 yr	10	Japan (23.0 yr)
White women	19.8 yr	10	
All men	16.8 yr	9	Iceland (18.1 yr)
White men	16.9 yr	9	

*The number in parentheses is the value for the indicated health-status measure.

†OECD data for five countries are missing.

‡OECD data for six countries are missing.

The Case of Tobacco

The prevalence of smoking in the United States declined among men from 57% in 1955 to 23% in 2005 and among women from 34% in 1965 to 18% in 2005.[14,15] Why did tobacco use fall so rapidly? The 1964 report of the surgeon general, which linked smoking and lung cancer, was followed by multiple reports connecting active and passive smoking to myriad other diseases. Early antismoking advocates, initially isolated, became emboldened by the cascade of scientific evidence, especially with respect to the risk of exposure to secondhand smoke. Counter-marketing—first in the 1960s and more recently by several states and the American Legacy Foundation's "truth®" campaign—linked the creativity of Madison Avenue with messages about the duplicity of the tobacco industry to produce compelling antismoking messages[16] (an antismoking advertisement is available with the full text of this article at www.nejm.org). Laws, regulations, and litigation, particularly at the state and community levels, led to smoke-free public places and increases in the tax on cigarettes—two of the strongest evidence-based tobacco-control measures.[14,17,18] In this regard, local governments have been far ahead of the federal government, and they have inspired European countries such as Ireland and the United Kingdom to make public places smoke-free.[14,19] In addition, new medications have augmented face-to-face and telephone counseling techniques to increase the odds that clinicians can help smokers quit.[15,20,21]

It is tempting to be lulled by this progress and shift attention to other problems, such as the obesity epidemic. But there are still 44.5 million smokers in the United States, and each year

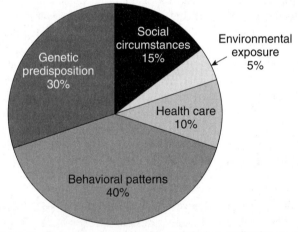

Figure 1 Determinants of health and their contribution to premature death.

Adapted from McGinnis et al.[10]

tobacco use kills 435,000 Americans, who die up to 15 years earlier than nonsmokers and who often spend their final years ravaged by dyspnea and pain.[14,20] In addition, smoking among pregnant women is a major contributor to premature births and infant mortality.[20] Smoking is increasingly concentrated in the lower socioeconomic classes and among those with mental illness or problems with substance abuse.[15,22,23] People with chronic mental illness die an average of 25 years earlier than others, and a large percentage of those years are lost because of smoking.[24] Estimates from the Smoking Cessation Leadership Center at the University of California at San Francisco, which are based on

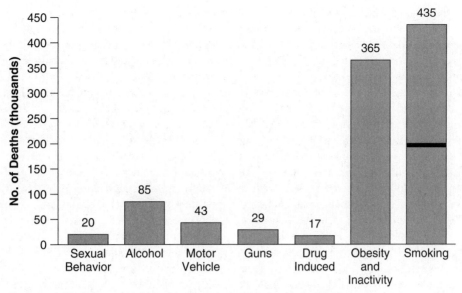

Figure 2 Numbers of U.S. deaths from behavioral causes, 2000.

Among the deaths from smoking, the horizontal bar indicates the approximately 200,000 people who had mental illness or a problem with substance abuse. Adapted from Mokdad et al.[12]

Table 2 Similarities and Differences between Tobacco Use and Obesity

Characteristic	Tobacco	Obesity
High prevalence	Yes	Yes
Begins in youth	Yes	Yes
20th-century phenomenon	Yes	Yes
Major health implications	Yes	Yes
Heavy and influential industry promotion	Yes	Yes
Inverse relationship to socioeconomic class	Yes	Yes
Major regional variations	Yes	Yes
Stigma	Yes	Yes
Difficult to treat	Yes	Yes
Clinician antipathy	Yes	Yes
Relative and debatable definition	No	Yes
Cessation not an option	No	Yes
Chemical addictive component	Yes	No
Harmful at low doses	Yes	No
Harmful to others	Yes	No
Extensively documented industry duplicity	Yes	No
History of successful litigation	Yes	No
Large cash settlements by industry	Yes	No
Strong evidence base for treatment	Yes	No
Economic incentives available	Yes	Yes
Economic incentives in place	Yes	No
Successful counter-marketing campaigns	Yes	No

The United States is approaching a "tobacco tipping point"—a state of greatly reduced smoking prevalence. There are already low rates of smoking in some segments of the population, including physicians (about 2%), people with a postgraduate education (8%), and residents of the states of Utah (11%) and California (14%).[25] When Kaiser Permanente of northern California implemented a multisystem approach to help smokers quit, the smoking rate dropped from 12.2% to 9.2% in just 3 years.[25] Two basic strategies would enable the United States to meet its Healthy People 2010 tobacco-use objective of 12% population prevalence: keep young people from starting to smoke and help smokers quit. Of the two strategies, smoking cessation has by far the larger short-term impact. Of the current 44.5 million smokers, 70% claim they would like to quit.[20] Assuming that one half of those 31 million potential non-smokers will die because of smoking, that translates into 15.5 million potentially preventable premature deaths.[20,26] Merely increasing the baseline quit rate from the current 2.5% of smokers to 10%—a rate seen in placebo groups in most published trials of the new cessation drugs—would prevent 1,170,000 premature deaths. No other medical or public health intervention approaches this degree of impact. And we already have the tools to accomplish it.[14,27]

Is Obesity the Next Tobacco?

Although there is still much to do in tobacco control, it is nevertheless touted as a model for combating obesity, the other major, potentially preventable cause of death and disability in the United States. Smoking and obesity share many characteristics (Table 2). Both are highly prevalent, start in childhood or adolescence, were relatively uncommon until the first (smoking) or second (obesity) half of the 20th century, are major risk factors for chronic disease, involve intensively marketed products, are more common in low socioeconomic classes, exhibit major regional variations (with higher rates in

the high rates and intensity (number of cigarettes per day plus the degree to which each is finished) of tobacco use in these populations, indicate that as many as 200,000 of the 435,000 Americans who die prematurely each year from tobacco-related deaths are people with chronic mental illness, substance-abuse problems, or both.[22,25] Understanding why they smoke and how to help them quit should be a key national research priority. Given the effects of smoking on health, the relative inattention to tobacco by those federal and state agencies charged with protecting the public health is baffling and disappointing.

southern and poorer states), carry a stigma, are difficult to treat, and are less enthusiastically embraced by clinicians than other risk factors for medical conditions.

Nonetheless, obesity differs from smoking in many ways (Table 2). The binary definition of smoking status (smoker or nonsmoker) does not apply to obesity. Body-mass index, the most widely used measure of obesity, misclassifies as overweight people who have large muscle mass, such as California governor Arnold Schwarzenegger. It is not biologically possible to stop eating, and unlike moderate smoking, eating a moderate amount of food is not hazardous. There is no addictive analogue to nicotine in food. Nonsmokers mobilize against tobacco because they fear injury from secondhand exposure, which is not a peril that attends obesity. The food industry is less concentrated than the tobacco industry, and although its advertising for children has been criticized as predatory and its ingredient-labeling practices as deceptive, it has yet to fall into the ill repute of the tobacco industry. For these reasons, litigation is a more problematic strategy, and industry payouts—such as the Master Settlement Agreement between the tobacco industry and 46 state attorneys general to recapture the Medicaid costs of treating tobacco-related diseases—are less likely.[14] Finally, except for the invasive option of bariatric surgery, there are even fewer clinical tools available for treating obesity than there are for treating addiction to smoking.

Several changes in policy have been proposed to help combat obesity.[28-30] Selective taxes and subsidies could be used as incentives to change the foods that are grown, brought to market, and consumed, though the politics involved in designating favored and penalized foods would be fierce.[31] Restrictions could also apply to the use of food stamps. Given recent data indicating that children see from 27 to 48 food advertisements for each 1 promoting fitness or nutrition, regulations could be put in place to shift that balance or to mandate support for sustained social-marketing efforts such as the "truth®" campaign against smoking.[16,32] Requiring more accurate labeling of caloric content and ingredients, especially in fast-food outlets, could make customers more aware of what they are eating and induce manufacturers to alter food composition. Better pharmaceutical products and counseling programs could motivate clinicians to view obesity treatment more enthusiastically. In contrast to these changes in policy, which will require national legislation, regulation, or research investment, change is already under way at the local level. Some schools have banned the sale of soft drinks and now offer more nutritionally balanced lunches. Opportunities for physical activity at work, in school, and in the community have been expanded in a small but growing number of locations.

Nonbehavioral Causes of Premature Death

Improving population health will also require addressing the nonbehavioral determinants of health that we can influence: social, health care, and environmental factors. (To date, we lack tools to change our genes, although behavioral and environmental factors can modify the expression of genetic risks such as obesity.) With respect to social factors, people with lower socio-economic status die earlier and have more disability than those with higher socioeconomic status, and this pattern holds true in a stepwise fashion from the lowest to the highest classes.[33-38] In this context, class is a composite construct of income, total wealth, education, employment, and residential neighborhood. One reason for the class gradient in health is that people in lower classes are more likely to have unhealthy behaviors, in part because of inadequate local food choices and recreational opportunities. Yet even when behavior is held constant, people in lower classes are less healthy and die earlier than others.[33-38] It is likely that the deleterious influence of class on health reflects both absolute and relative material deprivation at the lower end of the spectrum and psychosocial stress along the entire continuum. Unlike the factors of health care and behavior, class has been an "ignored determinant of the nation's health."[33] Disparities in health care are of concern to some policymakers and researchers, but because the United States uses race and ethnic group rather than class as the filter through which social differences are analyzed, studies often highlight disparities in the receipt of health care that are based on race and ethnic group rather than on class.

But aren't class gradients a fixture of all societies? And if so, can they ever be diminished? The fact is that nations differ greatly in their degree of social inequality and that—even in the United States—earning potential and tax policies have fluctuated over time, resulting in a narrowing or widening of class differences. There are ways to address the effects of class on health.[33] More investment could be made in research efforts designed to improve our understanding of the connection between class and health. More fundamental, however, is the recognition that social policies involving basic aspects of life and well-being (e.g., education, taxation, transportation, and housing) have important health consequences. Just as the construction of new buildings now requires environmental-impact analyses, taxation policies could be subjected to health-impact analyses. When public policies widen the gap between rich and poor, they may also have a negative effect on population health. One reason the United States does poorly in international health comparisons may be that we value entrepreneurialism over egalitarianism. Our willingness to tolerate large gaps in income, total wealth, educational quality, and housing has unintended health consequences. Until we are willing to confront this reality, our performance on measures of health will suffer.

One nation attempting to address the effects of class on health is the United Kingdom. Its 1998 Acheson Commission, which was charged with reducing health disparities, produced 39 policy recommendations spanning areas such as poverty, income, taxes and benefits, education, employment, housing, environment, transportation, and nutrition. Only 3 of these 39 recommendations pertained directly to health care: all policies that influence health should be evaluated for their effect on the disparities in health resulting from differences in socioeconomic status; a high priority should be given to the health of families with children; and income inequalities should be reduced and living standards among the poor improved.[39] Although implementation of these recommendations has been incomplete, the mere fact of their existence means more attention is paid to the effects of social policies on health. This element is missing in

U.S. policy discussions—as is evident from recent deliberations on income-tax policy.

Although inadequate health care accounts for only 10% of premature deaths, among the five determinants of health (Fig. 1), health care receives by far the greatest share of resources and attention. In the case of heart disease, it is estimated that health care has accounted for half of the 40% decline in mortality over the past two decades.[40] (It may be that exclusive reliance on international mortality comparisons shortchanges the results of America's health care system. Perhaps the high U.S. rates of medical-technology use translate into comparatively better function. To date, there are no good international comparisons of functional status to test that theory, but if it could be substantiated, there would be an even more compelling claim for expanded health insurance coverage.) U.S. expenditures on health care in 2006 were an estimated $2.1 trillion, accounting for 16% of our gross domestic product.[41] Few other countries even reach double digits in health care spending.

There are two basic ways in which health care can affect health status: quality and access. Although qualitative deficiencies in U.S. health care have been widely documented,[42] there is no evidence that its performance in this dimension is worse than that of other OECD nations. In the area of access, however, we trail nearly all the countries: 45 million U.S. citizens (plus millions of immigrants) lack health insurance, and millions more are seriously underinsured. Lack of health insurance leads to poor health.[43] Not surprisingly, the uninsured are disproportionately represented among the lower socioeconomic classes.

Environmental factors, such as lead paint, polluted air and water, dangerous neighborhoods, and the lack of outlets for physical activity, also contribute to premature death. People with lower socioeconomic status have greater exposure to these health-compromising conditions. As with social determinants of health and health insurance coverage, remedies for environmental risk factors lie predominantly in the political arena.[44]

The Case for Concentrating on the Less Fortunate

Since all the actionable determinants of health—personal behavior, social factors, health care, and the environment—disproportionately affect the poor, strategies to improve national health rankings must focus on this population. To the extent that the United States has a health strategy, its focus is on the development of new medical technologies and support for basic biomedical research. We already lead the world in the per capita use of most diagnostic and therapeutic medical technologies, and we have recently doubled the budget for the National Institutes of Health. But these popular achievements are unlikely to improve our relative performance on health. It is arguable that the status quo is an accurate expression of the national political will—a relentless search for better health among the middle and upper classes. This pursuit is also evident in how we consistently outspend all other countries in the use of alternative medicines and cosmetic surgeries and in how frequently health "cures" and "scares" are featured in the popular media.[45] The result is that only when the middle class feels threatened by external menaces

(e.g., secondhand tobacco smoke, bioterrorism, and airplane exposure to multidrug-resistant tuberculosis) will it embrace public health measures. In contrast, our investment in improving population health—whether judged on the basis of support for research, insurance coverage, or government-sponsored public health activities—is anemic.[46-48] Although the Department of Health and Human Services periodically produces admirable population health goals—most recently, the Healthy People 2010 objectives[49]—no government department or agency has the responsibility and authority to meet these goals, and the importance of achieving them has yet to penetrate the political process.

Why Don't Americans Focus on Factors That Can Improve Health?

The comparatively weak health status of the United States stems from two fundamental aspects of its political economy. The first is that the disadvantaged are less well represented in the political sphere here than in most other developed countries, which often have an active labor movement and robust labor parties. Without a strong voice from Americans of low socioeconomic status, citizen health advocacy in the United States coalesces around particular illnesses, such as breast cancer, human immunodeficiency virus infection and the acquired immunodeficiency syndrome (HIV–AIDS), and autism. These efforts are led by middle-class advocates whose lives have been touched by the disease. There have been a few successful public advocacy campaigns on issues of population health—efforts to ban exposure to secondhand smoke or to curtail drunk driving—but such efforts are relatively uncommon.[44] Because the biggest gains in population health will come from attention to the less well off, little is likely to change unless they have a political voice and use it to argue for more resources to improve health-related behaviors, reduce social disparities, increase access to health care, and reduce environmental threats. Social advocacy in the United States is also fragmented by our notions of race and class.[33] To the extent that poverty is viewed as an issue of racial injustice, it ignores the many whites who are poor, thereby reducing the ranks of potential advocates.

The relatively limited role of government in the U.S. health care system is the second explanation. Many are familiar with our outlier status as the only developed nation without universal health care coverage.[50] Less obvious is the dispersed and relatively weak status of the various agencies responsible for population health and the fact that they are so disconnected from the delivery of health services. In addition, the American emphasis on the value of individual responsibility creates a reluctance to intervene in what are seen as personal behavioral choices.

How Can the Nation's Health Improve?

Given that the political dynamics of the United States are unlikely to change soon and that the less fortunate will continue to have weak representation, are we consigned to a low-tier status when it comes to population health? In my view, there

11

is room for cautious optimism. One reason is that despite the epidemics of HIV–AIDS and obesity, our population has never been healthier, even though it lags behind so many other countries. The gain has come from improvements in personal behavior (e.g., tobacco control), social and environmental factors (e.g., reduced rates of homicide and motor-vehicle accidents and the introduction of fluoridated water), and medical care (e.g., vaccines and cardiovascular drugs). The largest potential for further improvement in population health lies in behavioral risk factors, especially smoking and obesity. We already have tools at hand to make progress in tobacco control, and some of these tools are applicable to obesity. Improvement in most of the other factors requires political action, starting with relentless measurement of and focus on actual health status and the actions that could improve it. Inaction means acceptance of America's poor health status.

Improving population health would be more than a statistical accomplishment. It could enhance the productivity of the workforce and boost the national economy, reduce health care expenditures, and most important, improve people's lives. But in the absence of a strong political voice from the less fortunate themselves, it is incumbent on health care professionals, especially physicians, to become champions for population health. This sense of purpose resonates with our deepest professional values and is the reason why many chose medicine as a profession. It is also one of the most productive expressions of patriotism. Americans take great pride in asserting that we are number one in terms of wealth, number of Nobel Prizes, and military strength. Why don't we try to become number one in health?

References

1. OECD health data 2006 (2001 figures). Paris: Organisation for Economic Cooperation and Development, October 2006.
2. Infant, neonatal, and postneonatal deaths, percent of total deaths, and mortality rates for the 15 leading causes of infant death by race and sex: United States, 2001. Hyattsville, MD: National Center for Health Statistics. (Accessed August 24, 2007, at http://www.cdc.gov/search.do?action=search&queryText=infant+mortality+rate+2001&x=18&y=15.)
3. Hoyert DL. Maternal mortality and related concepts. Vital Health Stat 3 2007; 33:4.
4. Chartbook on trends in the health of Americans. Table 27: life expectancy at birth, at age 65 years of age, and at age 75 years of age, by race and sex: United States, selected years 1900–2004:193. Hyattsville, MD: National Center for Health Statistics. (Accessed August 24, 2007, at http://www.cdc.gov/nchs/fastats/lifexpec.htm.)
5. WHO core health indicators. Geneva: World Health Organization. (Accessed August 24, 2007, at http://www3.who.int/whosis/core/core_select_process.cfm.)
6. Minino AM, Heron M, Smith BL. Deaths: preliminary data for 2004. Health E-Stats. Released April 19, 2006. (Accessed August 24, 2007, at http://www.cdc.gov/nchs/products/pubs/pubd/hestats/prelimdeaths04/preliminarydeaths04.htm.)
7. Harper S, Lynch J, Burris S, Davey Smith G. Trends in the black-white life expectancy gap in the United States, 1983–2003. JAMA 2007;297:1224–32.
8. Murray JL, Kulkarni SC, Michaud C, et al. Eight Americas: investigating mortality disparities across races, counties, and race-counties in the United States. PLoS Med 2006;3(9):e260.
9. Woolf SH, Johnson RE, Phillips RL, Philipsen M. Giving everyone the health of the educated: an examination of whether social change would save more lives than medical advances. Am J Public Health 2007;97:679–83.
10. McGinnis JM, Williams-Russo P, Knickman JR. The case for more active policy attention to health promotion. Health Aff (Millwood) 2002;21(2):78–93.
11. McGinnis JM, Foege WH. Actual causes of death in the United States. JAMA 1993;270:2207–12.
12. Mokdad AH, Marks JS, Stroup JS, Gerberding JL. Actual causes of death in the United States, 2000. JAMA 2004;291: 1238–45. [Errata, JAMA 2005;293:293–4, 298.]
13. Seldin DW. The boundaries of medicine. Trans Assoc Am Phys 1981;38:lxxvlxxxvi.
14. Schroeder SA. Tobacco control in the wake of the 1998 Master Settlement Agreement. N Engl J Med 2004;350:293–301.
15. Idem. What to do with the patient who smokes? JAMA 2005;294:482–7.
16. Farrelly MC, Healton CH, Davis KC, et al. Getting to the truth: evaluating national tobacco countermarketing campaigns. Am J Public Health 2002;92:901–7. [Erratum, Am J Public Health 2003;93:703.]
17. Warner KE. Tobacco policy research: insights and contributions to public health policy. In: Warner KE, ed. Tobacco control policy. San Francisco: Jossey-Bass, 2006:3–86.
18. Schroeder SA. An agenda to combat substance abuse. Health Aff (Millwood) 2005;24:1005–13.
19. Koh HK, Joossens LX, Connolly GN. Making smoking history worldwide. N Engl J Med 2007;356:1496–8.
20. Fiore MC, Bailey WC, Cohen SJ, et al. Treating tobacco use and dependence: clinical practice guideline. Rockville, MD: Public Health Service, 2000.
21. Schroeder SA, Sox HC. Trials that matter: varenicline—a new designer drug to help smokers quit. Ann Intern Med 2006;145:784–5.
22. Lasser K, Boyd JW, Woolhandler S, Himmelstein DU, McCormick D, Bor DH. Smoking and mental illness: a population-based prevalence study. JAMA 2000;284: 2606–10.
23. Zeidonis DM, Williams JM, Steinberg ML, et al. Addressing tobacco dependence among veterans with a psychiatric disorder: a neglected epidemic of major clinical and public health concern. In: Isaacs SL, Schroeder SA, Simon JA, eds. VA in the vanguard: building on success in smoking cessation. Washington, DC: Department of Veterans Affairs, 2005: 141–70. (Accessed, August 24, 2007, at http://smokingcessationleadership.ucsf.edu/AboutSCLC_vanguard.html.)
24. Colton CW, Manderscheid RW. Congruencies in increased mortality rates, years of potential life lost, and causes of death among public mental health clients in eight states. Prev Chronic Dis 2006;3:April (online only). (Accessed August 24, 2007, at http://www.cdc.gov/pcd/issues/2006/apr/05_0180.htm.)
25. Smoking Cessation Leadership Center. Partner highlights. (Accessed August 24, 2007, at http://smokingcessationleadership.ucsf.edu/PartnerFeatured.html.)
26. Doll R, Peto R, Boreham J, Sutherland I. Mortality in relation to smoking: 50 years' observations on male British doctors. BMJ 2004;328:1519–27.
27. Fiore MC, Croyle RT, Curry SJ, et al. Preventing 3 million premature deaths and helping 5 million smokers quit: a national action plan for tobacco cessation. Am J Public Health 2004;94:205–10.
28. Nestle M. Food marketing and childhood obesity—a matter of policy. N Engl J Med 2006;354:2527–9.
29. Mello MM, Studdert DM, Brennan TA. Obesity—the new frontier of public health law. N Engl J Med 2006;354:2601–10.
30. Gostin LO. Law as a tool to facilitate healthier lifestyles and prevent obesity. JAMA 2007;297:87–90.

31. Pollan M. You are what you grow. New York Times Sunday Magazine. April 22, 2007:15–8.

32. Food for thought: television food advertising to children in the United States. Menlo Park, CA: Kaiser Family Foundation, March 2007:3.

33. Isaacs SL, Schroeder SA. Class—the ignored determinant of the nation's health. N Engl J Med 2004;351:1137–42.

34. Adler NE, Boyce WT, Chesney MA, Folkman S, Syme SL. Socioeconomic inequalities in health: no easy solution. JAMA 1993;269:3140–5.

35. McDonough P, Duncan GJ, Williams DR, House J. Income dynamics and adult mortality in the United States, 1972 through 1989. Am J Public Health 1997;87:1476–83.

36. Marmot M. Inequalities in health. N Engl J Med 2001;345:134–6.

37. Williams DR, Collins C. US socioeconomic and racial differences in health: patterns and explanations. Annu Rev Sociol 1995;21:349–86.

38. Minkler M, Fuller-Thomson E, Guralnik JM. Gradient of disability across the socioeconomic spectrum in the United States. N Engl J Med 2006;355:695–703.

39. Independent inquiry into inequalities in health report. London: Stationery Office, 1998 (Accessed August 24, 2007, at http://www.archive.official-documents.co.uk/document/doh/ih/contents.htm.)

40. Ford ES, Ajani UA, Croft JB, et al. Explaining the decrease in U.S. deaths from coronary disease, 1980–2000. N Engl J Med 2007;356:2388–98.

41. Poisal JA, Truffer C, Smith S, et al. Health spending projections through 2016: modest changes obscure Part D's impact. Health Aff (Millwood) 2007;26:w242-w253 (Web only). (Accessed August 24, 2007, at http://content.healthaffairs.org/cgi/content/full/26/2/w242.)

42. Institute of Medicine. To err is human: building a safer health system. Washington, DC: National Academy Press, 2000.

43. *Idem.* Hidden costs, value lost: uninsurance in America. Washington, DC: National Academy of Sciences, 2003.

44. Isaacs SL, Schroeder SA. Where the public good prevailed: lessons from success stories in health. The American Prospect. June 4, 2001:26–30.

45. Gawande A. Annals of medicine: the way we age now. The New Yorker. April 30, 2007:50–9.

46. McGinnis JM. Does proof matter? Why strong evidence sometimes yields weak action. Am J Health Promot 2001;15:391–6.

47. Kindig DA. A pay-for-population health performance system. JAMA 2006; 296:2611–3.

48. Woolf SH. Potential health and economic consequences of misplaced priorities. JAMA 2007;297:523–6.

49. Healthy People 2010: understanding and improving health. Washington, DC: Department of Health and Human Services, 2001.

50. Schroeder SA. The medically uninsured—will they always be with us? N Engl J Med 1996;334:1130–3.

From the Department of Medicine, University of California at San Francisco, San Francisco. Address reprint requests to Dr. Schroeder at the Department of Medicine, University of California at San Francisco, 3333 California St., Suite 430, San Francisco, CA 94143, or at schroeder@medicine.ucsf.edu.

Supported in part by grants from the Robert Wood Johnson and American Legacy Foundations. The sponsors had no role in the preparation of the Shattuck Lecture.

No potential conflict of interest relevant to this article was reported.

I thank Stephen Isaacs for editorial assistance; Michael McGinnis, Harold Sox, Stephen Shortell, and Nancy Adler for comments on an earlier draft; and Kristen Kekich and Katherine Kostrzewa for technical support.

From *The New England Journal of Medicine*, September 20, 2007. Copyright © 2007 by Massachusetts Medical Society. All rights reserved. Reprinted by permission.

On the Road to Wellness

Lawmakers want Americans to eat better, stop smoking, exercise and relax.

AMY WINTERFELD

Dave Barry was kidding, but he was way ahead of the curve in 1985, when he advised everyone to "stay fit and healthy until you're dead." U.S. Secretary of Health and Human Services Mike Leavitt, however, was dead serious when he said, in October 2006, that he wants to make Americans healthier.

"Emphasis on the four pillars of the HealthierUS initiative—physical activity, good diet, healthy choices and preventive screening—is crucial for the nation's health," says Leavitt. "Changing the culture from one of treating sickness to staying healthy calls for small steps and good choices to be made each and every day. [The department's] physical activity guidelines will encourage the creation of a culture of wellness across America."

The California governor's plan for health care reform, announced last month, also gives a nod to wellness, leading off with a proposed Healthy Action Rewards/Incentives program for both publicly and privately insured Californians. It would provide incentives such as gym memberships, weight management programs and reductions in health insurance premiums to promote prevention, wellness and healthy lifestyles.

It's no wonder that Leavitt and other policymakers want to encourage Americans to adopt healthy habits and stay well. Treatment for chronic diseases accounts for 75 percent of what the country spends on health care each year. Rates continue to rise for one of the leading precursors to chronic disease, obesity. An estimated 66 million Americans are overweight or obese. More than 60 percent of American adults do not get enough physical activity, and 25 percent are not active at all.

Another 44.5 million U.S. adults continue to smoke cigarettes, even though this will result in death or disability for half of them.

Treatment for the consequences of these unhealthy behaviors is improving. But it costs—a lot. Preventing diseases and promoting good health for everyone can help control these costs. Making healthy food choices more available, designing environments to encourage physical activity, offering incentives for healthy behaviors and encouraging preventive screenings are strategies that work at lowering costs.

"We have a finite amount of resources to spend on health care," says Hawaii Representative Josh Green, an ER doctor who chairs the House Health Committee. "The only way to afford the things we must have is to focus on preventive health measures and screening. We'll always need trauma centers like the one where I work, but that means we need to be smart about other health costs."

Starting Young

During the past 30 years, obesity rates have more than quadrupled for children ages 6 to 11 and more than tripled for young people 12 to 19. Many lawmakers are enacting wellness policies for schools, where 98 percent of 5- to 17-year-olds can be found on any given school day in the United States.

Beginning this fall, federal law requires school districts participating in federally funded school meals programs—nearly every school district in the country—to establish a local wellness policy that includes goals for physical activity. School meals must meet nutrition standards set by the U.S. Department of Agriculture. And there must be a plan for measuring success.

Colorado, Florida, Illinois, Indiana, Kentucky, Mississippi, Ohio, Pennsylvania, Rhode Island, Tennessee and Washington have all enacted legislation in the past few years to support school and state wellness policies.

Legislators have worked to improve the nutritional quality of school foods, provide more opportunities for physical activity, and ensure that nutrition is part of the school curriculum. At the local level, 92 of the nation's

Paying for Prevention for the Publicly Insured

States have recently begun to structure public insurance programs to cover more preventive care to help ward off chronic conditions, which account for 96 percent of Medicare spending and about 83 percent of Medicaid spending. Examples include the following:

- **Coverage for obesity prevention services.** In Connecticut, the state's Medicaid managed care plans pay for obesity related services if they are medically necessary. Nutritional counseling, exercise programs and behavioral health services are covered under Medicaid and SCHIP if they meet the necessity criteria. The state also covers gastric bypass surgery through Medicaid, if medically necessary.
- **Coverage for smoking cessation treatments.** In 2005, 38 states covered some tobacco-dependence counseling or medication for all Medicaid recipients. Four more states offered coverage only for pregnant women. Oregon is the single state offering all smoking cessation medication and counseling treatments recommended by the U.S. Public Health Service.
- **Wellness incentives.** West Virginia has some of the nation's highest rates of obesity, diabetes, heart disease and smoking. In three pilot counties, Medicaid patients will be asked to sign contracts agreeing to do their best to stay healthy by attending health improvement programs as directed, having routine checkups and health screenings, taking prescribed medicine, keeping appointments and limiting emergency room use. As an incentive, they will receive antismoking and weight loss classes, home health visits as needed, mental health counseling, diabetes management assistance, cardiac rehabilitation and additional prescription medications. Over future years, Medicaid beneficiaries who stick to the plan will qualify for extra benefits, possibly orthodontic or other dental care. Medicaid recipients who do not sign or adhere to the contract will be limited to the standard benefits determined by the state. Critics say the plan may limit access to the enhanced benefits by those most likely to need them, for example, people with existing mental health or substance abuse problems that create difficulties in keeping scheduled appointments. It may also put doctors in an awkward position as administrative enforcers of factors that may be beyond patient control and may interfere with effective doctor-patient relationships.
- **Preventive services for those on Medicare.** In January, Medicare increased payments to doctors for face-to-face doctor-patient consultations about a patient's health and what needs to be done to maintain or improve health. The hope is to encourage more discussions about preventive services like controlling diabetes and get doctors to refer more patients to diabetes self-management training and medical nutrition therapy. Medicare will also now cover these services at federally qualified health centers, increasing access in rural and underserved areas.

100 largest school districts—which educate 23 percent of American students—have developed a wellness policy.

Lawmakers are also looking at ways to encourage kids to get more exercise on the way to school. The federal Safe Routes to School program includes $612 million for grants over five years for communities to build bike lanes, sidewalks and trails that will make it safer and easier for children to bike and walk to school.

Getting Workers Healthy

Investing in employee health also pays off. Healthy workers are more productive. An analysis of 32 studies of workplace wellness initiatives found 28 with an average return on investment of $3.48 per $1 in program costs, as reported in 2001 in the American Journal of Public Health. Citibank saved $8.9 million over two years after investing $1.9 million for wellness initiatives, translating into a return of $4.70 for each dollar spent on the wellness program. Motorola saw a return of $3.93 for every dollar spent on its wellness program, and saved nearly $10.5 million annually in disability expenses for program participants compared to non-participants.

State governments and other public employers are initiating workplace wellness programs as well. The U.S. Department of Health and Human Services awarded Hawaii an innovation in prevention award last November for promoting physical activity and nutrition at work. The state health department has outlined these ideas in an online Worksite Wellness Toolkit, so that other employers can start similar programs.

Delaware, Kentucky, Oklahoma, Rhode Island and South Dakota have launched health promotion initiatives for state employees. And Arkansas, North Dakota, Ohio and Vermont have statewide wellness programs for the whole population. In 2005, Nevada's legislature established a State Program for Fitness and Wellness and a state advisory council to raise awareness and create programs for physical fitness, nutrition and the prevention of obesity and chronic diseases. In Arizona, an executive order created a State Employee Wellness Advisory Council in 2005 that organizes wellness fairs and health screenings for state employees, including blood pressure screenings, cholesterol checks, smoking cessation, weight management and diabetes screenings.

States have also had success by starting on a small scale, building on pilot programs. North Carolina's HealthSmart program started with nine local programs that identified employees with specific health conditions and provided them with intensive health advice on lifestyle changes. It was expanded to all state employees in 2005. Delaware launched the Health Rewards pilot study program for state employees in 2003, offering comprehensive health assessments, guidance, and fitness advice to state employees through their group health insurance programs.

State efforts to improve workplace wellness have also included smoking bans that cover all workplaces, including bars and restaurants. Hawaii's ban, effective in November 2006, is "essentially the end of the issue of secondhand smoke in public places," says Representative Green.

Building Healthy Communities

The way we design our communities can influence our health. Decisions about zoning, community design and land use affect the daily choices people make, whether it is to drive or walk to the store, exercise, or the buy healthy foods. Creating incentives can encourage cities and developers to take health and livability into account when retrofitting old developments or building new ones. The design of neighborhoods, transportation systems and biking or walking paths can encourage physical activity.

Healthy foods, such as fresh fruits and vegetables, which are accessible and affordable, are part of the equation. Encouraging schools and government agencies to buy local produce, providing fiscal incentives for locating grocery stores in all communities—especially underserved urban or rural communities—and setting school nutrition standards and school wellness policies can have a big impact on people's health.

Incentives for Wellness

Indiana Senator Beverly Gard wants to give employers incentives to create wellness programs. She sponsored legislation last year that will allow Indiana employers to offer financial incentives to reduce employee tobacco use.

"This seemed like something we could do that would give employers an opportunity to provide employees with incentives for healthy behavior," Gard says. Rather than penalize smokers, Indiana amended its smokers' bill of rights to allow employers to implement financial incentives related to employer-provided health benefits that are intended to reduce employee tobacco use. "We wanted to take a more positive approach," Gard says.

States have looked at a number of different ways to provide incentives for wellness and healthy behavior for individuals and for businesses, large and small. Some of the most popular are:

- **Insurance incentives such as premium discounts or rebates.** Michigan enacted legislation in 2006 that requires insurers, HMOs and nonprofits that offer group health insurance coverage to give premium rebates when a majority of employees or health plan members enroll and maintain participation in group wellness programs. The rebate applies for individuals and families with their own policies who participate in approved wellness programs too.

- **Insurance rating incentives.** New Hampshire lawmakers in 2004 permitted small group and individual insurers to use a rating factor to discount premium rates for plans, giving monetary incentives for participants in wellness or disease management programs.

- **Tax credits.** Over the past few years, wellness tax credits have been proposed in at least seven states including Hawaii, Iowa, Mississippi, New Jersey, New York, Rhode Island and Wisconsin. The idea is to provide employers—especially smaller businesses—with income, franchise or corporate tax credits for wellness programs such as nutrition, weight management, smoking cessation or substance abuse counseling, or purchasing or maintaining fitness equipment.

- **Insurance benefits for screenings and early treatment.** According to Blue Cross-Blue Shield's "Survey of Health Plans" for 2005, specific preventive or screening benefits currently required by states include alcoholism treatment (44 states), blood lead screening (7 states), bone density screening (15 states), cervical cancer screening (29 states), colorectal cancer screening (24 states), diabetic supplies or education (47 states), mammography screening (50 states), morbid obesity care (4 states), prostate cancer screening (28 states) and well child care (32 states).

- **Task forces, advisory committees or studies.** States have considered creating task forces or advisory committees, or conducting studies exploring the benefits and feasibility of wellness programs or health promotion activities.

- **Raising awareness.** Legislators are sponsoring or participating in wellness events. For example, the Legislature declared May 2006 as Fitness Month in California and encouraged all Californians to enrich their lives through proper diet and exercise. Kentucky established the Governor's Council on Wellness and Physical Activity specifically to raise public awareness and promote citizen engagement.

Something Must Be Done

What if Americans don't get healthier? The costs could be shocking. Future cost of health care and other benefits could reach between $600 billion and $1.3 trillion for the nation's estimated 24.5 million active and retired state and local public employees.

Moving U.S. health policy toward a more preventive approach is key to containing health care costs. "The burden of chronic disease is increasingly making the U.S. health system unaffordable and causing much unnecessary pain and suffering," says former U.S. Surgeon General David Satcher. The solution? According to health experts at the Robert Wood Johnson Foundation it is "Leadership that informs and motivates, economic incentives that encourage change, and science that moves the frontiers."

NCSL's health care expert **AMY WINTERFELD** tracks wellness and obesity.

From *State Legislatures*, February 2007, pp. 14–16. Copyright © 2007 by National Conference of State Legislatures. Reprinted by permission.

UNIT 2
Stress and Mental Health

Unit Selections

Key Points to Consider

- How have humankind's stressors changed over the last 5,000 years?

- What are the major stressors in your life? How do you manage your stress?

- What roles do religion, love, and spirituality play in curing disease?

- Give examples that demonstrate the interaction between mental and physical health.

- Explain how worry can be both a positive and a negative force in shaping one's life.

- Why were there many predictions made about post traumatic stress disorders after the September 11 attacks?

- How does the presence or absence of sunlight affect mental health?

- What causes obsessive compulsive disorder?

Student Website
www.mhcls.com

Internet References

The American Institute of Stress
   http://www.stress.org
National Mental Health Association (NMHA)
   http://www.nmha.org/index.html
Self-Help Magazine
   http://www.selfhelpmagazine.com/index.html

The brain is one organ that still mystifies and baffles the scientific community. While more has been learned about this organ in the last decade than in all the rest of recorded history, our understanding of the brain is still in its infancy. What has been learned, however, has spawned exciting new research, and has contributed to the establishment of new disciplines, such as psychophysiology and psychoneuroimmunology (PNI).

Traditionally, the medical community has viewed health problems as either physical or mental, and has treated each type separately. This dichotomy between the psyche (mind) and soma (body) is fading in the light of scientific data that reveal profound physiological changes associated with mood shifts. What are the physiological changes associated with stress? Hans Selye, the father of stress research, described stress as a nonspecific physiological response to anything that challenges the body. He demonstrated that this response could be elicited by both mental and physical stimuli. Stress researchers have come to regard this response pattern as the "flight or fight" response, perhaps an adaptive throwback to our primitive ancestors. Researchers now believe that repeated and prolonged activation of this response can trigger destructive changes in our bodies and contribute to the development of several chronic diseases. So profound is the impact of emotional stress on the body that current estimates suggest that approximately 90 percent of all doctor visits are for stress-related disorders. If emotional stress elicits a generalized physiological response, why are there so many different diseases associated with it? Many experts believe that the answer may best be explained by what has been termed "the weak-organ theory." According to this theory, every individual has one organ system that is most susceptible to the damaging effects of prolonged stress.

Mental illness, which is generally regarded as a dysfunction of normal thought processes, has no single identifiable etiology. One may speculate that this is due to the complex nature of the organ system involved. There is also mounting evidence to suggest that there is an organic component to the traditional forms of mental illness such as schizophrenia, chronic depression, and manic depression. The fact that certain mental illnesses tend to occur within families has divided the mental health community into two camps: those who believe that there is a genetic factor operating and those who see the family tendency as more of a learned behavior. In either case, the evidence supports mental illness as another example of the weak-organ theory. The reason one person is more susceptible to the damaging effects of stress than another may not be altogether clear, but evidence is mounting that one's perception or attitude plays a key role in the stress equation. A prime example demonstrating this relationship comes from the research that relates cardiovascular disease to stress. The realization that our attitude has such a significant impact on our health has led to a burgeoning

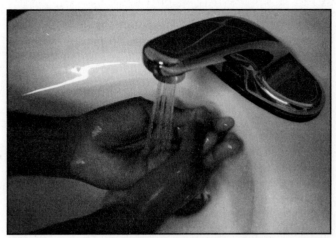

© McGraw-Hill Companies, Inc./Gary He, photographer

new movement in psychology termed "positive psychology." Dr. Martin Segilman, professor of psychology at the University of Pennsylvania and father of the positive psychology movement, believes that optimism is a key factor in maintaining not only our mental health, but our physical health as well. Dr. Segilman notes that while some people are naturally more optimistic than others, optimism can be learned.

One area in particular that appears to be influenced by the "positive psychology movement" is the area of stress management. Traditionally, stress management programs have focused on the elimination of stress, but that is starting to change as new strategies approach stress as an essential component of life and a potential source of health. It is worth noting that this concept, of stress serving as a positive force in a person's life, was presented by Dr. Hans Selye in 1974 in his book *Stress Without Distress*. Dr. Selye felt that there were three types of stress: negative stress (distress), normal stress, and positive stress (eustress). He maintained that positive stress not only increases a person's self-esteem but also serves to inoculate the person against the damaging effects of distress. Only time will tell if this change of focus in the area of stress management, will make any real difference in patient outcome. In "Stressed Out Nation," author Zak Stambor indicates that though most people experience stress, not all know how to manage it. He claims that negative responses to stress, such as overeating, smoking, or alcohol abuse can lead to health problems that will actually increase stress.

The causes of stress are many, but for some individuals, the coming of winter is a very difficult time for them. Many of these folks experience periods of depression during the shorter days of winter. Workplace stress is another form of distress affects the economy to the tune of billions of dollars per year due to sick leave and loss of productivity.

Researchers have made significant strides in their understanding of the mechanisms that link emotional stress to physical ailments, but they are less clear on the mechanisms by which positive emotions bolster one's health.

Two new articles in this section address mental health issues including depression and obsessive compulsive disorders. In "Redefining Depression as Mere Sadness," Ronald Pies believes it's valuable to treat individuals with profound sadness as depressed and to provide whatever therapeutic approaches that make the patient feel better. In "Are Your Rituals Driving You Crazy?", Ginny Graves discusses obsessive compulsive disorder and how it's managed. Most people with the condition are diagnosed before age 36 and the earlier the illness is identified, the more difficult it is to manage.

Although significant gains have been made in our understanding of the relationship between body and mind, much remains to be learned. What is known indicates that perception and one's attitude are the key elements in shaping our responses to stressors.

Redefining Depression as Mere Sadness

RONALD PIES, MD

Let's say a patient walks into my office and says he's been feeling down for the past three weeks. A month ago, his fiancée left him for another man, and he feels there's no point in going on. He has not been sleeping well, his appetite is poor and he has lost interest in nearly all of his usual activities.

Should I give him a diagnosis of clinical depression? Or is my patient merely experiencing what the 14th-century monk Thomas à Kempis called "the proper sorrows of the soul"? The answer is more complicated than some critics of psychiatric diagnosis think.

To these critics, psychiatry has medicalized normal sadness by failing to consider the social and emotional context in which people develop low mood—for example, after losing a job or experiencing the breakup of an important relationship. This diagnostic failure, the argument goes, has created a bogus epidemic of increasing depression.

A debate over when and how to treat a patient reeling from a loss.

In their recent book "The Loss of Sadness" (Oxford, 2007), Allan V. Horwitz and Jerome C. Wakefield assert that for thousands of years, symptoms of sadness that were "with cause" were separated from those that were "without cause." Only the latter were viewed as mental disorders.

With the advent of modern diagnostic criteria, these authors argue, doctors were directed to ignore the context of the patient's complaints and focus only on symptoms—poor appetite, insomnia, low energy, hopelessness and so on. The current criteria for major depression, they say, largely fail to distinguish between "abnormal" reactions caused by "internal dysfunction" and "normal sadness" brought on by external circumstances. And they blame vested interests—doctors, researchers, pharmaceutical companies—for fostering this bloated concept of depression.

But while this increasingly popular thesis contains a kernel of truth, it conceals a bushel basket of conceptual and scientific problems.

For one thing, if modern diagnostic criteria were converting mere sadness into clinical depression, we would expect the number of new cases of depression to be skyrocketing compared with rates in a period like the 1950s to the 1970s. But several new studies in the United States and Canada find that the incidence of serious depression has held relatively steady in recent decades.

Second, it may seem easy to determine that someone with depressive complaints is reacting to a loss that touched off the depression. Experienced clinicians know this is rarely the case.

Most of us can point to recent losses and disappointments in our lives, but it is not always clear that they are causally related to our becoming depressed. For example, a patient who had a stroke a month ago may appear tearful, lethargic and depressed. To critics, the so-called depression is just "normal sadness" in reaction to a terrible psychological blow. But strokes are also known to disrupt chemical pathways in the brain that directly affect mood.

What is the "real" trigger for this patient's depression? Perhaps it is a combination of psychological and neurological factors. In short, the notion of "reacting" to adverse life events is complex and problematic.

Third, and perhaps most troubling, is the implication that a recent major loss makes it more likely that the person's depressive symptoms will follow a benign and limited course, and therefore do not need medical treatment. This has never been demonstrated, to my knowledge, in any well-designed studies. And what *has* been demonstrated, in a study by Dr. Sidney Zisook, is that antidepressants may help patients with major depressive symptoms occurring just after the death of a loved one.

Yes, most psychiatrists would concede that in the space of a brief "managed care" appointment, it's very hard to understand much about the context of the patient's depressive complaints. And yes, under such conditions, some doctors are tempted to write that prescription for Prozac or Zoloft and move on to the next patient.

But the vexing issue of when bereavement or sadness becomes a disorder, and how it should be treated, requires much more study. Most psychiatrists believe that undertreatment of severe depression is a more pressing problem than overtreatment of "normal sadness." Until solid research persuades me otherwise, I will most likely see people like my jilted patient as clinically depressed, not just "normally sad"—and I will provide him with whatever psychiatric treatment he needs to feel better.

RONALD PIES is a professor of psychiatry at Tufts and SUNY Upstate Medical Center in Syracuse.

From *The New York Times*, June 16, 2008. Copyright © 2008 by The New York Times Company. Reprinted by permission via PARS International.

Stressed Out Nation

Many Americans resort to unhealthy habits to help manage extreme stress, a new survey suggests.

ZAK STAMBOR

More than half of working adults—and 47 percent of all Americans—say they are concerned with the amount of stress in their lives, according to a new telephone survey conducted Jan. 12–24 by APA's Practice Directorate in partnership with the National Women's Health Resource Center and iVillage.com.

Moreover, the survey finds that people experiencing stress are more likely to report hypertension, anxiety, depression or obesity. The survey, which sampled 2,152 adults who are 18 years or older, is part of the Practice Directorate's "Mind/Body Health: For a Healthy Mind and Body, Talk to a Psychologist" campaign. The initiative aims to highlight psychology's role at the intersection between mental and physical well-being.

By focusing on the physical and mental toll of stress, the campaign is shining light on how many Americans react to both work- and family-related stress—by engaging in unhealthy behaviors, such as comfort eating, making poor diet choices, smoking and being inactive, says Helen Mitternight, assistant executive director of public relations in the Practice Directorate.

"Americans are stressed out, and they are dealing with that stress in an unhealthy way," says Mitternight.

However, on a positive note, she notes, nearly 20 percent of those most concerned about stress said that seeing a mental health professional could help them get back on track and relieve some of their stress.

Gender Differences

Stress is particularly prevalent for the primary decision-maker in the household for health issues, says Mitternight. Since 73 percent of women identify themselves as such, women feel the brunt of the health-care burden, she adds.

"Women are the health-care managers of their families," says Amber McCracken, director of communications for the National Women's Health Resource Center. "From taking care of their own health to serving as the caregivers for their children, partner and parents, each aspect of care brings stress. Unfortunately, too often women do not take the necessary steps to alleviate that stress, and their own physical health suffers."

Moreover, men and women exhibit their stress differently, the survey found. Women are more likely than men to report feelings of nervousness, wanting to cry or lacking energy. Men, 40 percent of whom consider themselves the primary health-care decision-maker, are prone to describing their stressed condition as sleepless, irritable or angry.

Those gender differences are magnified in men and women's coping mechanisms, the survey found. For instance, nearly 31 percent of women say they are comfort eaters, while only 19 percent of men report eating to deal with their problems. The urge to comfort-eat can have complex consequences, as the survey found that comfort eaters are more likely to exhibit higher levels of the most common stress symptoms, including fatigue, lack of energy, nervousness and sleeplessness.

The survey also found that 21 percent of participants who ate at a fast-food restaurant in the week prior to the survey reported being very concerned about stress, while only 13 percent of people who did not eat at a fast-food restaurant in the week prior to the survey were very concerned about stress. Not surprisingly, the fast-food-eaters were also more likely to experience more serious health problems like hypertension and high cholesterol.

Mind/Body Connection

The survey suggests that for most Americans stress results from a conglomeration of concerns. For instance, an office worker stressing out over a project deadline may quickly down a hamburger and fries while he or she works to save time. In turn, that stress-fueled decision may next lead to health worries.

"Everybody experiences stress," says Newman. "The key is how effectively people deal with and manage stress. People who turn to comfort food or smoking are starting a vicious cycle. Their attempts to reduce stress can actually lead to health problems that result in even more stress."

Russ Newman
APA Practice Directorate

The office worker's stressors are not unique, as more than half the survey respondents included concerns about money, work, family-member health problems or the state of the world today, as some of their leading sources of stress. More than 40 percent of participants also cited the health of immediate family members and caring for their children as common stressors.

An effective means of dealing with stress, suggests Russ Newman, PhD, JD, executive director of APA's Practice Directorate, is learning how to cope.

"Everybody experiences stress," says Newman. "The key is how effectively people deal with and manage stress. People who turn to comfort food or smoking are starting a vicious cycle. Their attempts to reduce stress can actually lead to health problems that result in even more stress."

To help break the cycle, Newman suggests that stressed people pay attention to their behaviors and lifestyle choices. Additionally, he notes that although some behaviors can be particularly difficult to change, working with a psychologist can help modify those actions.

The survey sponsors released the results at February press event in New York City that garnered national media attention on TV news shows such as "Good Morning America" and in newspapers such as *USA Today*. In addition to the media campaign, the sponsors are pairing the results with additional tips on how to manage stress. iVillage is also posting a Stress Smarts Quiz on its website to help readers understand the seriousness of their stress.

From *Monitor on Psychology* by Zak Stambor, April 2006, pp. 28–29. Copyright © 2006 by American Psychological Association. Reprinted by permission. No further distribution without permission from the American Psychological Association.

Seasonal Affective Disorder

Patients with seasonal affective disorder have episodes of major depression that tend to recur during specific times of the year, usually in winter. Like major depression, seasonal affective disorder probably is underdiagnosed in primary care settings. Although several screening instruments are available, such screening is unlikely to lead to improved outcomes without personalized and detailed attention to individual symptoms. Physicians should be aware of comorbid factors that could signal a need for further assessment. Specifically, some emerging evidence suggests that seasonal affective disorder may be associated with alcoholism and attention-deficit/hyperactivity disorder. Seasonal affective disorder often can be treated with light therapy, which appears to have a low risk of adverse effects. Light therapy is more effective if administered in the morning. It remains unclear whether light is equivalent to drug therapy, whether drug therapy can augment the effects of light therapy, or whether cognitive behavior therapy is a better treatment choice. (Am Fam Physician 2006;74:1521–24. Copyright © 2006 American Academy of Family Physicians.)

STEPHEN J. LURIE ET AL.

The *Diagnostic and Statistical Manual of Mental Disorders,* 4th ed., (DSM-IV) categorizes seasonal affective disorder (SAD) not as a unique mood disorder, but as a specifier of major depression.[1] Thus, patients with SAD experience episodes of major depression that tend to recur at specific times of the year. These seasonal episodes may take the form of major depressive or bipolar disorders.

Epidemiology

The overall lifetime prevalence of SAD ranges from 0 to 9.7 percent.[2] This estimate depends on the specific population studied, as well as whether SAD is diagnosed by a screening questionnaire or a more rigorous clinical interview. In one U.S. study that used DSM-IV-based criteria, the lifetime prevalence of major depression with a seasonal pattern was 0.4 percent.[3] Prevalence may be higher at northern latitudes, and it may vary within ethnic groups at the same latitude.[4]

Patients with SAD are more likely to have family members with SAD, although this may be subject to reporting bias.[5] Twin studies have found that there may be a genetic component to susceptibility. Several genes code for serotonin transport, but the overall pattern of heritability likely is complex and polygenomic.[6]

Patients with SAD have more outpatient visits, more diagnostic testing, more prescriptions, and more referrals throughout the year compared with age- and sex-matched controls.[7] Patients with SAD visit their primary care physician more often in the winter than other patients, but rates between the groups are similar the rest of the year.[8]

Screening for SAD

Primary care physicians routinely fail to diagnose nearly one half of all patients who present with depression and other mental health problems.[9] Because SAD is a subtype of major depression, screening for depression should theoretically help identify patients with this disorder. The U.S. Preventive Services Task Force (USPSTF) concluded that there is good evidence that screening improves the accurate identification of patients with depression in primary care settings, and that treatment decreases clinical morbidity. The USPSTF concluded that the benefits of screening likely outweigh any potential harms.[10]

There are several instruments for detecting depression in primary care, ranging in length from one to 30 items with an average administration time of two to six minutes. Typically, the reading level of these instruments is between the third- and fifth-grade levels.[11] Some standardized instruments focus more narrowly on SAD. Reports on the sensitivity and specificity of these instruments can be difficult to interpret because of the small sizes and heterogeneity of patient samples tested, the possibility of differential recall bias (depending on the time of year the test is administered), and ongoing controversy over the criteria standard for SAD.

The Seasonal Pattern Assessment Questionnaire (SPAQ) is perhaps the most widely studied tool. It has been reported to have a high specificity (94 percent) for SAD but a low sensitivity (41 percent).[12] Other authors, however, have reported a much lower specificity.[13] The Seasonal Health Questionnaire has been reported to have higher specificity and sensitivity than the SPAQ,[14] but these results must be confirmed in larger and more diverse patient groups.

Sort: Key Recommendations for Practice

Clinical Recommendation	Evidence Rating	References
Standardized screening instruments for SAD probably are not sensitive enough to be used for routine screening.	C	12
Light therapy may be used for treating SAD, with effect sizes similar to those for antidepressant medications in treating depression. The total daily dosage should be approximately 5,000 lux, administered in the morning over 30 to 120 minutes.	A	23
Cognitive behavior therapy may be considered as an alternative to light therapy in the treatment of SAD.	B	28

SAD = seasonal affective disorder.
A = consistent, good-quality patient-oriented evidence; B = inconsistent or limited-quality patient-oriented evidence; C = consensus, disease-oriented evidence, usual practice, expert opinion, or case series. For information about the SORT evidence rating system, see page 1463 or http://www.aafp.org/afpsort.xml.

Although benefits from screening are less likely to be achieved without an accurate diagnostic work-up, effective treatment interventions, and close follow-up, it is unclear whether screening ultimately improves the care and outcomes of patients with major depression. When deciding to implement a screening instrument in a practice, office personnel should consider the administration time, scoring ease, reading level, and usefulness in identifying major depression and assessing change in the depression scores over time.[15]

Once patients have been identified as having major depression, questions must be asked to determine if the depression is linked to SAD. These questions concern the relationship between depression and time of year (if remission occurs during certain times of the year) and whether the depression has occurred at the same time during the past two years.

Associated Diagnoses

Because SAD is associated with serotonergic dysregulation and possibly with noradrenergic mechanisms, it may overlap with other diagnoses that share similar mechanisms, including generalized anxiety disorder, panic disorder, bulimia nervosa, late luteal phase dysphoric disorder, and chronic fatigue syndrome.[16] SAD also may be associated with attention-deficit/hyperactivity disorder (ADHD). Both conditions have been described as "disorders of central underarousal coupled with a heightened sensitivity to stimuli from the physical environment," and both are more common in women with a particular genotype for *HTR2A,* a gene that codes for a serotonin receptor.[17,18]

A pattern of seasonal alcohol use also may be associated with SAD. A summary of current research findings concluded that some patients with alcoholism may be self-medicating an underlying depression with alcohol or manifesting a seasonal pattern to alcohol-induced depression.[19] Such patterns appear to have a familial component and, like the link between ADHD and SAD, may be related to serotonergic functioning.

Treatment

Treatment options for SAD include light therapy, cognitive behavior therapy, and pharmacotherapy. Each option has been proven beneficial in treating SAD, but no large studies have found any treatment to be superior.

Light Therapy

Among susceptible persons, decreased seasonal exposure to light may mediate SAD through phase shifts in circadian rhythms, with resulting alterations in several aspects of serotonin metabolism. Thus, light replacement has been the most widely studied treatment for SAD.[20] In a review of studies of light therapy, an average dosage of 2,500 lux daily for one week was superior to placebo, as indicated by improvements on a depression rating scale.[21] The dosage most often found to be effective is 5,000 lux per day, given as 2,500 lux for two hours or 10,000 lux for 30 minutes.[22] A recent meta-analysis of 23 studies of light therapy found that the odds ratio for remission was 2.9 (95% confidence interval, 1.6 to 5.4); this ratio is similar to those of many pharmaceutical treatments for depression.[23] Like drug therapy for depression, light therapy carries some risk of precipitating mania.[24]

Light therapy generally is most effective when administered earlier in the day.[21,25,26] Early morning light therapy regulates the circadian pattern of melatonin secretion, whereas the use of light in the evening delays the normal melatonin phase shift.[27]

To ensure adequate response, patients should be treated with light therapy units that are specifically designed to treat SAD. Units that are not specifically designed for SAD treatment may not provide adequate brightness and may not have appropriate ultraviolet light filtration.[22]

Cognitive Behavior Therapy

Although cognitive behavior therapy (CBT) has some effectiveness in improving dysfunctional automatic thoughts and attitudes, behavior withdrawal, low rates of positive reinforcement, and ruminations in patients with major depression, few studies have assessed its effectiveness in the treatment of SAD. In one small clinical trial, patients with SAD were randomized to six weeks of treatment with CBT or light therapy, or CBT plus light therapy.[28] At the end of treatment, all three groups had significantly decreased levels of depression, but there was no difference between groups. However, this study only enrolled 26 subjects. To date, there have been no studies large enough to establish the effectiveness of CBT in the treatment of SAD.

Pharmacotherapy

Because patients with SAD also must fulfill criteria for depression, several randomized trials have assessed the use of antidepressants for this condition.[29–33] Most of these studies have compared pharmacotherapy with placebo rather than light therapy, making it difficult to determine if one treatment is superior. In the largest of these trials, patients with SAD had significantly better response on several measures of depression after eight weeks of sertraline (Zoloft) therapy compared with control patients.[29] Patients were excluded if they were receiving light therapy or other psychoactive medications, or if they had a history of alcoholism, drug abuse, or "emotional or intellectual problems."

A smaller study found that, in some statistical analyses, fluoxetine (Prozac) was better than placebo in the treatment of SAD.[30] Another small study found that the monoamine oxidase inhibitor moclobemide (not available in the United States) was similar to placebo in terms of changes on several general depression scales.[31]

Small trials of other agents (i.e., carbidopa/levodopa [Sinemet] and vitamin B_{12}) found no benefit over placebo.[34,35] Although there may be some theoretical justification for these treatments, there have not been trials of sufficient size to assess their effects.

Few randomized trials have assessed the effect of light therapy compared with pharmacotherapy.[32,36] These trials failed to find a difference between the effect of 6,000 lux and that of 20 mg of fluoxetine daily,[32] or between 10,000 lux and 20 mg of fluoxetine daily.[36] Larger trials will be required to establish whether there is a difference in effect size between light therapy and pharmacotherapy.

It is also possible that pharmacotherapy may preserve an initial therapeutic response to light therapy. Among 168 patients who had a positive response to light therapy, citalopram (Celexa) was found to be no more effective than placebo at preventing relapse; however, it was superior in terms of some secondary measures of depression.[33] In general, current evidence does not provide clear guidance as to whether antidepressant treatment is superior to light therapy, or whether antidepressants are useful as an adjunct to light therapy.

References

1. American Psychiatric Association. Task Force on DSM-IV. Diagnostic and Statistical Manual of Mental Disorders. 4th ed. Washington, D.C.: American Psychiatric Association, 1994.
2. Magnusson A. An overview of epidemiological studies on seasonal affective disorder. Acta Psychiatr Scand 2000;101:176–84.
3. Blazer DG, Kessler RC, Swartz MS. Epidemiology of recurrent major and minor depression with a seasonal pattern. The National Comorbidity Survey. Br J Psychiatry 1998;172:164–7.
4. Mersch PP, Middendorp HM, Bouhuys AL, Beersma DG, van den Hoofdakker RH. Seasonal affective disorder and latitude: a review of the literature. J Affect Disord 1999;53:35–48.
5. Sher L, Goldman D, Ozaki N, Rosenthal NE. The role of genetic factors in the etiology of seasonal affective disorder and seasonality. J Affect Disord 1999;53:203–10.
6. Sher L. Genetic studies of seasonal affective disorder and seasonality. Compr Psychiatry 2001;42:105–10.
7. Eagles JM, Howie FL, Cameron IM, Wileman SM, Andrew JE, Robertson C, et al. Use of health care services in seasonal affective disorder. Br J Psychiatry 2002;180:449–54.
8. Andrew JE, Wileman SM, Howie FL, Cameron IM, Naji SA, Eagles JM. Comparison of consultation rates in primary care attenders with and without seasonal affective disorder. J Affect Disord 2001;62:199–205.
9. Higgins ES. A review of unrecognized mental illness in primary care. Prevalence, natural history, and efforts to change the course. Arch Fam Med 1994;3:908–17.
10. U.S. Preventive Services Task Force. Screening for depression: recommendations and rationale. Ann Intern Med 2002;136:760–4.
11. Williams JW Jr, Pignone M, Ramirez G, Perez Stellato C. Identifying depression in primary care: a literature synthesis of case-finding instruments. Gen Hosp Psychiatry 2002;24:225–37.
12. Mersch PP, Vastenburg NC, Meesters Y, Bouhuys AL, Beersma DG, van den Hoofdakker RH, et al. The reliability and validity of the Seasonal Pattern Assessment Questionnaire: a comparison between patient groups. J Affect Disorder 2004;80:209–19.
13. Raheja SK, King EA, Thompson C. The Seasonal Pattern Assessment Questionnaire for identifying seasonal affective disorders. J Affect Disord 1996;41:193–9.
14. Thompson C, Thompson S, Smith R. Prevalence of seasonal affective disorder in primary care; a comparison of the seasonal pattern assessment questionnaire. J Affect Disord 2004;78:219–26.
15. Nease DE Jr, Malouin JM. Depression screening: a practical strategy. J Fam Pract 2003;52:118–24.
16. Partonen T, Magnusson A. Seasonal Affective Disorder: Practice and Research. New York, N.Y.: Oxford University Press, 2001.
17. Levitan RD, Masellis M, Basile VS, Lam RW, Jain U, Kaplan AS, et al. Polymorphism of the serotonin-2A receptor gene (HTR2A) associated with childhood attention deficit hyperactivity disorder (ADHD) in adult women with seasonal affective disorder. J Affect Disord 2002;71:229–33.
18. Levitan RD, Jain UR, Katzman MA. Seasonal affective symptoms in adults with residual attention-deficit hyperactivity disorder. Compr Psychiatry 1999;40:261–7.
19. Sher L. Alcoholism and seasonal affective disorder. Compr Psychiatry 2004;45:51–6.
20. Partonen T, Lonnqvist J. Seasonal affective disorder. Lancet 1998;352:1369–74.
21. Terman M, Terman JS, Quitkin FM, McGrath PJ, Stewart JW, Rafferty B. Light therapy for seasonal affective disorder. A review of efficacy. Neuropsychopharmacology 1989;2:1–22.
22. Levitan RD. What is the optimal implementation of bright light therapy for seasonal affective disorder (SAD)? J Psychiatry Neurosci 2005;30:72.
23. Golden RN, Gaynes BN, Ekstrom RD, Hamer RM, Jacobsen FM, Suppes T, et al. The efficacy of light therapy in the treatment of mood disorders: a review and meta-analysis of the evidence. Am J Psychiatry 2005;162:656–62.
24. Sohn CH, Lam RW. Treatment of seasonal affective disorder: unipolar versus bipolar differences. Curr Psychiatry Rep 2004;6:478–85.
25. Eastman CI, Young MA, Fogg LF, Liu L, Meaden PM. Bright light treatment of winter depression: a placebo-controlled trial. Arch Gen Psychiatry 1998;55:883–9.
26. Terman M, Terman JS, Ross DC. A controlled trial of timed bright light and negative air ionization for treatment of winter depression. Arch Gen Psychiatry 1998;55:875–82.
27. Terman JS, Terman M, Lo ES, Cooper TB. Circadian time of morning light administration and therapeutic response in winter depression. Arch Gen Psychiatry 2001;58:69–75.
28. Rohan KJ, Lindsey KT, Roecklein KA, Lacy TJ. Cognitive-behavioral therapy, light therapy, and their combination in treating seasonal affective disorder. J Affect Disord 2004;80:273–83.

29. Moscovitch A, Blashko CA, Eagles JM, Darcourt G, Thompson C, Kasper S, et al., for the International Collaborative Group on Sertraline in the Treatment of Outpatients with Seasonal Affective Disorders. A placebo-controlled study of sertraline in the treatment of outpatients with seasonal affective disorder. Psychopharmacology (Berl) 2004;171:390–7.

30. Lam RW, Gorman CP, Michalon M, Steiner M, Levitt AJ, Corral MR, et al. Multicenter, placebo-controlled study of fluoxetine in seasonal affective disorder. Am J Psychiatry 1995;152:1765–70.

31. Lingjaerde O, Reichborn-Kjennerud T, Haggag A, Gartner I, Narud K, Berg EM. Treatment of winter depression in Norway. II. A comparison of the selective monoamine oxidase A inhibitor moclobemide and placebo. Acta Psychiatr Scand 1993;88:372–80.

32. Ruhrmann S, Kasper S, Hawellek B, Martinez B, Hoflich G, Nickelsen T, et al. Effects of fluoxetine versus bright light in the treatment of seasonal affective disorder. Psychol Med 1998;28:923–33.

33. Martiny K, Lunde M, Simonsen C, Clemmensen L, Poulsen DL, Solstad K, et al. Relapse prevention by citalopram in SAD patients responding to 1 week of light therapy. A placebo-controlled study. Acta Psychiatr Scand 2004;109:230–4.

34. Oren DA, Moul DE, Schwartz PJ, Wehr TA, Rosenthal NE. A controlled trial of levodopa plus carbidopa in the treatment of winter seasonal affective disorder: a test of the dopamine hypothesis. J Clin Psychopharmacol 1994;14:196–200.

35. Oren DA, Teicher MH, Schwartz PJ, Glod C, Turner EH, Ito YN, et al. A controlled trial of cyanocobalamin (vitamin B12) in the treatment of winter seasonal affective disorder. J Affect Disord 1994;32:197–200.

36. Lam RW, Levitt AJ, Levitan RD, Enns MW, Morehouse R, Michalek EE, et al. The Can-SAD study: a randomized controlled trial of the effectiveness of light therapy and fluoxetine in patients with winter seasonal affective disorder. Am J Psychiatry 2006;163:805–12.

STEPHEN J. LURIE, MD, PhD, is assistant professor of family medicine at the University of Rochester (N.Y.) School of Medicine and Dentistry. BARBARA GAWINSKI, PhD, is director of psychosocial curriculum in the Department of Family Medicine at the University of Rochester School of Medicine and Dentistry. DEBORAH PIERCE, MD, MPH, is clinical associate professor of family medicine at the University of Rochester School of Medicine and Dentistry. SALLY J. ROUSSEAU, MSW, is administrator of the Family Medicine Research Center at the University of Rochester School of Medicine and Dentistry.

Address correspondence to Stephen J. Lurie, MD, PhD, Dept. of Family Medicine, University of Rochester School of Medicine and Dentistry, 1381 South Ave., Rochester, NY 14620 (e-mail: Stephen_Lurie @urmcrochester.edu). Reprints are not available from the authors.

From *American Family Physician*, November 1, 2006, pp. 1521–1524. Copyright © 2006 by American Academy of Family Physicians. Reprinted by permission.

Dealing with the Stressed

Workplace stress costs the economy more than $30 billion a year, and yet nobody knows what it is or how to deal with it.

KEN MacQUEEN

Life is hard. You work in a "fabric-covered box," as Dilbert puts it. Some troll in the IT department monitors your every keystroke. Lunch is a greasy slab of *pizza al desko,* eaten under heavy email fire. Your eyesight is shot, you're going to flab, you've vowed to make this just a 50-hour week because your spouse—toiling in another cubicle across town—needs every night and the weekend to meet her ridiculous deadline. It's 4:59 p.m., and if you're late again the daycare's gonna dump the kid on the street and call Children's Aid. Grab the cell. Grab the BlackBerry. You just know the boss is going to tug your electronic leash if he sees you leaving this early. Yeah, yeah, life is hard.

It's, you know, stressful. Whatever that means.

Stress is part of an explosion in workplace mental health issues now costing the Canadian economy an estimated $33 billion a year in lost productivity, as well as billions more in medical costs. It's become a political priority for Prime Minister Stephen Harper, who recently announced a new Mental Health Commission of Canada. With almost one million Canadians suffering from a mental health disorder, "it's now the fastest-growing category of disability insurance claims in Canada," Harper said. The cause is unclear. "Some blame the hectic pace of modern life, the trend to smaller and fragmented families, often separated by great distances, or the mass migration from small stable communities to huge, impersonal cities," he said. If there was a false note in his speech, it was his optimistic view of society's comprehension of the issue. "We now understand," he said, "that mental illness is not a supernatural phenomenon, or a character flaw."

Well, maybe. Such understanding is hardly universal in the workplace, where, as Harper noted, "stress or worse" exacts a heavy toll. It's as likely that stress-related maladies will be viewed with a combination of cynicism, incomprehension, and a skepticism bordering on hostility. To critics—a field that includes many employers, some academics, and co-workers resentful at picking up the slack—stress is the new whiplash, except bigger, more expensive, harder to define, and even more difficult to prove. Or to disprove.

"Stress," says U.S. author and workplace counsellor Scott Sheperd, "is probably the most overused and misused word in the English language—with the possible exception of love." It means everything and nothing. It is, he argues in *Attacking the Stress Myth,* "The Great Excuse." Look at the numbers: stress leaves are off the charts and some of the zombies who do show up accomplish little more than draining the company coffee pot.

The cause of this growing hit on productivity is indeed a mystery. Did the world get harder, or did people get softer? Or are employers stuck with an addled labour force of their own creation? It's not as if today's children will be sent to work in the mines. Women aren't struggling to raise six kids, while mourning several more who died in infancy. Men aren't spending 12 hours a day plowing fields behind a mule, or sweating over some mechanical monster of the Industrial Revolution, waiting for an arm or a leg to be dragged into its innards. No, odds are you've got indoor work, no heavy lifting, a 40-hour week (in theory), holiday time, and a big-screen TV waiting at home. How hard can life be?

Well, one person's dream job can be another's nightmare.

Nights, weekends, Janie Toivanen, an employee on the Burnaby campus of video game giant Electronic Arts (Canada) Ltd., gave her all to her job. She was part of the team producing EA's wildly popular NHL game series. EA prides itself on being a work-hard/play-hard kind of place. The complex looks like a workers' paradise, complete with a sand-covered beach volleyball court, an artificial turf soccer pitch, a full-on fitness centre, massage, yoga classes and a steam room. There's a gourmet cafeteria, and an employee concierge service to look after such mundanities as dry cleaning and car washing. In exchange, EA expects a huge degree of worker commitment.

Toivanen, an employee since 1996, earned strong performance ratings in her early years, regular bonuses and stock options. She rose through the ranks, often using what downtime she had to catch up on her sleep. "Ms. Toivanen's career was her life," says a decision last year by the British Columbia Human Rights Tribunal. But life caught up with her. By 2002, at age 47, she was carrying a heavy load, and looming deadlines preyed on her mind and ruined her sleep. Dealings with co-workers were strained, questions from supervisors were met with tears or anger.

She resisted her doctor's urging to take stress leave, fearing it would hurt her career. Finally, on the edge of a breakdown in September 2002, she handed her doctor's note to a supervisor and requested leave, only to be told EA had already decided to fire her. Big mistake. The failure to investigate her deteriorating condition or to accommodate her medical condition violated the provincial human rights code, the tribunal concluded. "She thought that EA was a company that prided itself on looking after employees," it said. "Instead of investing any time and energy in bringing her back, healthy, to her workplace, it fired her." She spiralled into depression and was placed on long-term disability by her former employer's insurer. At the time of the ruling in 2006 she was still on paid disability. The tribunal ordered EA to pay almost $150,000 in costs, severance, stock option losses and damages, "for injury to her dignity, feelings and self-respect."

Chronic job stress has emerged in epidemic terms. Our job is to make a business case for mental health.

Employers neglect the work environment at their peril, warns Bill Wilkerson, a former insurance company president and now CEO of the Global Business and Economic Roundtable on Addiction and Mental Health. "Chronic job stress has emerged in what you might call epidemic terms," he says. He co-founded the group 10 years ago, as private insurers grew alarmed at the runaway impact of mental health issues.

The first indicator was the spiralling costs of prescription drugs for maladies that were "imprecise in their nature," says Wilkerson, who also now serves as chairman of the workplace advisory board of the Canadian Mental Health Commission. Depression, insomnia, hypertension were all part of the mix. "As a business guy I was focused on how we tackled these as costs," he says. After a decade immersed in the science, Wilkerson has no doubt stress is a trigger for mental health issues, and such physical ailments as hypertension and heart attack. But there remains, he concedes, skepticism in boardrooms and corner offices. "We have to talk tough love to business leaders all the time," he says. "Our job isn't to make a case for business, it's to make a business case for mental health."

Still, the skepticism remains. In the case of politicians, for example, some think stress leave is just an excuse to escape political problems. Consider some examples: veteran NDP MP Svend Robinson walked into a public auction in 2004 and stole an expensive ring. Days later, he turned himself in, held a tearful news conference and embarked on stress leave. He was subsequently diagnosed with a bipolar disorder. A year

later, Conservative Gurmant Grewal, then an MP from Surrey, B.C., took stress leave after being embroiled in a scandal over secretly recording conversations with senior Liberal officials, among other bizarre incidents. "One of the things that makes me pretty cynical is when I hear a politician or a CEO who's gotten into trouble leave to spend more time with his family, or to take stress leave," says stress researcher Donna Lero of the University of Guelph.

Even when companies think they have clear evidence of malingering, they may find the courts decide otherwise. James Symington, a Halifax police officer and aspiring actor, left work June 11, 2001, citing an elbow injury. He was found fit for duty; instead, he booked off on stress leave. Months later, still on leave, Symington took his service dog to New York to help search for bodies after the terror attacks of Sept. 11. He also worked acting gigs. Symington was fired in early 2005, while still on leave, after the force said he wouldn't co-operate with attempts to get him back to work. This August, the Nova Scotia Court of Appeal cleared the way for Symington to sue the police for malicious prosecution for conducting a fraud investigation into his alleged misuse of stress leave. He's also suing his union, claiming it failed to protect him from a hostile work environment.

Understandably, many employers have become highly skeptical of complaints about excessive stress, and they vent their frustration to people like employment law specialist Howard Levitt, a Toronto-based lawyer for Lang Michener. He says stress issues have mushroomed during his 28 years in the field. "It's become for most employers the single biggest bugaboo in terms of workplace law issues," he says. Companies are "infuriated" by doctors who recommend stress leaves "without any real substantiation." For one thing, the family doctor isn't diagnosing the problem behind the alleged stress. Nor does the doctor know if there are other jobs in the workplace the patient is still capable of doing. The end result, ironically, is a more stressful workplace. "It's a bad motivation for other employees who see these employees getting away with it, and then have to work harder to pick up the slack," says Levitt. "So, often they say, 'Why shouldn't I participate in this scam?' And everybody works a little less hard."

A vocal minority of academics and others share a view that stress is a bogus concept. British author and former Fulbright Scholar Angela Patmore took on the "stress industry" in her 2006 book, *The Truth About Stress*. She doesn't buy that life in Britain is more stressful than it was, for instance, during the war years or the disease-ridden Victorian era. "The concept of mitigating stress is bollocks," she told *Maclean's*. "Everywhere in the West we see this message, 'you will drop dead, you will go mad, avoid negative emotions, avoid emotional situations.' None of our ancestors would have understood a word of this." She has an ally in Bob Briner, an occupational psychologist teaching at London University's Birkbeck College. He considers stress a meaningless concept; one that is creating a generation of "emotional hypochondriacs." As he writes, "One of the main explanations for the popularity of stress is that people like simple catch-all ways of 'explaining' why bad things happen, particularly illness."

The concept of mitigating stress is bollocks. Our ancestors wouldn't have understood a word of this.

Whether you believe stress is a real condition with debilitating effects, or the product of a generation of weak-minded workers, this much is indisputable: the costs are real, and spectacular. "Today, our estimate is that mental health conditions—with stress a risk factor—clearly cost the economy $33 billion per annum in lost industrial output," says Wilkerson. Those losses, he adds, "are excessively higher than the cost of health care associated with treating these conditions."

But one of the central problems with treating the apparent stress epidemic is that it remains exceptionally difficult to cure a problem that can't be easily defined. If you ask experts for a definition of stress, you often get a pause and then something like this: it is a highly individualistic, multi-faceted response to a set of circumstances that place a demand on physical or mental energy. There is "distress," a negative response to disturbing circumstances. And there is "eustress," so-called good stress. Eustress might come on the day you marry the love of your life. Distress might come on the day the love of your life marries someone else. Stress is a kind of personal weather system, ever changing, its components unique to the individual. It may consist of overwork and job insecurity, combined with colicky children and a sickly mother. It may be an unrealistic deadline, vague expectations and hostile co-workers. It may be the thing that gets you up in the morning, the challenge that makes work bearable, the risk of failure that makes success sweeter. Stress is bad. Stress is good. Stress is a mess. It is also a constantly moving target.

"Is stress quantitatively growing, I don't know," says Shannon Wagner, a clinical psychologist and a specialist in workplace stress research at the University of Northern British Columbia. "What we do know is it is qualitatively changing." Jobs may not be as physically laborious as they were but they're more relentless, she says. "A lot of people now are identifying techno-stress and the 24/7 workday, which we didn't have even 10 or 15 years ago, this feeling of being constantly plugged in, of checking email 500 times a day."

There is ample evidence that people are working longer and harder, skimping on holidays, and paying a price. The work-life balance is out of whack, says Donna Lero, who holds the Jarislowsky Chair in Families and Work at the University of Guelph. She says the stresses today's families face are different, and come from all directions. Workdays are longer, and for most families, including three-quarters of those with children, both parents work. "What used to be three people's work is being done by two, with nobody home when the child is sick," she says. Families are smaller, but they're also scattered. The sandwich generation is often simultaneously handling both child and elder care. "At a time when employers and certainly individuals are voicing concerns about work-family conflict, we're seeing things go in the opposite direction we'd like them to."

Consider the impact on the federal public service. A newly released Treasury Board study of remuneration for some 351,000 public servants notes that disability claims for its two main insurance plans have more than doubled between 1990 and 2002. "Much of the increase," the report concludes, "resulted from growth in cases relating to depression and anxiety." In fact, more than 44 per cent of all new public service disability claims were for depression and anxiety—up from less than 24 per cent a decade earlier. Stress and mental health issues are now the leading reason for long-term disability claims, ahead of cancer. The problem seems to be especially acute in Quebec, where civil servants are off the job an average of 14 days a year, an increase of 33 per cent since 2001, according to a recent report.

Nationally, an estimated 35 million workdays are lost to mental conditions among our 10 million workers. A six-year-old Health Canada report estimates the annual cost of just depression and distress at $14.4 billion: $6.3 billion in treatment and $8.1 billion in lost productivity. And all that only measures the number of people who actually miss time at work. Just as serious may be "presenteeism"— the phenomenon of stressed-out workers who show up to work anyway and accomplish little. It's estimated to cost Canadian employers $22 billion a year. "It's the silent scourge of productivity," says Paul Hemp, who wrote a definitive article on the subject for *The Harvard Business Review* in 2004. A U.S. study of 29,000 adults calculated the total cost of presenteeism at more than US$150 billion.

So what is an enlightened, conscientious employer to do? That's a quandary: in some cases, a generous benefits plan actually *increases* the likelihood of workers booking off. A study on sick leave published last year by Statistics Canada found unionized workers with disability insurance are far more likely to take extended leaves. The recent federal public service pay study uncovered an interesting fact: prison guards, dockyard workers, heating plant operators and hospital service groups consistently used the most sick leave per capita during the 13-year period under examination. It's understandable that those in "difficult environments like penitentiaries or dockyards" would make more claims, the study notes. But their consistent use of leave over the years "suggests that cultural and management factors may also play a role in the level of demand for sick leave." Translation: some workers take stress leave simply because they can.

Nationally, an estimated 35 million workdays are lost each year due to mental and emotional distress.

It seems the key is to strike a difficult balance between compassion and coddling. It's not easy, but for those who get it right, the results are dramatic. For example, the Vancouver City Savings Credit Union—Vancity—has been repeatedly ranked among *Maclean's* Top 100 employers, in part because of an ingrained employee assistance program and management training in spotting employee problems before they reach a crisis.

Few jobs are as stressful as front-line tellers, especially in Vancouver, with an average 237 bank robberies a year, about the highest rate in Canada. Ann Leckie, Vancity's director of human resources, concedes "one of the greatest negative situations we can face is robbery." Vancity set out in the mid-1980s to limit the personal and financial fallout by contracting Daniel Stone & Associates Inc., its employee assistance provider, to design a robbery recovery program. Branch employees who wish to gather after a robbery can meet with Stone, a clinical counsellor, and others of his staff. Those who wish can have one-on-one sessions later. All have access to a 24-hour help line. Managers keep watch for delayed signs of stress: absenteeism, increased mistakes or mood swings. These workers are urged to seek help.

If it all seems too touchy-feely, consider the results. In B.C., the average post-robbery absence per branch—as paid out by the Workers Compensation Board—is 62 days. "In Vancity [in 2005] 17 of our 19 robberies had no days absent," says Leckie. The other two robberies had an average absence of two days. Leckie does a quick calculation: "That's 1,054 days not lost," she says. "There's a big financial incentive to doing it right."

Doing it right means building mutual trust and respect between employer and employee. It means heading off problems in advance and believing in those employees who need help. "The sense that there are non-sick people obtaining benefits fraudulently is an urban myth," Leckie says. The Vancity program is much copied, but rarely duplicated. "I have seen the program fail," she says. "In a cynical organization you get comments like, 'Well, the only time I get to talk to anyone important is when I have a gun to my head.'"

Sometimes the gun is real, more often it's a metaphor. Maybe bad stress is exactly that: a robbery. It steals joy and purpose and health; and it takes from the bottom line. In that sense it is real, no matter how it is defined, or how cynically it is viewed.

With Martin Patriquin and John Intini.

From *Maclean's*, October 15, 2007. Copyright © 2007 by Macleans. Reprinted by permission.

UNIT 3
Nutritional Health

Unit Selections

Key Points to Consider

- What are the foods that are considered healthy? What are the foods that are considered unhealthy?

- What dietary changes could you make to improve your diet? What is keeping you from making these changes?

- Do you think that fast food restaurants should be forced to limit the amount of fat and sodium they use in the food items they sell? Why or why not?

- What are the facts and details that you check on a food label?

- What are the nutritional advantages of breastfeeding?

- What are the functions of vitamin D? What effect does it have on health?

- Why is it important to eat breakfast?

- How can you eat healthy on a budget?

Student Website
www.mhcls.com

Internet References

The American Dietetic Association
   http://www.eatright.org
Center for Science in the Public Interest (CSPI)
   http://www.cspinet.org/
Food and Nutrition Information Center
   http://www.nalusda.gov/fnic/index.html

For years, the majority of Americans paid little attention to nutrition, other than to eat three meals a day and, perhaps, take a vitamin supplement. While this dietary style was generally adequate for the prevention of major nutritional deficiencies, medical evidence began to accumulate linking the American diet to a variety of chronic illnesses. In an effort to guide Americans in their dietary choices, the U.S. Dept. of Agriculture and the U.S. Public Health Service review and publish Dietary Guidelines every 5 years. The year 2000 Dietary Guidelines' recommendations are no longer limited to food choices; they include advice on the importance of maintaining a healthy weight and engaging in daily exercise. In addition to the Dietary Guidelines, the Department of Agriculture developed the *Food Guide Pyramid* to show the relative importance of food groups.

Despite an apparent ever-changing array of dietary recommendations from the scientific community, five recommendations remain constant: 1) eat a diet low in saturated fat, 2) eat whole grain foods, 3) drink plenty of fresh water daily, 4) limit your daily intake of sugar and salt, and 5) eat a diet rich in fruits and vegetables. These recommendations, while general in nature, are seldom heeded and in fact many Americans don't eat enough fruits and vegetables and eat too much sugar and saturated fat.

Of all the nutritional findings, the link between dietary fat and coronary heart disease remains the most consistent throughout the literature. The article "Fat City" addresses the recent New York City restaurant ban on trans fat. These fats occur naturally in limited amounts in some meats and dairy products. The majority of these fats, however, enter the diet via a process known as hydrogenation. Hydrogenation causes liquid oils to harden into products such as vegetable shortening and margarine. In addition to these products, trans fats are found in many commercially prepared and restaurant foods. Current recommendations suggest that the types of fats consumed may play a much greater role in disease processes than the total amount of fat consumed. As it currently stands, most experts agree that it is prudent to limit our intake of trans fat which appears to raise LDLs, the bad cholesterol, and lower HDLs, the good cholesterol, and thus increases the risk of heart disease. There's also evidence that trans fats increase the risk of diabetes.

While the basic advice on eating healthy remains fairly constant, many Americans are still confused over exactly what to eat. Should their diet be low carbohydrate, high protein, or low fat? When people turn to standards such as the *Food Guide Pyramid,* even here there is some confusion. The *Pyramid,*

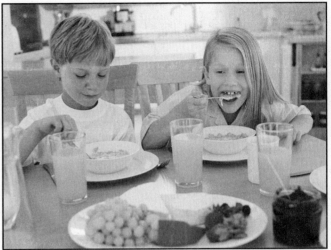

© BananaStock/PunchStock

designed by the Department of Agriculture over 20 years ago, recommends a diet based on grains, fruits, and vegetables with several servings of meats and dairy products. It also restricts the consumption of fats, oils, and sweets. While the pyramid offers guidelines as to food groups, individual nutrients are not emphasized. One nutrient, vitamin D, has been in the news recently. New research on the "sunshine" vitamin suggests current recommendations may not be adequate especially for senior citizens. The data also indicate that vitamin D may help lower the incidence of cancers, type 1 diabetes, and multiple sclerosis.

In "Suck on This," Pat Thomas addresses the benefits of breastfeeding on an infant's nutritional status. Formula increases the risks of babies developing diabetes, eczema, and certain cancers as well as twice the overall risk of dying in the first six weeks of life.

Of all the topic areas in health, food and nutrition is certainly one of the most interesting, if for no other reason than the rate at which dietary recommendations change. One recommendation that hasn't changed is the adage that a good breakfast is the best way to start the day. In "What Good Is Breakfast," author Amanda Fortini addresses the relationship between breakfast and a reduced risk of obesity. She also discusses the link between better grades and breakfast among school children. Despite all the controversy and conflict, the one message that seems to remain constant is the importance of balance and moderation in everything we eat.

Fat City

Banning trans fats probably makes sense from a public-health standpoint—but will the doughnut survive?

CORBY KUMMER

In December, to the delight of many cardiologists and the dismay of many doughnut lovers, the New York City Board of Health voted to ban artificial trans fats from restaurants, school cafeterias, pushcarts, and almost every other food-service establishment it oversees, which includes most everything except hospitals. Trans fats don't occur naturally in the things people like but feel guilty eating, or at least not at high levels (there are small proportions in the fat in meat and dairy products). But artificial ones are plentiful in commercial foods, because they are easy to use, cheaper than natural fats, and keep practically forever. Trans fats are made by pumping hydrogen gas into liquid fats usually in the presence of nickel so that they will remain solid at room temperature, like butter and lard; and they have the same wonderful properties in pie crusts, cookies, and cakes. Crisco, still generic for solid shortening made by partial hydrogenation (of cottonseed oil), soon became the "sanitary" choice for pie crust and fried chicken, making pastry almost as flaky and skin almost as crisp as lard does.

But starting in the 1970s, a time of general fat panic related to heart disease, trans fats began to look as bad for cholesterol levels as the dreaded saturated fats, and in the 1990s the picture got worse. Trans fats, long-term studies reported, not only raise "bad" cholesterol (LDL); they also lower "good" cholesterol (HDL)—which not even saturated fats do. They look about as bad for the arteries as a fat can be. A 2002 consensus report from the National Academies of Sciences' Institute of Medicine called the relationship between trans-fat consumption and coronary heart disease "linear" and stated that the only acceptable level of trans fats in the diet was zero. The next year the Food and Drug Administration required food processors to list trans-fat levels on nutrition labels along with saturated fat. When the rule went into effect, in January 2006, public awareness of trans fats went up, and the stage was set for the New York City ban.

Thomas Frieden, New York's health commissioner, was already unpopular among libertarians. An epidemiologist and doctor whose speciality is infectious disease, he advocates the blunt instrument of regulation, often over the current public-health approach to most problems, which emphasizes education programs that encourage people to make healthy choices. Frieden made international news by leading the charge to pass the city's comprehensive smoking ban, which has been duplicated across the country and the world. He believes that government should make the healthful choice the default, and that eliminating trans fats will do that, just as fluoridating water and getting the lead out of paint did.

Why an outright ban? Asking nicely didn't work. Starting in June of 2005, the city sent information on why and how to avoid trans fats to 30,000 restaurants and food-service establishments and to 200,000 clinics and community centers; it also provided training to 7,800 restaurant operators. A year later, the share of food-service establishments using trans fats—half—hadn't budged. With the support of Michael Bloomberg, Frieden's health-conscious boss, the city's board of health passed the proposed ban.

Libertarians were newly displeased, as legislators in California and Massachusetts began calling for similar bans. Chicago, which last summer enacted a widely ridiculed (and flouted) ban on foie gras, was also said to have trans fats in its sights. Columnists began asking exasperated what-next questions: Salt, a perennial runner-up to fat in the sin sweepstakes? Sugar? Whole milk? Alcohol, again?

Boston, with a similarly activist commissioner and a bold, public-healthminded mayor, Thomas M. Menino, was reported to be the next large city considering a ban. That commissioner, John Auerbach, is my spouse, so I followed the debate closely. I attended a meeting of the Boston Public Health Commission board (a meeting open to the public and press) and listened to the drafters of the New York ban narrate a PowerPoint presentation by conference call. The board was interested in the practicalities of enforcing the ban. I was interested in the practicalities of how small-business owners could follow the new rules—and how cooks could give customers the flavors and textures they were used to.

The New York presenters were reassuring, if short on details. Restaurant inspectors would simply add questions about trans fats to their normal checklist, scanning menus for items likely to contain them—say, cake mixes and frozen french fries—and asking to see labels for all cooking fats. It would add just a few

Doughnut Heaven

Since he began frying doughnuts in his East Village basement twelve years ago, using his North Carolina baker grandfather's recipe, Mark Isreal has made himself and his doughnuts New York City landmarks, selling to carriage-trade shops like Dean & Deluca and Zabar's and coyly (and correctly) refusing to ship them anywhere. What sets his doughnuts apart is the quality of the ingredients, particularly the butter—yes, doughnut batter has a lot of it—and the flavorings.

These days practically the first thing a visitor sees at the Doughnut Plant, Isreal's utilitarian Lower East Side shop, is a sign: NO TRANS FATS. Liquid oil (he fries in corn oil) is no problem for yeast doughnuts—airy, if very large, delights, which he makes in flavors like Valrhona chocolate and pistachio. But cake doughnuts are hard to make without trans-fat shortening, which thickens when it cools and gives Dunkin' Donuts' and other good commercial cake doughnuts the velvety, mouth-coating texture that virtuous corn oil can't quite match.

Isreal is as secretive about his recipes as he is talkative, so he wouldn't tell me which three milks he uses for "Tres Leches, the best of his cake doughnuts. But I suspect that condensed or evaporated milk, sweet and very thick, is his workaround for the mouthfeel challenge. None of his doughnuts ore ascetic, but these are lush.

Doughnut Plant, 379 Grand Street, New York City, 212-505-3700.

---

minutes to the usual hour-long inspection. As for telling restaurants how to substitute other fats and where to buy them, the health department planned to contract with culinary educators to teach at workshops and to staff technical-assistance help lines.

It seemed clear that restaurants would be left with plenty of questions, and I had a few of my own. I made an appointment to talk to Frieden, and to see several cooks whose businesses would be significantly affected by the ban. I also learned a lot about doughnuts—including that I like them more than can be good for me, whatever the fat.

A youthful forty-six, and thin, as you would expect, Frieden is both plainspoken and sure he is right. The morning I visited him, in the health department's WPA-era headquarters in Lower Manhattan, he told me that he and his communications director, Geoffrey Cowley, had just been wondering why his initiatives were so frequently "mis-spun" as the work of the "nanny state." He presents himself more as an emergency repairman. Little of what he does, he said, "would be necessary if our healthcare system worked—if every person had a doctor, continuity of care, and that doctor had access to their records." Better labels are all well and good, but "we don't want to exhort people to look at labels for trans fat," he said. "We want people to walk into a restaurant and not worry there's

an artificial chemical in their food" that is killing them. A city trans-fat ban, he says, could prevent 500 premature deaths a year from heart disease.

I asked Frieden if he was trying to do what the federal government would not: force fast-food chains to remove trans fats. Kentucky Fried Chicken has already replaced its trans fats, as has Wendy's; Disney, Starbucks, and other companies have also gotten on the bandwagon. But McDonald's has been dragging its heels. It loudly announced, in 2002, that it would remove trans fats from all its food, but never got around to taking them out of its french fries—by far the biggest source, and the greatest challenge for texture (the original fat in McDonald's french fries was the lard-like beef tallow). Now it and every other chain unwilling to abandon the New York City market will have to reformulate their menus, and given research costs and economies of scale, the changes are likely to be national, not just regional. "Nothing like a deadline to focus the mind," Frieden said.

Wasn't New York's ban a case of governing the country from one city—and wasn't it really aimed at obesity? Frieden emphatically rejected the idea, saying that his fiduciary responsibility was solely to the citizens of New York City. The ban was meant to reduce premature deaths from heart disease, no more and no less. And he wasn't depriving people of pleasure. "We're not going to desalinate New York," he said, although he sounded as if he'd like to. "We're not going to ban eggs and ham." The science on trans fats, he said, had come clear slowly, as had the science on the effects of secondhand smoke. But once it did, it did decisively, and he had to act.

So far, the chains that have initiated trans-fat removal have been the ones whose image depends on health or whose owners are concerned with health: the Tennessee-based Ruby Tuesday; the Boston-based Legal Sea Foods (whose owner, Roger Berkowitz, has long been ahead of every health curve); and Au Bon Pain, another Boston-based chain.

When I visited Au Bon Pain's headquarters and test kitchen, the head baker, Harold Midttun, told me that he had sold his family bakery after a heart attack at age thirty-nine. Once he got to Au Bon Pain, he took immediate interest in its mission to find substitutes for trans fats in cookies, muffins, and bagels; with Thomas John, the executive chef, and John Billingsley, the chief operating officer, he organized many tastings to sample new formulations alongside the originals. What were the tastings like? I asked the three men. Fattening, Billingsley replied.

Breads and even muffins were relatively simple; cookies were not. Chocolate-chip cookies, for instance, need the snap and solid texture that butter—or shortening, its much less expensive substitute—gives them when they cool. The company intended to "be zero trans fat" by April of this year, but not all the strudel problems (or the cream-soup ones, for that matter) had been solved.

I realized that saying trans fats are "totally replaceable," as Frieden repeatedly does—asserting that they are merely used for texture, not taste—is easier for a health official than for a product developer. It should be simple, yes, to get rid of an entirely artificial ingredient that is used mostly for the convenience of industry. Researchers have been working for decades on substitutes, which should by now be as plentiful and as cheap as trans fats.

But they're not. Midttun and John gave the example of their blueberry muffins, which used to be the highest in trans fats, as a challenge they had finally met. They did it by using a new fat and adding several other ingredients to mask its taste and still get the same mouthfeel. The ingredients, they told me, included oat bran, ground golden flaxseed, soy protein, and emulsifiers. Individual bakers, I thought, were sunk: They'd never be able to figure all that out, even with frequent calls to a city help line.

And the substitute fats have problems of their own. Earth Balance, a blend that Au Bon Pain uses, includes some palm-fruit oil, which is 50 percent saturated. Very highly saturated tropical oils, like coconut, were the target of a widely publicized 1994 expose of movie popcorn by the Center for Science in the Public Interest. Now, the current thinking runs, saturated fats are not quite as bad for you as trans fats—but they're still bad, and the American Heart Association has expressed concern about using them as a substitute for trans fats.

Dunkin' Donuts, another national chain based in the Boston area, says that it has tried twenty-two different fats in sixty-seven tests, hoping to get the same texture its doughnuts now have. Recognizing the difficulty posed by doughnuts and other fried doughs, New York modified its regulation to give doughnut makers eighteen months to come up with suitable alternatives. If Dunkin' has found a good substitute, it isn't saying.

Doughnut Plant, a cult fry shop on Manhattan's Lower East Side, is a poster child for the ban: It proudly announces that it fries only in corn oil (see "Doughnut Heaven," page 122). Mark Isreal, the eccentric, garrulous owner, certainly doesn't compromise on quality or expertise with his doughnuts. When I went to see him, I found myself following Frieden's example: He told me that at a health-department staff gathering after the ban was passed, he "couldn't stop eating" Isreal's doughnuts.

But when I tried similar favors at Dunkin' Donuts, I saw why lard and solid shortening have always been best for deep frying (Dunkin' has never used lard): The resolidified fat gives the interior a texture that oil simply cannot. Yeast-raised doughnuts are less problematic, because they should remain airy. But in a cake doughnut, the right texture is as unmistakable as the firm crumble of a butter cake—which, of course, requires a fat that solidifies at room temperature. A good cake doughnut has the substance of pound cake. It won't get that from corn or canola oil.

It's a confusing picture. Looking into trans fats got me hooked on an extremely fatty food I hadn't eaten since childhood (positively unpatriotic, as John T. Edge's monograph *Donuts: An American Passion* engagingly makes clear). Frieden readily admits that banning trans fats won't help reduce obesity. Posting calorie counts where you pay for your food—a less-noticed regulation he got passed at the same time as the trans-fat ban—might help. Or it might just make people eat more doughnuts: A Dunkin' Donuts glazed yeast doughnut has 180 calories, a glazed cake doughnut has 350, a reduced-fat blueberry muffin has 400, and a corn muffin has 510. Getting people to eat less fat and more fresh and unprocessed food—the real path to health—can't be done by any regulation yet proposed by the "food police."

Still, it does seem like a good idea to remove artificial substances from the food supply, especially if trans fats result in thousands of needless deaths a year. And the international headlines the initiative produced will most likely make people think more about the healthfulness of the food they eat, and restaurateurs about what they put into their food, all for a relatively modest expenditure on the city's part. As my spouse points out, regulations get headlines; education programs on the dangers of saturated fats and how to find, buy, and cook better food—programs in which his department invests heavily—get yawns. I'll be watching follow-up studies to see whether the cure for trans fats, which in many cases is to replace them with highly saturated fats, is worse than the disease.

And when the beleaguered cooks at Dunkin' Donuts finally solve the riddle of removing trans fats, as New York City says they must by July of next year, I'll be eager to learn how they did it. At the risk of revealing a rival's trade secret, may I suggest oat bran and golden flaxseed?

CORBY KUMMER is an *Atlantic* senior editor.

From *The Atlantic*, March 2007, pp. 121–124. Copyright © 2007 by Corby Kummer. Reprinted by permission of the author.

Eating Well on a Downsized Food Budget

JANE E. BRODY

Now may be a good time to bring back the basics—the nutritious and affordable foods that have been all but forgotten by many affluent families since the Great Depression.

I'm not going to suggest a nightly diet of stone soup or the cheap fat- and sugar-rich menus of the urban poor. But many people who once gave little thought to dining on steak, lobster, asparagus, baby spinach or crème brûlée are now having to spend less on just about everything, including food.

Those who have lost jobs may be able to turn some of their unwanted spare time toward the grocery and kitchen. Others, like families with two working parents or working single parents, have to carve out time to provide economical, nourishing meals.

Not only is it possible, but it can improve the health and reduce the girth of Americans, regardless of socioeconomic status.

A Little Effort Goes a Long Way

"We need to look at real foods for real people, the foods that got us through the last depression," said Adam Drewnowski, an epidemiologist at the University of Washington's Center for Public Health Nutrition. "We must avoid the temptation to turn to cheap, empty calories—the refined grains, added sugars and added fats that give you the most calories you can get for your food dollar."

Instead, Dr. Drewnowski said, "there are many foods that are affordable and nutrient-rich and not loaded with empty calories."

And eating for good health does not have to mean eating less. "If you have equal portions of foods that are nutrient-dense, you will end up eating fewer calories," he said.

For families accustomed to eating out and ordering in, shopping for and preparing meals can take more time. According to the Economic Research Service of the United States Department of Agriculture, low-income women who work full time spend just over 40 minutes a day on meal preparation. With a little planning, another 20 or 30 minutes can provide healthy, economical fare.

Households not accustomed to home cooking may have to make small investments in kitchen equipment and ingredients that can speed food preparation and will remain useful long after the economy improves. Even families using food stamps can afford the foods discussed below to make recipes like those posted with this column at nytimes.com/health. And no one need go hungry.

Value-Added Foods

To assess which foods provide the best value of balanced nutrients for less money, Dr. Drewnowski said, "we need to calculate nutrients per calorie and nutrients per dollar and make those foods part of the mainstream diet."

Researchers at the State University of New York at Buffalo who studied families in a program for overweight children found that basing the family diet on low-calorie, high-nutrient foods not only improved the health of the entire family but also reduced the amount spent on food.

One myth to dispel is that fruits and vegetables must be fresh to be nutritious. Not only do canned and frozen versions usually cost less and require less preparation, but nutrient value is as good or better and less food is wasted. Fresh produce is often harvested before it is fully ripe and so comes to the consumer with fewer than optimal nutrients. But fruits and vegetables that are canned or frozen are picked at the peak of ripeness. There is more vitamin C in a glass of orange juice made from frozen concentrate than in freshly squeezed juice.

So let's welcome back to the American table meals made from potatoes, eggs, beans, low-fat or nonfat yogurt and milk (including reconstituted powdered milk), carrots, kale or collards, onions, bananas, apples, peanut butter, almonds, lean ground beef, chicken and turkey, along with canned or frozen corn, peas, tomatoes, broccoli and fish. For nutrient-dense beverages, Dr. Drewnowski suggests 100 percent fruit juice blends and fruit-and-vegetable juice blends.

To his suggestions I would add pasta and rice (the whole-wheat kinds cost just pennies more), which can be a base for many quick, nutritious meals. Combining leftover vegetables and meat or poultry with a pot of pasta or rice takes just minutes, and has the added benefit of reducing potential waste.

For dessert, try frozen yogurt or low-fat ice cream topped with seasonal fruit for the best nutrient-to-calorie ratio and value.

Potatoes: One of the Good Guys

Some perfectly good foods have been unfairly smeared by a broad brush. Potatoes are an example, deplored by nutrition advocates for how they are most often consumed—fried and heavily salted—and by the low-carb set for their high glycemic index.

In fact, potatoes are highly versatile, they are easily prepared in many delicious ways with little or no added fat, and they are nearly always consumed with other foods, which greatly reduces their effect on blood sugar. And they are nutritious. A five-ounce potato provides just 100 calories, for which you get 35 percent of a day's recommended vitamin C, 20 percent of the vitamin B6, 15 percent of the iodine, 10 percent each of niacin, iron and copper, and 6 percent of the protein.

Try potatoes baked, boiled or steamed and topped with low-fat yogurt or sour cream seasoned with your favorite herbs or spices.

Beans, whether prepared from scratch (soaked overnight and then cooked) or taken from a can, are a low-cost nutritional powerhouse. They are low in fat, rich sources of B vitamins and iron, and richer in protein than any other plant food. When combined in a meal with a grain like rice (preferably brown), bulgur or whole-wheat bread, the protein quality is as good as that of meat.

Cabbage, too, gives you more than your money's worth of nutrients, including vitamin C and potassium, at only 17 calories a cup eaten shredded and raw, 29 calories a cup when cooked. Collards are high in vitamins A and C, potassium, calcium (cup for cup, on a par with milk), iron, niacin and protein, and yet low in sodium and calories. Kale has only 43 calories a cup when cooked.

In the fruit category, it's hard to beat apples for year-round, economical, nutritious and versatile fare that can be a part of any meal or served as a snack or dessert (as in baked apples). Bananas are also handy; even when overripe, they can be mashed and used to make banana bread or a smoothie.

Here are some other tips for busy cooks concerned about nutrition and cost:

- Buy family-size packages of meat or poultry; divide them up and freeze meal-size portions, labeled and dated.
- Choose the less expensive store brands of canned and frozen produce.
- Use powdered reconstituted milk for cooking.
- Cook in batches, enough for two or more meals, and freeze single portions for lunch.
- Use meat, poultry and fish as a condiment, in small amounts added to main-dish salads, soups and sauces.
- Try main-dish soups and salad for filling yet low-calorie meals. Soups can also be made in large amounts and frozen.
- Consider buying a slow cooker for efficient, one-dish meals.

From *The New York Times*, March 3, 2009. Copyright © 2009 by The New York Times Company. Reprinted by permission via PARS International.

Suck on This

The human species has been breastfeeding for nearly half a million years. It's only in the last 60 years that we have begun to give babies the highly processed convenience food called 'formula'. The health consequences— twice the risk of dying in the first six weeks of life, five times the risk of gastroenteritis, twice the risk of developing eczema and diabetes and up to eight times the risk of developing lymphatic cancer—are staggering. With UK formula manufacturers spending around £20 per baby promoting this 'baby junk food', compared to the paltry 14 pence per baby the government spends promoting breastfeeding, can we ever hope to reverse the trend? Pat Thomas uncovers a world where predatory baby milk manufacturers, negligent health professionals and an ignorant, unsympathetic public all conspire to keep babies off the breast and on the bottle.

PAT THOMAS

All mammals produce milk for their young, and the human species has been nurturing its babies at the breast for at least 400,000 years. For centuries, when a woman could not feed her baby herself, another lactating woman, or 'wet nurse', took over the job. It is only in the last 60 years or so that we have largely abandoned our mammalian instincts and, instead, embraced a bottlefeeding culture that not only encourages mothers to give their babies highly processed infant formulas from birth, but also to believe that these breastmilk substitutes are as good as, if not better than, the real thing.

Infant formulas were never intended to be consumed on the widespread basis that they are today. They were conceived in the late 1800s as a means of providing necessary sustenance for foundlings and orphans who would otherwise have starved. In this narrow context— where no other food was available—formula was a lifesaver.

However, as time went on, and the subject of human nutrition in general—and infant nutrition, in particular—became more 'scientific', manufactured breastmilk substitutes were sold to the general public as a technological improvement on breastmilk.

'If anybody were to ask 'which formula should I use?' or 'which is nearest to mother's milk?', the answer would be 'nobody knows' because there is not one single objective source of that kind of information provided by anybody,' says Mary Smale, a breastfeeding counsellor with the National Childbirth Trust (NCT) for 28 years. 'Only the manufacturers know what's in their stuff, and they aren't telling. They may advertise special 'healthy' ingredients like oligosaccharides, long-chain fatty acids or, a while ago, beta-carotene, but they never actually tell you what the basic product is made from or where the ingredients come from.'

There can be no food more locally produced, more sustainable or more environmentally friendly than a mother's breastmilk, the only food required by an infant for the first six months of life. It is a naturally renewable resource, which requires no packaging or transport, results in no wastage and is free.

The known constituents of breastmilk were and are used as a general reference for scientists devising infant formulas. But, to this day, there is no actual 'formula' for formula. In fact, the process of producing infant formulas has, since its earliest days, been one of trial and error.

Within reason, manufacturers can put anything they like into formula. In fact, the recipe for one product can vary from batch to batch, according to the price and availability of ingredients. While we assume that formula is heavily regulated, no transparency is required of manufacturers: they do not, for example, have to log the specific constituents of any batch or brand with any authority.

Most commercial formulas are based on cow's milk. But before a baby can drink cow's milk in the form of infant formula, it needs to be severely modified. The protein and mineral content must be reduced and the carbohydrate content increased, usually by adding sugar. Milk fat, which is not easily absorbed by the human body, particularly one with an immature digestive system, is removed and substituted with vegetable, animal or mineral fats.

Vitamins and trace elements are added, but not always in their most easily digestible form. (This means that the claims that formula is 'nutritionally complete' are true, but only in the crudest sense of having had added the full complement of vitamins and mineral to a nutritionally inferior product.)

Many formulas are also highly sweetened. While most infant formulas do not contain sugar in the form of sucrose, they can contain high levels of other types of sugar such as lactose (milk sugar), fructose (fruit sugar), glucose (also known as dextrose, a simple sugar found in plants) and maltodextrose (malt sugar). Because of a loophole in the law, these can still be advertised as 'sucrose free'.

Formula may also contain unintentional contaminants introduced during the manufacturing process. Some may contain traces of genetically engineered soya and corn.

The bacteria *Salmonella* and aflatoxins—potent toxic, carcinogenic, mutagenic, immunosuppressive agents produced by species of the fungus *Aspergillus*—have regularly been detected in commercial formulas, as has *Enterobacter sakazakii*, a devastating foodborne pathogen that can cause sepsis (overwhelming bacterial infection in the bloodstream), meningitis (inflammation of the lining of the brain) and necrotising enterocolitis (severe infection and inflammation of the small intestine and colon) in newborn infants.

The packaging of infant formulas occasionally gives rise to contamination with broken glass and fragments of metal as well as industrial chemicals such as phthalates and bisphenol A (both carcinogens) and, most recently, the packaging constituent isopropyl thioxanthone (ITX; another suspected carcinogen).

Infant formulas may also contain excessive levels of toxic or heavy metals, including aluminum, manganese, cadmium and lead.

Soya formulas are of particular concern due to the very high levels of plant-derived oestrogens (phytoestrogens) they contain. In fact, concentrations of phytoestrogens detected in the blood of infants receiving soya formula can be 13,000 to 22,000 times greater than the concentrations of natural oestrogens. Oestrogen in doses above those normally found in the body can cause cancer.

Killing Babies

For years, it was believed that the risks of illness and death from bottlefeeding were largely confined to children in developing countries, where the clean water necessary to make up formula is sometimes scarce and where poverty-stricken mothers may feel obliged to dilute formula to make it stretch further, thus risking waterborne illnesses such as diarrhoea and cholera as well as malnutrition in their babies. But newer data from the West clearly show that babies in otherwise affluent societies are also falling ill and dying due to an early diet of infant convenience food.

Because it is not nutritionally complete, because it does not contain the immune-boosting properties of breastmilk and because it is being consumed by growing babies with vast, ever-changing nutritional needs—and not meeting those needs—the health effects of sucking down formula day after day early in life can be devastating in both the short and long term.

Bottlefed babies are twice as likely to die from any cause in the first six weeks of life. In particular, bottlefeeding raises the risk of SIDS (sudden infant death syndrome) by two to five times.

Bottlefed babies are also at a significantly higher risk of ending up in hospital with a range of infections. They are, for instance, five times more likely to be admitted to hospital suffering from gastroenteritis.

Even in developed countries, bottlefed babies have rates of diarrhoea twice as high as breastfed ones. They are twice as likely (20 per cent vs 10 per cent) to suffer from otitis media (inner-ear infection), twice as likely to develop eczema or a wheeze if there is a family history of atopic disease, and five times more likely to develop urinary tract infections. In the first six months of life, bottlefed babies are six to 10 times more likely to develop necrotising enterocolitis—a serious infection of the intestine, with intestinal tissue death—a figure that increases to 30 times the risk after that time.

Even more serious diseases are also linked with bottlefeeding. Compared with infants who are fully breastfed even for only three to four months, a baby drinking artificial milk is twice as likely to develop juvenile-onset insulin-dependent (type 1) diabetes. There is also a five- to eightfold risk of developing lymphomas in children under 15 who were formulated, or breastfed for less than six months.

In later life, studies have shown that bottlefed babies have a greater tendency towards developing conditions such as childhood inflammatory bowel disease, multiple sclerosis, dental malocclusion, coronary heart disease, diabetes, hyperactivity, autoimmune thyroid disease and coeliac disease.

For all of these reasons, formula cannot be considered even 'second best' compared with breastmilk. Officially, the World Health Organization (WHO) designates formula milk as the last choice in infant-feeding: Its first choice is breastmilk from the mother; second choice is the mother's own milk given via cup or bottle; third choice is breastmilk from a milk bank or wet nurse and, finally, in fourth place, formula milk.

And yet, breastfed babies are becoming an endangered species. In the UK, rates are catastrophically low and have been that way for decades. Current figures suggest that only 62 per cent of women in Britain even attempt to breastfeed (usually while in hospital). At six weeks, just 42 per cent are breastfeeding. By four months, only 29 per cent are still breastfeeding and, by six months, this figure drops to 22 per cent.

Breastmilk vs Formula: No Contest

Breastmilk is a 'live' food that contains living cells, hormones, active enzymes, antibodies and at least 400 other unique components. It is a dynamic substance, the composition of which changes from the beginning to the end of the feed and according to the age and needs of the baby. Because it also provides active immunity, every time a baby breastfeeds it also receives protection from disease.

Compared to this miraculous substance, the artificial milk sold as infant formula is little more than junk food. It is also the only manufactured food that humans are encouraged to consume exclusively for a period of months, even though we know that no human body can be expected to stay healthy and thrive on a steady diet of processed food.

Breast Milk	Formula	Comments
Fats		
Rich in brain-building omega-3s, namely, DHA and AA. Automatically adjusts to infant's needs; levels decline as baby gets older. Rich in cholesterol; nearly completely absorbed. Contains the fat-digesting enzyme lipase	No DHA Doesn't adjust to infant's needs No cholesterol Not completely absorbed No lipase	The most important nutrient in breastmilk; the absence of cholesterol and DHA may predispose a child to adult heart and CNS diseases. Leftover, unabsorbed fat accounts for unpleasant smelling stools in formula-fed babies
Protein		
Soft, easily digestible whey. More completely absorbed; higher in the milk of mothers who deliver preterm. Lactoferrin for intestinal health. Lysozyme, an antimicrobial. Rich in brain- and body-building protein components. Rich in growth factors. Contains sleep-inducing proteins	Harder-to-digest casein curds Not completely absorbed, so more waste, harder on kidneys Little or no lactoferrin No lysozyme. Deficient or low in some brain and body-building proteins Deficient in growth factors Contains fewer sleep-inducing proteins	Infants aren't allergic to human milk proteins
Carbohydrates		
Rich in oligosaccharides, which promote intestinal health	No lactose in some formulas Deficient in oligosaccharides	Lactose is important for brain development
Immune-boosters		
Millions of living white blood cells, in every feeding Rich in immunoglobulins	No live white blood cells or any other cells. Has no immune benefit	Breastfeeding provides active and dynamic protection from infections of all kinds. Breastmilk can be used to alleviate a range of external health problems such as nappy rash and conjunctivitis
Vitamins & Minerals		
Better absorbed Iron is 50–75 per cent absorbed Contains more selenium (an antioxidant)	Not absorbed as well Iron is 5–10 per cent absorbed Contains less selenium (an antioxidant)	Nutrients in formula are poorly absorbed. To compensate, more nutrients are added to formula, making it harder to digest
Enzymes & Hormones		
Rich in digestive enzymes such as lipase and amylase. Rich in many hormones such as thyroid, prolactin and oxytocin. Taste varies with mother's diet, thus helping the child acclimatise to the cultural diet	Processing kills digestive enzymes Processing kills hormones, which are not human to begin with Always tastes the same	Digestive enzymes promote intestinal health; hormones contribute to the biochemical balance and wellbeing of the baby
Cost		
Around £350/year in extra food for mother if she was on a very poor diet to begin with	Around £650/year. Up to £1300/year for hypoallergenic formulas. Cost for bottles and other supplies. Lost income when parents must stay home to care for a sick baby	In the UK, the NHS spends £35 million each year just treating gastroenteritis in bottlefed babies. In the US, insurance companies pay out $3.6 billion for treating diseases in bottlefed babies

These figures could come from almost any developed country in the world and, it should be noted, do not necessarily reflect the ideal of 'exclusive' breastfeeding. Instead, many modern mothers practice mixed feeding—combining breastfeeding with artificial baby milks and infant foods. Worldwide, the WHO estimates that only 35 per cent of infants are getting any breastmilk at all by age four months and, although no one can say for sure because research into exclusive breastfeeding is both scarce and incomplete, it is estimated that only 1 per cent are exclusively breastfed at six months.

Younger women in particular are the least likely to breastfeed, with over 40 per cent of mothers under 24 never even trying. The biggest gap, however, is a socioeconomic one. Women who live in low-income households or who are poorly educated are many times less likely to breastfeed, even though it can make an enormous difference to a child's health.

In children from socially disadvantaged families, exclusive breastfeeding in the first six months of life can go a long way towards cancelling out the health inequalities between being born into poverty and being born into affluence. In essence, breastfeeding takes the infant out of poverty for those first crucial months and gives it a decent start in life.

So Why Aren't Women Breastfeeding?

Before bottles became the norm, breastfeeding was an activity of daily living based on mimicry, and learning within the family and community. Women became their own experts through the trial and error of the experience itself. But today, what should come more or less naturally has become extraordinarily complicated—the focus of global marketing strategies and politics, lawmaking, lobbying support groups, activists and the interference of a well-intentioned, but occasionally ineffective, cult of experts.

According to Mary Smale, it's confidence and the expectation of support that make the difference, particularly for socially disadvantaged women.

'The concept of 'self efficacy'—in other words, whether you think you can do something—is quite important. You can say to a woman that breastfeeding is really a good idea, but she's got to believe various things in order for it to work. First of all, she has to think it's a good idea—that it will be good for her and her baby. Second, she has to think: 'I'm the sort of person who can do that'; third—and maybe the most important thing—is the belief that if she does have problems, she's the sort of person who, with help, will be able to sort them out.

'Studies show, for example, that women on low incomes often believe that breastfeeding hurts, and they also tend to believe that formula is just as good. So from the start, the motivation to breastfeed simply isn't there. But really, it's the thought that if there were any problems, you couldn't do anything about them; that, for instance, if it hurts, it's just the luck of the draw. This mindset is very different from that of a middle-class mother who is used to asking for help to solve things, who isn't frightened of picking up the phone, or saying to her midwife or health visitor, 'I want you to help me with this'.'

Nearly all women—around 99 per cent—can breastfeed successfully and make enough milk for their babies to not simply grow, but to thrive. With encouragement, support and help, almost all women are willing to initiate breastfeeding, but the drop-off rates are alarming: 90 per cent of women who give up in the first six weeks say that they would like to have continued. And it seems likely that long-term exclusive breastfeeding rates could be improved if consistent support were available, and if approval within the family and the wider community for breastfeeding, both at home and in public, were more obvious and widespread.

Clearly, this social support isn't there, and the bigger picture of breastfeeding vs bottlefeeding suggests that there is, in addition, a confluence of complex factors—medical, socioeconomic, cultural and political—that regularly undermine women's confidence, while reinforcing the notion that feeding their children artificially is about lifestyle rather than health, and that the modern woman's body is simply not up to the task of producing enough milk for its offspring.

'Breastfeeding is a natural negotiation between mother and baby and you interfere with it at your peril,' says Professor Mary Renfrew, Director of the Mother and Infant Research Unit, University of York. "But, in the early years of the last century, people were very busy interfering with it. In terms of the ecology of breastfeeding, what you have is a natural habitat that has been disturbed. But it's not just the presence of one big predator—the invention of artificial milk—that is important. It is the fact that the habitat was already weakened by other forces that made it so vulnerable to disaster.

Are infant formula manufacturers simply clever entrepreneurs doing their jobs or human-rights violators of the worst kind?

'If you look at medical textbooks from the early part of the 20th century, you'll find many quotes about making breastfeeding scientific and exact, and it's out of these that you can see things beginning to fall apart.' This falling apart, says Renfrew, is largely due to the fear and mistrust that science had of the natural process of breastfeeding. In particular, the fact that a mother can put a baby on the breast and do something else while breastfeeding, and have the baby naturally come off the breast when it's had enough, was seen as disorderly and inexact. The medical/scientific model replaced this natural situation with precise measurements—for instance, how many millilitres of milk a baby should ideally have at each sitting—which skewed the natural balance between mother and baby, and established bottlefeeding as a biological norm.

Breastfeeding rates also began to decline as a consequence of women's changed circumstances after World War I, as more women left their children behind to go into the workplace as a consequence of women's emancipation—and the loss of men in the 'killing fields'—and to an even larger extent with the advent of World War II, when even more women entered into employment outside of the home.

'There was also the first wave of feminism,' says Renfrew, 'which stamped into everyone's consciousness in the 60s, and encouraged women get away from their babies and start living their lives. So the one thing that might have helped—women supporting each other—actually created a situation where even the intellectual, engaged, consciously aware women who might have questioned this got lost for a while. As a consequence, we ended up with a widespread and declining confidence in breastfeeding, a declining understanding of its importance and a declining ability of health professionals to support it. And, of course, all this ran along the same timeline as the technological development of artificial milk and the free availability of formula.'

Medicalised Birth

Before World War II, pregnancy and birth—and, by extension, breastfeeding—were part of the continuum of normal life. Women gave birth at home with the assistance and support of trained midwives, who were themselves part of the community, and afterwards they breastfed with the encouragement of family and friends.

Taking birth out of the community and relocating it into hospitals gave rise to the medicalisation of women's reproductive lives. Life events were transformed into medical problems, and traditional knowledge was replaced with scientific and technological solutions. This medicalisation resulted in a cascade of interventions that deeply undermined women's confidence in their abilities to conceive and grow a healthy baby, give birth to it and then feed it.

The cascade falls something like this: Hospitals are institutions; they are impersonal and, of necessity, must run on schedules and routines. For a hospital to run smoothly, patients must ideally be sedate and immobile. For the woman giving birth, this meant lying on her back in a bed, an unnatural position that made labour slow, unproductive and very much more painful.

To 'fix' these iatrogenically dysfunctional labours, doctors developed a range of drugs (usually synthetic hormones such as prostaglandins or syntocinon), technologies (such as forceps and vacuum extraction) and procedures (such as episiotomies) to speed the process up. Speeding up labour artificially made it even more painful and this, in turn, led to the development of an array of pain-relieving drugs. Many of these were so powerful that the mother was often unconscious or deeply sedated at the moment of delivery and, thus, unable to offer her breast to her newborn infant.

All pain-relieving drugs cross the placenta, so even if the mother were conscious, her baby may not have been, or may have been so heavily drugged that its natural rooting instincts (which help it find the nipple) and muscle coordination (necessary to latch properly onto the breast) were severely impaired.

While both mother and baby were recovering from the ordeal of a medicalised birth, they were, until the 1970s and 1980s, routinely separated. Often, the baby wasn't 'allowed' to breastfeed until it had a bottle first, in case there was something wrong with its gastrointestinal tract. Breastfeeding, when it took place at all, took place according to strict schedules. These feeding schedules—usually on a three- or four-hourly basis—were totally unnatural for human newborns, who need to feed 12 or more times in any 24-hour period. Babies who were inevitably hungry between feeds were routinely given supplements of water and/or formula.

'There was lots of topping up,' says Professor Renfrew. 'The way this 'scientific' breastfeeding happened in hospital was that the baby would be given two minutes on each breast on day one, then four minutes on each breast on day two, seven minutes on each on day three, and so on. This created enormous anxiety since the mother would then be watching the clock instead of the baby. The babies would then get topped-up after every feed, then topped-up again throughout the night rather than brought to their mothers to feed. So you had a situation where the babies were crying in the nursery, and the mothers were crying in the postnatal ward. That's what we called 'normal' all throughout the 60s and 70s.'

Breastmilk is produced on a supply-and-demand basis, and these topping-up routines, which assuaged infant hunger and lessened demand, also reduced the mother's milk supply. As a result, women at the mercy of institutionalised birth experienced breastfeeding as a frustrating struggle that was often painful and just as often unsuccessful.

When, under these impossible circumstances, breastfeeding 'failed', formula was offered as a 'nutritionally complete solution' that was also more 'modern', 'cleaner' and more 'socially acceptable'.

At least two generations of women have been subjected to these kinds of damaging routines and, as a result, many of today's mothers find the concept of breastfeeding strange and unfamiliar, and very often framed as something that can and frequently does not 'take', something they might 'have a go' at but, equally, something that they shouldn't feel too badly about if it doesn't work out.

Professional Failures

The same young doctors, nurses and midwives who were pioneering this medical model of reproduction are now running today's health services. So, perhaps not surprisingly, modern hospitals are, at heart, little different from their predecessors. They may have TVs and CD players, and prettier wallpaper, and the drugs may be more sophisticated, but the basic goals and principles of medicalised birth have changed very little in the last 40 years—and the effect on breastfeeding is still as devastating.

In many cases, the healthcare providers' views on infant-feeding are based on their own, highly personal experiences. Surveys show, for instance, that the most important factor influencing the effectiveness and accuracy of a doctor's breastfeeding advice is whether the doctor herself, or the doctor's wife, had breastfed her children. Likewise, a midwife, nurse or health visitor formulated her own children is unlikely to be an effective advocate for breastfeeding.

Women do not fail to breastfeed. Health professionals, health agencies and governments fail to educate and support women who want to breastfeed.

More worrying, these professionals can end up perpetuating damaging myths about breastfeeding that facilitate its failure. In some hospitals, women are still advised to limit the amount of time, at first, that a baby sucks on each breast, to 'toughen up' their nipples. Or they are told their babies get all the milk they 'need' in the first 10 minutes and sucking after this time is unnecessary. Some are still told to stick to four-hour feeding schedules. Figures from the UK's Office of National Statistics show that we are still topping babies up. In 2002, nearly 30 per cent of babies in UK hospitals were given supplemental bottles by hospital staff, and nearly 20 per cent of all babies were separated from their mothers at some point while in hospital.

Continued inappropriate advice from medical professionals is one reason why, in 1991, UNICEF started the Baby Friendly Hospital Initiative (BFHI)—a certification system for hospitals meeting certain criteria known to promote successful breastfeeding. These criteria include: training all healthcare staff on how to facilitate breastfeeding; helping mothers start breastfeeding within one hour of birth; giving newborn infants no food or drink other than breastmilk, unless medically indicated; and the hospital not accepting free or heavily discounted formula and supplies. In principle, it is an important step in the promotion of breastfeeding, and studies show that women who give birth in Baby Friendly hospitals do breastfeed for longer.

In Scotland, for example, where around 50 per cent of hospitals are rated Baby Friendly, breastfeeding initiation rates have increased dramatically in recent years. In Cuba, where 49 of the country's 56 hospitals and maternity facilities are Baby Friendly, the rate of exclusive breastfeeding at four months almost tripled in six years—from 25 per cent in 1990 to 72 per cent in 1996. Similar increases have been found in Bangladesh, Brazil and China.

Unfortunately, interest in obtaining BFHI status is not universal. In the UK, only 43 hospitals (representing just 16 per cent of all UK hospitals) have achieved full accreditation—and none are in London. Out of the approximately 16,000 hospitals worldwide that have qualified for the Baby Friendly designation, only 32 are in the US. What's more, while Baby Friendly hospitals achieve a high initiation rate, they cannot guarantee continuation of breastfeeding once the woman is back in the community. Even among women who give birth in Baby Friendly hospitals, the number who exclusively breastfeed for six months is unacceptably low.

The Influence of Advertising

Baby Friendly hospitals face a daunting task in combatting the laissez-faire and general ignorance of health professionals, mothers and the public at large. They are also fighting a difficult battle with an acquiescent media which, through politically correct editorialising aimed at assuaging mothers' guilt if they bottlefeed and, more influentially, through advertising, has helped redefine formula as an acceptable choice.

Although there are now stricter limitations on the advertising of infant formula, for years, manufacturers were able, through advertising and promotion, to define the issue of infant-feeding in both the scientific world (for instance, by providing doctors with growth charts that established the growth patterns of bottlefed babies as the norm) and in its wider social context, reframing perceptions of what is appropriate and what is not.

As a result, in the absence of communities of women talking to each other about pregnancy, birthing and mothering, women's choices today are more directly influenced by commercial leaflets, booklets and advertising than almost anything else.

Baby-milk manufacturers spend countless millions devising marketing strategies that keep their products at the forefront of public consciousness. In the UK, formula companies spend at least £12 million per year on booklets, leaflets and other promotions, often in the guise of 'educational materials'. This works out at approximately £20 per baby born. In contrast, the UK government spends about 14 pence per newborn each year to promote breastfeeding.

It's a pattern of inequity that is repeated throughout the world—and not just in the arena of infant-feeding. The food-industry's global advertising budget is $40 billion, a figure greater than the gross domestic product (GDP) of 70 per cent of the world's nations. For every $1 spent by the WHO on preventing the diseases caused by Western diets, more than $500 is spent by the food industry to promote such diets.

Since they can no longer advertise infant formulas directly to women (for instance, in mother and baby magazines or through direct leafleting), or hand out free samples in hospitals or clinics, manufacturers have started to exploit other outlets, such as mother and baby clubs, and Internet sites that purport to help busy mothers get all the information they need about infant-feeding. They also occasionally rely on subterfuge. Manufacturers are allowed to advertise follow-on milks, suitable for babies over six months, to parents. But, sometimes, these ads feature a picture of a much younger baby, implying the product's suitability for infants.

The impact of these types of promotions should not be underestimated. A 2005 NCT/UNICEF study in the UK determined that one third of British mothers who admitted to seeing formula advertisements in the previous six months believed that infant formula was as good or better than breastmilk. This revelation is all the more surprising since advertising of infant formula to mothers has been banned for many years in several countries, including the UK.

To get around restrictions that prevent direct advertising to parents, manufacturers use a number of psychological strategies that focus on the natural worries that new parents have about the health of their babies. Many of today's formulas, for instance, are conceived and sold as solutions to the 'medical' problems of infants such as lactose intolerance, incomplete digestion and being 'too hungry'—even though many of these problems can be caused by inappropriately giving cow's milk formula in the first place.

> **Helmut Maucher, a powerful corporate lobbyist and honorary chairman of Nestlé—the company that claims 40 percent of the global baby-food market—has gone on record as saying: 'Ethical decisions that injure a firm's ability to compete are actually immoral'.**

The socioeconomic divide among breastfeeding mothers is also exploited by formula manufacturers, as targeting low-income women (with advertising as well as through welfare schemes) has proven very profitable.

When presented with the opportunity to provide their children with the best that science has to offer, many low-income mothers are naturally tempted by formula. This is especially true if they receive free samples, as is still the case in many developing countries.

But the supply-and-demand nature of breastmilk is such that, once a mother accepts these free samples and starts her baby on formula, her own milk supply will quickly dry up. Sadly, after these mothers run out of formula samples and money-off coupons, they will find themselves unable to produce breastmilk and have no option but to spend large sums of money on continuing to feed their child with formula.

Even when manufacturers 'promote' breastfeeding, they plant what Mary Smale calls 'seeds of 'conditionality' that can lead to failure. 'Several years ago, manufacturers used to produce these amazing leaflets for women, encouraging women to breastfeed and reassuring them that they only need a few extra calories a day. You couldn't fault them on the words, but the pictures which were of things like Marks & Spencer yoghurt and whole fish with their heads on, and wholemeal bread—but not the sort of wholemeal bread that you buy in the corner shop, the sort of wholemeal bread you buy in specialist shops.

The underlying message was clear: a healthy pregnancy and a good supply of breastmilk are the preserve of the middle classes, and that any women who doesn't belong to that group will have to rely on other resources to provide for her baby.

A quick skim through any pregnancy magazine or the 'Bounty' pack—the glossy information booklet with free product samples given to new mothers in the UK—shows that these subtle visual messages, which include luxurious photos of whole grains and pulses, artistically arranged bowls of muesli, artisan loaves of bread and wedges of deli-style cheeses, exotic mangoes, grapes and kiwis, and fresh vegetables artistically arranged as crudités, are still prevalent.

Funding Research

Manufacturers also ply their influence through contact with health professionals (to whom they can provide free samples for research and 'educational purposes') as middlemen. Free gifts, educational trips to exotic locations and funding for research are just some of the ways in which the medical profession becomes 'educated' about the benefits of formula.

According to Patti Rundall, OBE, policy director for the UK's Baby Milk Action group, which has been lobbying for responsible marketing of baby food for over 20 years, 'Throughout the last two decades, the baby-feeding companies have tried to establish a strong role for themselves with the medical profession, knowing that health and education services represent a key marketing opportunity. Companies are, for instance, keen to fund the infant-feeding research on which health policies are based, and to pay for midwives, teachers, education materials and community projects.'

They are also keen to fund 'critical' NGOs—that is, lay groups whose mandate is to inform and support women. But this sort of funding is not allowed by the International Code of Marketing of Breastmilk Substitutes (see below) because it prejudices the ability of these organisations to provide mothers with independent information about infant feeding. Nevertheless, such practices remain prevalent—if somewhat more discreet than in the past—and continue to weaken health professionals' advocacy for breastfeeding.

Fighting Back

When it became clear that declining breastfeeding rates were affecting infant health and that the advertising of infant formula had a direct effect on a woman's decision not to breastfeed, the International Code of Marketing of Breastmilk Substitutes was drafted and eventually adopted by the World Health Assembly (WHA) in 1981. The vote was near-unanimous, with 118 member nations voting in favour, three abstaining and one—the US—voting against. (In 1994, after years of opposition, the US eventually joined every other developed nation in the world as a signatory to the Code.)

The Code is a unique instrument that promotes safe and adequate nutrition for infants on a global scale by trying to protect breastfeeding and ensuring the appropriate marketing of breastmilk substitutes. It applies to all products marketed as partial or total replacements for breastmilk, including infant formula, follow-on formula, special formulas, cereals, juices, vegetable mixes and baby teas, and also applies to feeding bottles and teats. In addition, it maintains that no infant food may be marketed in ways that undermine breastfeeding. Specifically, the Code:

- Bans all advertising or promotion of these products to the general public
- Bans samples and gifts to mothers and health workers
- Requires information materials to advocate for breastfeeding, to warn against bottlefeeding and to not contain pictures of babies or text that idealises the use of breastmilk substitutes
- Bans the use of the healthcare system to promote breast-milk substitutes
- Bans free or low-cost supplies of breastmilk substitutes
- Allows health professionals to receive samples, but only for research purposes
- Demands that product information be factual and scientific
- Bans sales incentives for breastmilk substitutes and direct contact with mothers
- Requires that labels inform fully on the correct use of infant formula and the risks of misuse
- Requires labels not to discourage breastfeeding.

This document probably couldn't have been created today. Since the founding of the World Trade Organization (WTO) and its 'free trade' ethos in 1995, the increasing sophistication of corporate power strategies and aggressive lobbying of health organisations has increased to the extent that the Code would have been binned long before it reached the voting stage.

However, in 1981, member states, corporations and NGOs were on a somewhat more equal footing. By preventing industry from advertising infant formula, giving out free samples, promoting their products in healthcare facilities or by way of mother-and-baby 'goody bags', and insisting on better labelling, the Code acts to regulate an industry that would otherwise be given a free hand to pedal an inferior food product to babies and infants.

Unfortunately . . .

Being a signatory to the Code does not mean that member countries are obliged to adopt its recommendations wholesale. Many countries, the UK included, have adopted only parts of it—for instance, the basic principle that breastfeeding is a good thing—while ignoring the nuts-and-bolts strategies that limit advertising and corporate contact with mothers. So, in the UK, infant formula for 'healthy babies' can be advertised to mothers through hospitals and clinics, though not via the media.

> **"Breastfeeding is a natural negotiation between mother and baby and you interfere with it at your peril."**
>
> Professor Mary Renfrew,
> University of York

What's more, formula manufacturers for their part continue to argue that the Code is too restrictive and that it stops them from fully exploiting their target markets. Indeed, Helmut Maucher, a powerful corporate lobbyist and honorary chairman of Nestlé—the company that claims 40 per cent of the global baby-food market—has gone on record as saying: 'Ethical decisions that injure a firm's ability to compete are actually immoral'.

And make no mistake, these markets are big. The UK baby milk market is worth £150 million per year and the US market around $2 billion. The worldwide market for baby milks and foods is a staggering $17 billion and growing by 12 per cent each year. From formula manufacturers' point of view, the more women breastfeed, the more profit is lost. It is estimated that, for every child exclusively breastfed for six months, an average of $450 worth of infant food will not be bought. On a global scale, that amounts to billions of dollars in lost profits.

What particularly worries manufacturers is that, if they accept the Code without a fight, it could set a dangerous precedent for other areas of international trade—for instance, the pharmaceutical, tobacco, food and agriculture industries, and oil companies. This is why the focus on infant-feeding has been diverted away from children's health and instead become a symbolic struggle for a free market.

While most manufacturers publicly agree to adhere to the Code, privately, they deploy enormous resources in constructing ways to reinterpret or get round it. In this endeavour, Nestlé has shown a defiance and tenacity that beggars belief.

In India, for example, Nestlé lobbied against the Code being entered into law and when, after the law was passed, it faced criminal charges over its labelling, it issued a writ petition against the Indian government rather than accept the charges.

Years of aggressive actions like this, combined with unethical advertising and marketing practices, has led to an ongoing campaign to boycott the company's products that stretches back to 1977.

The Achilles' heel of the Code is that it does not provide for a monitoring office. This concept was in the original draft, but was removed from subsequent drafts. Instead, monitoring of the Code has been left to 'governments acting individually and collectively through the World Health Organization'.

But, over the last 25 years, corporate accountability has slipped lower down on the UN agenda, far behind free trade, self-regulation and partnerships. Lack of government monitoring means that small and comparatively poorly funded groups like the International Baby Food Action Network (IBFAN), which has 200 member groups working in over 100 countries, have taken on the job of monitoring Code violations almost by default. But while these watchdog groups can monitor and report Code violations to the health authorities, they cannot stop them.

In 2004, IBFAN's bi-annual report *Breaking the Rules, Stretching the Rules,* analysed the promotional practices of 16 international baby-food companies, and 14 bottle and teat companies, between January 2002 and April 2004. The researchers found some 2,000 violations of the Code in 69 countries.

On a global scale, reinterpreting the Code to suit marketing strategies is rife, and Nestlé continues to be the leader of the pack. According to IBFAN, Nestlé believes that only one of its products—infant formula—comes within the scope of the Code. The company also denies the universality of the Code, insisting that it only applies to developing nations. Where Nestlé, and the Infant Food Manufacturers Association that it dominates, leads, other companies have followed, and when companies like Nestlé are caught breaking the Code, the strategy is simple, but effective—initiate complex and boring discussions with organisations at WHO or WHA level about how best to interpret the Code in the hopes that these will offset any bad publicity and divert attention from the harm caused by these continual infractions.

According to Patti Rundall, it's important not to let such distractions divert attention from the bottom line: 'There can be no food more locally produced, more sustainable or more environmentally friendly than a mother's breastmilk, the only food required by an infant for the first six months of life. It is a naturally renewable resource, which requires no packaging or transport, results in no wastage and is free. Breastfeeding can also help reduce family poverty, which is a major cause of malnutrition.'

So perhaps we should be further simplifying the debate by asking: Are the companies who promote infant formula as the norm simply clever entrepreneurs doing their jobs or human-rights violators of the worst kind?

Not Good Enough

After more than two decades, it is clear that a half-hearted advocacy of breastfeeding benefits multinational formula manufacturers, not mothers and babies, and that the baby-food industry has no intention of complying with UN recommendations on infant-feeding or with the principles of the International Code for Marketing of Breastmilk Substitutes—unless they are forced to do so by law or consumer pressure or, more effectively, both.

Women do not fail to breastfeed. Health professionals, health agencies and governments fail to educate and support women who want to breastfeed.

Without support, many women will give up when they encounter even small difficulties. And yet, according to Mary Renfrew, 'Giving up breastfeeding is not something that women do lightly. They don't just stop breastfeeding and walk away from it. Many of them fight very hard to continue it and they fight with no support. These women are fighting society—a society that is not just bottle-friendly, but is deeply breastfeeding-unfriendly.'

To reverse this trend, governments all over the world must begin to take seriously the responsibility of ensuring the good health of future generations. To do this requires deep and profound social change. We must stop harassing mothers with simplistic 'breast is best' messages and put time, energy and money into reeducating health professionals and society at large.

We must also stop making compromises. Government health policies such as, say, in the UK and US, which aim for 75 per cent of women to be breastfeeding on hospital discharge, are little more than paying lip service to the importance of breastfeeding.

Most of these women will stop breastfeeding within a few weeks, and such policies benefit no one except the formula manufacturers, who will start making money the moment breastfeeding stops.

To get all mothers breastfeeding, we must be prepared to:

- Ban all advertising of formula including follow-on milks
- Ban all free samples of formula, even those given for educational or study purposes
- Require truthful and prominent health warnings on all tins and cartons of infant formula
- Put substantial funding into promoting breastfeeding in every community, especially among the socially disadvantaged, with a view to achieving 100-per-cent exclusive breastfeeding for the first six months of life
- Fund advertising and education campaigns that target fathers, mothers-in-law, schoolchildren, doctors, midwives and the general public
- Give women who wish to breastfeed in public the necessary encouragement and approval
- Make provisions for all women who are in employment to take at least six months paid leave after birth, without fear of losing their jobs.

Such strategies have already proven their worth elsewhere. In 1970, breastfeeding rates in Scandinavia were as low as those in Britain. Then, one by one, the Scandinavian countries banned all advertising of artificial formula milk, offered a year's maternity leave with 80 per cent of pay and, on the mother's return to work, an hour's breastfeeding break every day. Today, 98 per cent of Scandinavian women initiate breastfeeding, and 94 per cent are still breastfeeding at one month, 81 per cent at two months, 69 per cent at four months and 42 per cent at six months. These rates, albeit still not optimal, are nevertheless the highest in the world, and the result of a concerted, multifaceted approach to promoting breastfeeding.

Given all that we know of the benefits of breastfeeding and the dangers of formula milk, it is simply not acceptable that we have allowed breastfeeding rates in the UK and elsewhere in the world to decline so disastrously.

The goal is clear—100 per cent of mothers should be exclusively breastfeeding for at least the first six months of their babies' lives.

From *The Ecologist*, May 2006, pp. 22–32. Copyright © 2006 by The Ecologist. Reprinted by permission.

An Oldie Vies for Nutrient of the Decade

Jane E. Brody

The so-called sunshine vitamin is poised to become the nutrient of the decade, if a host of recent findings are to be believed. Vitamin D, an essential nutrient found in a limited number of foods, has long been renowned for its role in creating strong bones, which is why it is added to milk.

Now a growing legion of medical researchers have raised strong doubts about the adequacy of currently recommended levels of intake, from birth through the sunset years. The researchers maintain, based on a plethora of studies, that vitamin D levels considered adequate to prevent bone malformations like rickets in children are not optimal to counter a host of serious ailments that are now linked to low vitamin D levels.

To be sure, not all medical experts are convinced of the need for or the desirability of raising the amount of vitamin D people should receive, either through sunlight, foods, supplements or all three. The federal committee that establishes daily recommended levels of nutrients has resisted all efforts to increase vitamin D intake significantly, partly because the members are not convinced of assertions for its health-promoting potential and partly because of time-worn fears of toxicity.

This column will present the facts as currently known, but be forewarned. In the end, you will have to decide for yourself how much of this vital nutrient to consume each and every day and how to obtain it.

Where to Obtain It

Through most of human history, sunlight was the primary source of vitamin D, which is formed in skin exposed to ultraviolet B radiation (the UV light that causes sunburns). Thus, to determine how much vitamin D is needed from food and supplements, take into account factors like skin color, where you live, time of year, time spent out of doors, use of sunscreens and coverups and age.

Sun avoiders and dark-skinned people absorb less UV radiation. People in the northern two-thirds of the country make little or no vitamin D in winter, and older people make less vitamin D in their skin and are less able to convert it into the hormone that the body uses. In addition, babies fed just breast milk consume little vitamin D unless given a supplement.

In addition to fortified drinks like milk, soy milk and some juices, the limited number of vitamin D food sources include oily fish like salmon, mackerel, bluefish, catfish, sardines and tuna, as well as cod liver oil and fish oils. The amount of vitamin D in breakfast cereals is minimal at best. As for supplements, vitamin D is found in prenatal vitamins, multivitamins, calcium-vitamin D combinations and plain vitamin D. Check the label, and select brands that contain vitamin D3, or cholecalciferol. D2, or ergocalciferol, is 25 percent less effective.

Vitamin D content is listed on labels in international units (I.U.). An eight-ounce glass of milk or fortified orange juice is supposed to contain 100 I.U. Most brands of multivitamins provide 400 a day. Half a cup of canned red salmon has about 940, and three ounces of cooked catfish about 570.

Myriad Links to Health

Let's start with the least controversial role of vitamin D—strong bones. Last year, a 15-member team of nutrition experts noted in The American Journal of Clinical Nutrition that "randomized trials using the currently recommended intakes of 400 I.U. vitamin D a day have shown no appreciable reduction in fracture risk."

"In contrast," the experts continued, "trials using 700 to 800 I.U. found less fracture incidence, with and without supplemental calcium. This change may result from both improved bone health and reduction in falls due to greater muscle strength."

A Swiss study of women in their 80s found greater leg strength and half as many falls among those who took 800 I.U. of vitamin D a day for three months along with 1,200 milligrams of calcium, compared with women who took just calcium. Greater strength and better balance have been found in older people with high blood levels of vitamin D.

In animal studies, vitamin D has strikingly reduced tumor growth, and a large number of observational studies in people have linked low vitamin D levels to an increased risk of cancer, including cancers of the breast, rectum, ovary, prostate, stomach, bladder, esophagus, kidney, lung, pancreas and uterus, as well as Hodgkin's lymphoma and multiple myeloma.

Researchers at Creighton University in Omaha conducted a double-blind, randomized, placebo-controlled trial (the most reliable form of clinical research) among 1,179 community-living, healthy postmenopausal women. They reported last year in The American Journal of Clinical Nutrition that over the course of four years, those taking calcium and 1,100 I.U. of vitamin D3 each day developed about 80 percent fewer cancers than those who took just calcium or a placebo.

Vitamin D seems to dampen an overactive immune system. The incidence of autoimmune diseases like Type 1 diabetes and multiple sclerosis has been linked to low levels of vitamin D. A study published on Dec. 20, 2006, in The Journal of the American Medical Association examined the risk of developing multiple sclerosis among more than seven million military recruits followed for up to 12 years. Among whites, but not blacks or Hispanics, the risk of developing M.S. increased with ever lower levels of vitamin D in their blood serum before age 20.

A study published in Neurology in 2004 found a 40 percent lower risk of M.S. in women who took at least 400 I.U. of vitamin D a day.

Likewise, a study of a national sample of non-Hispanic whites found a 75 percent lower risk of diabetes among those with the highest blood levels of vitamin D.

Vitamin D is a fat-soluble vitamin that when consumed or made in the skin can be stored in body fat. In summer, as little as five minutes of sun a day on unprotected hands and face can replete the body's supply. Any excess can be stored for later use. But for most people during the rest of the year, the body needs dietary help.

Furthermore, the general increase in obesity has introduced a worrisome factor, the tendency for body fat to hold on to vitamin D, thus reducing its overall availability.

As for a maximum safe dose, researchers like Bruce W. Hollis, a pediatric nutritionist at the Medical University of South Carolina in Charleston, maintain that the current top level of 2,000 I.U. is based on shaky evidence indeed—a study of six patients in India. Dr. Hollis has been giving pregnant women 4,000 I.U. a day, and nursing women 6,000, with no adverse effects. Other experts, however, are concerned that high vitamin D levels (above 800 I.U.) with calcium can raise the risk of kidney stones in susceptible people.

From *The New York Times*, February 19, 2008. Copyright © 2008 by The New York Times Company. Reprinted by permission via PARS International.

What Good Is Breakfast?

The New Science of the Loneliest Meal

How I learned to Love breakfast (or at Least What to Eat for It).

AMANDA FORTINI

As meals go, breakfast is something of a celebrity. It is one of the most studied, analyzed, parsed, discussed, and advised-about subjects of nutritional science. Never more so than today, as doctors, and nutritionists, and countless articles and academic papers prescribe breakfast as both prophylactic and cure-all: The morning meal is said to stoke metabolism, stop late-night grazing, thwart obesity, reduce diabetes risk, improve nutritional intake, sharpen concentration—even increase longevity. In March, a new study more conclusively linked breakfast with body-mass index, with weight increasing as the frequency of breakfast consumption decreased. Breakfast, it seems, is highly influential: the power broker of repasts.

Are we making ourselves hungrier, dumber, shorter-lived, slow metabolizers by not eating a proper breakfast?

Yet despite all the fussing over and fetishizing of breakfast, most of us have only the vaguest notion of what we should be ingesting. Each new study of breakfast seems to contradict the last. Are eggs advisable, or will they raise one's cholesterol? Is a meal of toast anemic or adequate? What is a whole grain, anyway? And most important, are we really making ourselves fatter, hungrier, dumber, shorter-lived, slow metabolizers by not eating a so-called proper breakfast? As the experts continue to debate, most of us shrug and make choices not out of any real knowledge but for lack of time. If we don't slurp down a bowl of cereal at home, or succumb to the buxom muffin beckoning from the glass case at the deli, then an enormous caffeinated drink with a hyphenated name becomes our de facto morning meal.

Or we have nothing at all. National survey data cited by the Breakfast Research Institute indicates that between 1965 and 1991, the number of adults who regularly skip breakfast increased from 14 to 25 percent. The attrition of breakfast-eaters is understandable. After all, what's to love about breakfast? The first meal of the day tends not to be celebratory or communal; unless we're talking about brunch, breakfast's fashionably late cousin, the morning meal is usually a solitary, functional affair. "Breakfast is the proper meal, the one that's usually prepared by oneself and eaten alone," David Heber, director of the UCLA Center for Human Nutrition, told me. "It's not as much fun as going out with friends for lunch or dinner. It's a chore. Breakfast is a meal people are ready to dump."

The multifarious reasons people cite for dumping breakfast shed some light on the psychology of the meal. Some simply don't like to eat in the morning; a handful of friends, none of them pregnant, tell me that even the smell of food before eleven makes them nauseated. Chronic dieters pass on breakfast with an eye toward shaving a few hundred calories off their day. Others can't seem to squeeze in a meal amid the chaos of their morning: the dog to walk, the children to dress, the in-box fires to extinguish, the enervating commute. Still others, and I count myself among this crowd, sometimes abstain because the received wisdom about breakfast seems possibly spurious—one of those persistent nutrition myths, like the notion that you need eight to ten glasses of water per day or that celery has negative calories: If breakfast is supposed to curb your appetite, then why, shortly after partaking, am I ravenous, unable to focus on anything but foraging for more food, hungrier than when I don't eat anything?

I am not the only breakfast skeptic out there (though this is, to be sure, a decidedly less populous camp). "I think it's a nonissue for adults," said Marion Nestle, professor of nutrition and food studies at New York University and a breakfast skipper herself. "I think people should eat when they're hungry. Some people are really hungry in the morning and some are not." In her book *What to Eat,* she writes, "I am well aware that everyone says breakfast is the most important meal of the day, but I am not convinced. What you eat—and how much—matters more to your health than when you eat."

But since so many researchers argue that breakfast does matter, I began to investigate. How, exactly, are we harming ourselves by failing to eat breakfast? The simplified answer is that it depends on how young you are. Even Nestle concedes that there is strong evidence that children who skip breakfast do not fare as well academically or physically as those who eat it. A study conducted by researchers at Tufts University found that children who consumed a breakfast of Quaker instant oatmeal displayed better spatial memory and an increased ability to stay on task (what the study called "vigilance attention") when performing a battery of cognitive tests than children who ate Cap'n Crunch, and, perhaps surprisingly, those who ate the sweetened cereal performed better than those who ate nothing. Another study, this one by researchers at the University of Reading, found that adolescents fed a sugary drink in the morning will subsequently display all the mental agility of a 70-year-old. It's not much of a leap to assume that an adult who skips breakfast will have the same difficulty concentrating at work as a kid sitting in a classroom—hunger is distracting whatever your age—but distracted office workers have not been a major concern for breakfast researchers.

Researchers are interested in breakfast because they are interested in obesity, and they suspect that skipping the former plays a role in fostering the latter. "The frequency of eating breakfast has declined over the past several decades, during which time the obesity epidemic has also unfolded," write researchers Maureen T. Timlin and Mark A. Pereira in an excellent meta-analysis of all the scientific literature on breakfast to date, published in the June 2007 issue of *Nutrition Reviews*. Timlin and Pereira—the pair appear to be the Boswells of breakfast—also conducted the study about breakfast and body-mass index (BMI) published in *Pediatrics* in March. They tracked 2,216 Minnesota adolescents for five years, and found that subjects who skipped breakfast were consistently heavier than those who did not.

The relationship appears to hold for adults as well. A 2003 study published in the *American Journal of Epidemiology* concluded that subjects who habitually skipped breakfast (at least 75 percent of the time) had a four and a half times higher risk of obesity than those who habitually consumed it. (Those who missed breakfast even once during the study had an increased risk of obesity.) And of the 5,000-plus members of the National Weight Control Registry—registrants have lost an average of 66 pounds and have kept it off for more than five years—78 percent claim to be regular breakfast eaters.

But breakfast-eating and weight management may not be connected in the way that we think: Despite what women's magazines, and pop health magazines, and legions of mothers say, the mere act of consuming breakfast does not miraculously speed up one's metabolism. In fact, it's hard to pinpoint exactly why eating breakfast tends to coincide with healthier weight. It may be that eating breakfast simply creates a feeling of satiety, which prevents trips to the vending machine or the drive-through in the afternoon or evening. (Eating at regular intervals maintains insulin and blood-sugar levels, preventing the peaks and valleys that cause voracity.) The *American Journal of Epidemiology* study found that adults consumed more calories on the days they eschewed a morning meal.

The real problem, from a researcher's point of view, is that breakfast consumption is a habit that tends to occur along with a constellation of other healthy behaviors—like exercising, not smoking, and maintaining a healthy diet—that may confound or influence the effect of breakfast on obesity. (Unhealthy behaviors, too, tend to stick together: Fewer than 5 percent of smokers eat breakfast daily.) In at least one study, when confounding variables were accounted for, the relationship between breakfast and body-mass index was not significant. The eating of breakfast was only an ancillary factor, one salubrious practice among several that contributed to slimness. Breakfasting and forgoing the gym will probably do little to reduce or control one's weight. In the *Pediatrics* study, for example, it seemed surprising the breakfast eaters often had a higher daily caloric intake and yet also a lower BMI than their breakfast-skipping peers, but when I asked Pereira what explained this finding—had eating a morning meal somehow increased the subjects' metabolism?—he emphasized that the eaters were exercisers as well.

This is all to say that it is not yet clear to researchers whether the relationship between breakfast and obesity is causal (i.e., breakfast consumption directly influences weight) or merely associational. Breakfast may play a supporting role in weight management, rather than a starring one. Few prospective studies (in which breakfast-eating subjects are followed over a period of time) or clinical trials (in which breakfast eating is tested as an interventional therapy, as a drug might be) have been done. This is why the *Pediatrics* study, conducted prospectively over the course of five years, was a significant contribution to the field of breakfast studies: We can observe the correlation between breakfast consumption and BMI over time, which approximates cause and effect.

If mere consumption is not itself transformative, the question remains: What are we to eat? People have been fretting about what constitutes an ideal breakfast since at least the 1800s. Sylvester Graham, of cracker fame, promoted his high-fiber, additive-free wheat flour as a remedy for the dyspepsia epidemic of the time, which he felt was caused by the meatcentric, multicourse American breakfast: an extravaganza of pancakes, biscuits, eggs, bacon, fried ham, salt pork, and potatoes. (Such hearty fare had been fuel for the farmer but was fattening to the more sedentary industrialist.) As Scott Bruce and Bill Crawford write in *Cerealizing America,* the ascetic Graham believed that "meat eating inflamed the 'baser properties,'" leading to masturbation—what he called "the vice"—and that "tea drinking led to delirium tremens." Sixty years later, John Harvey Kellogg, who breakfasted on graham crackers and apples himself, also peddled grains, in the form of the first flake cereal, as a vegetarian cure for digestive trouble. You might say that breakfast has a long history of having the fun drained out of it.

The warring of the diet factions continues today in a slightly more scientific fashion. A 2003 paper published in the *Journal of the American College of Nutrition* claimed that individuals who consumed ready-to-eat cereal, cooked cereal, or, oddly, "quick breads"—waffles, pancakes, pastries, and the like—had lower BMIs than those who ate meat and eggs or abstained from breakfast entirely. But a 2007 study found the opposite: Obese women who ate two eggs for breakfast daily for eight weeks lost 65 percent more weight than their bagel-fed counterparts. Like most prescriptive studies, however, these two must be taken with a grain of salt (or, in the case of the cereal study, a few granules of sugar): Kellogg funded the former; the American Egg Board funded the latter. Among those in the field of nutrition research, it is widely acknowledged that, for a variety of reasons ranging from flawed study design to buried negative results, industry-funded studies tend to find industry-favorable results. For instance: The Tufts study that found that Quaker instant oatmeal (and, to a lesser degree, Cap'n Crunch) improved cognitive performance was funded by Quaker, the maker of both products.

The studies and advice grow ever more specific and contradictory: If your aim is to optimize attention span and memory—especially in children—then, according to one study, the best breakfast is ham and hard cheese on whole-grain bread. If you want to prevent heart disease (and who doesn't?), try whole-grain cereal; one bowl per day is associated with a 28 percent lower risk of heart failure. If you're a woman hoping to conceive a boy, then, according to a recent study from the University of Exeter, you should increase your breakfast consumption by approximately 400 calories daily. (Women with the highest caloric intake had boys 56 percent of the time, compared with 45 percent with the lowest caloric intake.) It's enough to make one feel inclined to take refuge in Vonnegut's breakfast of champions: a morning martini.

And yet, even as they disagree on the specifics, the majority of researchers seem to agree that what we put into our bodies in the morning is a critical decision. Because it occurs after eight, ten, or even twelve hours of sleep, the breakfasting moment is physiologically unique. "The nature of the food we eat affects hormones in profound ways for many hours after a meal, and that's more important after breakfast," said Dr. David Ludwig, associate professor of pediatrics at Harvard Medical School and author of *Ending the Food Fight.* "We've been fasting and stress hormones are elevated and we're insulin-resistant, so we can use the properties of food at this time to our benefit or our detriment." A fasting body is particularly sensitive to, say, a sugary, refined-starch, low-fiber muffin; blood sugar will soar and then plummet, leaving you famished once again.

What's preferable, according to Ludwig, is to choose breakfast foods with a low glycemic index (GI). The term refers to the rate at which glucose is absorbed from carbohydrates—or, put another way, how rapidly carbohydrates affect blood sugar.

This is important because controlling insulin and blood-glucose levels in turn controls appetite and, ultimately, weight. In a 1999 study led by Ludwig, twelve obese teenage boys were fed at various occasions high-GI ("instant oatmeal"), medium-GI ("steel-cut oats"), and low-GI ("a vegetable omelette and fruit") breakfasts and lunches, and then were allowed to consume all the food they wanted for the rest of the day. The high-GI cohort, in a state of crashing blood sugar and surging adrenaline induced by the instant oatmeal, devoured 500 to 600 extra calories. (This phenomenon likely explains that postprandial ravenousness I often experience—my morning mainstays, toaster waffles and quick-cooking oats, rank fairly high on the GI list.) Low-glycemic foods may even help breakfasters achieve that dietary holy grail: speeding up metabolism. In another study, subjects kept on such a diet saw their metabolic rate shift slightly to burn approximately 80 more calories per day—not a lot, but every little bit helps.

How to tell if a food has a low glycemic index? A quick rule of thumb: The more processed the food, the higher its GI; the higher a food's fiber content, the lower its GI. Breakfast, in other words, should be a high-fiber affair. This means vegetables and fruits (but not juices—the fiber is in the pulp and skin) and whole grains. For the record, a whole grain is an intact, unrefined grain that retains the bran and germ, its nutrient- and fiber-rich components.

Eggs too may help to control blood sugar (protein stimulates the release of glucagon, a hormone that counterbalances insulin), but don't defect to the Atkins camp just yet. Eggs are also high in cholesterol. Many doctors, noting that sensitivity to dietary cholesterol varies, advise limiting eggs to several per week.

So what, then, to eat? The path of bread crumbs—or cereal flakes—through the thicket of breakfast suggestions is this: Breakfast is not dessert. Most muffins and bagels are out, as are those breakfast bars with the creepy strip of ersatz milk, and the many cereals that claim to be "whole grain" but are in fact sugary and fiberless. Out too are my beloved toaster waffles, unless I find a version containing the recommended five grams of fiber per serving. What remains are the foods that we probably should have been eating all along: unprocessed, low-GI, fiber-rich foods like fruits, vegetables (in omelettes if nowhere else), oatmeal (slow-cooking or steel-cut rather than instant), whole-grain breads and cereals (that are also high in fiber and low in sugar), protein in the form of low-fat dairy, and eggs in moderation. Nothing too exciting, but then, breakfast is all business. It you're looking for thrills, try dinner.

From *The New York Times*, June 9, 2008. Copyright © 2008 by The New York Times Company. Reprinted by permission via PARS International.

UNIT 4

Exercise and Weight Management

Unit Selections

Key Points to Consider

- What effect does exercise have on mental health and mental abilities?
- How important is exercise to achieving optimal health? Explain.

- Why should exercise be included in any weight control program?

- How do you feel about people who are overweight? Has your weight ever been a problem for you? If so, what have you done about it?

- Do you exercise on a regular basis? If not, explain why. What would it take to get you exercising on a regular basis?

- For young athletes, is there a need for balanced exercising? When does one begin to regard something as too much exercise?

- Should obesity be classified as a disease rather than the result of a lack of willpower?

- What are the factors that contribute to the development of eating disorders?

- Is it possible to diet on a limited food budget?

Student Website
www.mhcls.com

Internet References

American Society of Exercise Physiologists (ASEP)
http://www.asep.org
Cyberdiet
http://www.cyberdiet.com/reg/index.html
Shape Up America!
http://www.shapeup.org

Recently, a new set of guidelines, dubbed "Exercise Lite," has been issued by the U.S. Centers for Disease Control and Prevention in conjunction with the American College of Sports Medicine. These guidelines call for 30 minutes of exercise, 5 days a week, which can be spread over the course of a day. The primary focus of this approach to exercise is improving health, not athletic performance. Examples of activities that qualify under the new guidelines are walking your dog, playing tag with your kids, scrubbing floors, washing your car, mowing the lawn, weeding your garden, and having sex. From a practical standpoint, this approach to fitness will likely motivate many more people to become active and stay active. Remember, since the benefits of exercise can take weeks or even months before they become apparent, it is very important to choose an exercise program that you enjoy so that you will stick with it.

While a good diet cannot compensate for the lack of exercise, exercise can compensate for a less than optimal diet. Exercise not only makes people physically healthier, it also keeps their brains healthy. While the connection hasn't been proven, there is evidence that regular workouts may cause the brain to better process and store information which results in a smarter brain. While exercise and a nutritious diet can keep people fit and healthy, many Americans are not heeding this advice. For the first time in our history, the average American is now overweight when judged according to the standard height/weight tables. In addition, more than 25 percent of Americans are clinically obese, and the number appears to be growing. Why is this happening, given the prevailing attitude that Americans have toward fat? One theory that is currently gaining support suggests that while Americans have cut back on their consumption of fatty snacks and deserts, they have actually increased their total caloric intake by failing to limit their consumption of carbohydrates. The underlying philosophy goes something like this: fat calories make you fat, but you can eat as many carbohydrates as you want and not gain weight. The truth is that all calories count when it comes to weight gain, and if cutting back on fat calories prevents you from feeling satiated, you will naturally eat more to achieve that feeling. While this position seems reasonable enough, some groups, most notably supporters of the Atkins diet, have suggested that eating a high-fat diet will actually help people lose weight because of fat's high satiety value in conjunction with the formation of ketones (which suppress appetite). Whether people limit fat or carbohydrates, they will not lose weight unless their total caloric intake is less than their energy expenditure.

America's preoccupation with body weight has given rise to a billion-dollar industry. When asked why people go on diets, the predominant answer is for social reasons such as appearance and group acceptance, rather than concerns regarding health. Why do diets and diet aids fail? One of the major reasons lies in the mind-set of the dieter. Many dieters do not fully understand the biological and behavioral aspects of weight loss, and consequently they have unrealistic expectations regarding the process. While many people reasonably need to lose weight, many college women strive and compete with each other for the thinnest and most perfect body. This practice has led to an increase in the number of young women suffering from eating disorders. Hara Estroff Marano discusses this issue in "The Skinny Sweepstakes."

Being overweight not only causes health problems; it also carries with it a social stigma. Overweight people are often thought of as weak-willed individuals with little or no self-respect. The notion that weight control problems are the result of personality defects is being challenged by new research findings. Evidence is mounting that suggests that physiological and hereditary factors may play as great a role in

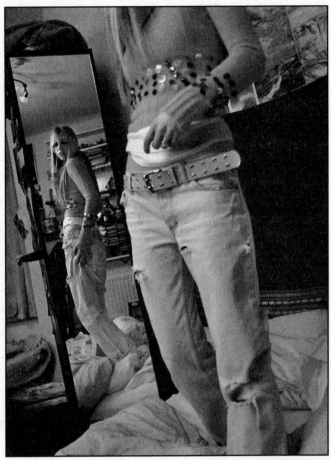

© BananaStock/PunchStock

obesity as do behavioral and environmental factors. Researchers now believe that gene tics dictate the base number of fat cells an individual will have, as well as the location and distribution of these cells within the body. The study of fat metabolism has provided additional clues as to why weight control is so difficult. These metabolic studies have found that the body seems to have a "setpoint," or desired weight, and it will defend this weight through alterations in basal metabolic rate and fat-cell activities. While this process is thought to be an adaptive throwback to primitive times when food supplies were uncertain, today, with our abundant food supply, this mechanism only contributes to the problem of weight control.

It should be apparent by now that weight control is both an attitudinal and a lifestyle issue. Fortunately, a new, more rational approach to the problem of weight control is emerging. This approach is based on the premise that you can be perfectly healthy and good looking without being pencil-thin. The primary focus of this approach to weight management is the attainment of your body's "natural ideal weight" and not some idealized, fanciful notion of what you would like to weigh. The concept of achieving your natural ideal body weight suggests that we need to take a more realistic approach to both fitness and weight control, and also serves to remind us that a healthy lifestyle is based on the concepts of balance and moderation. The negative side of exercise, especially in children, is addressed in "A Big-Time Injury Striking Little Players' Knees" by Gina Kolata.

A Big-Time Injury Striking Little Players' Knees

GINA KOLATA

Last year, when Collin Link was 11 years old, he was tackled as he went in for a touchdown in pee-wee football. "He didn't get up," his mother, Crystal Link, said. "He kept saying his knee hurt real bad." But Mrs. Link was not overly concerned, thinking it was just a sprain.

But the next morning when the family was getting ready to go to church near their home in The Woodlands, Tex., Collin said he could not walk. That Monday, a doctor told the Links what was wrong.

Torn ligament poses a greater risk for growing bones.

Collin had an injury that doctors used to think almost never occurred in children. He had torn the anterior cruciate ligament, or A.C.L., in his left knee, the main ligament that stabilizes the joint.

The standard and effective treatment for such an injury in adults is surgery. But the operation poses a greater risk for children and adolescents who have not finished growing because it involves drilling into a growth plate, an area of still-developing tissue at the end of the leg bone.

Although there are no complete or official numbers, orthopedists at leading medical centers estimate that several thousand children and young adolescents are getting A.C.L. tears each year, with the number being diagnosed soaring recently. Some centers that used to see only a few such cases a year are now seeing several each week.

And contrary to the old belief that boys are more prone to the injury than girls, as many as eight times more girls than boys are suffering the tears, doctors report.

It is not an overuse injury from playing one sport too intensively, like shoulder injuries in young pitchers. Instead, doctors say, the injury occurs simply from twisting the knee, and diagnoses are on the rise partly because it can now be easily detected and partly because the very nature of youth sports has changed.

In the old days, said Dr. Theodore J. Ganley, director of sports medicine at the Children's Hospital of Philadelphia and a spokesman for the American Academy of Orthopedic Surgeons, a child would develop a "trick knee" that made sports difficult, but the real reason was not understood. And most doctors, thinking children did not get A.C.L. tears, did not suspect the real reason.

Now that almost every child with a hurt knee gets a magnetic resonance imaging, doctors are finding the ligament tears on a regular basis.

The other reason for the reported surge in A.C.L. tears, doctors speculate, is that the best athletes are more or less constantly at risk. They play year-round and on multiple teams with frequent games, in which the risk of injury is higher than in practice because of the intensity of play.

"The kids are playing at really highly competitive levels at earlier and earlier ages," said Dr. Mininder S. Kocher, the associate director of the division of sports medicine at Children's Hospital in Boston.

Whatever the reason, the increase in diagnoses has created a new problem: what to do about the injury.

Every orthopedist is familiar with A.C.L. tears, but in adults. It is "the most common and most dreaded injury in professional sports," Dr. Kocher said. The well-established operation to repair it often results in a full return to function. And doctors often recommend that adults have the operation because without the ligament the knee is not stable.

After a tear, any sport, like soccer or basketball, that can twist the knee is dangerous. Without an anterior cruciate ligament, even everyday activities can injure the smooth, shock-absorbing cartilage that caps the knee joint. "Then you are on your way to arthritis," Dr. Kocher said.

But the standard A.C.L. repair operation, with its drilling into the growth plate, may cause permanent damage to the still-growing bones of young children. After drilling, surgeons replace the torn ligament with a tendon taken from elsewhere in the body, like the hamstring, or from a cadaver. But if the drilling damages a child's growth plate, the leg bone will not develop normally.

An injury once thought adults—only is a special problem for the young.

That happened recently to a 14-year-old boy who was referred to Dr. Freddie H. Fu, an orthopedic surgeon at the University of Pittsburgh. A year after the operation, Dr. Fu said, the leg with the repair was bowed 20 degrees on one side and was shorter than the other leg.

"I had to go in on the other side and stop the growth," Dr. Fu said. "Now, about six months later, the leg is still crooked. There still is a two-inch difference in length which I have to fix." The boy, he said, "will be a little bit shorter" as a result, although both legs will be the same length.

Doctors often suggest putting a brace on the injured knee and limiting a child's activities, delaying surgery until the child finishes growing. But the children who tear A.C.L.'s tend to be highly competitive athletes who chafe under the restrictions.

Ashley Hammond, owner of Soccer Domain, a domed facility in Montclair, N.J., said that parents of young soccer stars often wanted them to keep playing and that children were the type who would forget or resist instructions to wear a brace, putting their knees at risk.

"All kids feel they are indestructible," Mr. Hammond said. "The kids want to play no matter what we say." A result can be injuries to their knee cartilage and its attendant risk of arthritis in young adulthood.

Some surgeons are developing new and technically demanding methods to repair A.C.L. tears in children, drilling holes to create little tunnels in bone that is already finished growing and threading tendons around the growth plate. Different surgeons have different versions of the technique, Dr. Ganley said.

But the tendons are not anchored where they would normally be and the long-term effects of the operation are not known.

Dr. Kocher has perhaps the most extensive data, on 59 young patients. His results are encouraging; the implanted ligaments failed in only two patients and no patients had severe growth abnormalities. But the patients have been followed less than four years.

"We don't know the long-term results, 20, 30 years out," Dr. Willis said. "Are these people going to end up with arthritis? Some feel there's a chance of that, but we feel that surgery lessens the chance that will happen."

It is only with the new increase in diagnosed A.C.L. tears in children, orthopedists say, that they discovered how mistaken they once were about this injury.

Doctors used to think the tears did not occur or were extremely rare in children because children's ligaments were stronger than their bones. They thought an injury that would rip an adult's A.C.L. would, in children, result in a broken bone.

Another myth, Dr. Ganley said, is that A.C.L. tears arise mostly in contact injuries, like a tackle in football, and almost exclusively affect boys. Now, though, it appears that girls are more susceptible, although no one really knows why, said Dr. Baxter Willis, an orthopedist at Children's Hospital in Ottawa.

Doctors have also learned that contact injuries are not the most common cause of A.C.L. injuries. It turns out, Dr. Ganley said, that tears occur more often from twisting and jumping. A child can be running and step in a hole, twisting a leg. Or they can fall off a bike, like Malinda McCartney of Pembroke, Mass., who tore her ligament last year when she was 9.

Other times, a young athlete can tear an A.C.L. by coming down from a rebound in basketball or by accelerating and decelerating. Now, though, with doctors looking for the injury and surgeons finding new ways to repair it without touching the growth plate, parents often face difficult decisions, as Mrs. Link discovered. The first orthopedist told her that Collin should wear a knee brace and wait to have the operation until he stopped growing, which could take five years or more.

"He told Collin he was completely out of sports—soccer, basketball, baseball and football," Mrs. Link said. "They were his whole life. That was devastating to him."

So the Links took Collin to Children's Hospital in Dallas, where they saw another orthopedist. He said he could operate on Collin and that he had operated on a few children with A.C.L. tears, using one of the new methods that could avoid the growth plate. But first, he said, he wanted to put a brace on Collin's leg and see how he did before trying the surgery. The Links ended up traveling to Boston where Dr. Kocher operated on Collin. For the Links, it was the best of a bad set of choices. And the surgery and its aftermath were more difficult than they anticipated.

Collin was in intense pain and on a morphine drip after the operation and then spent much of the next six weeks lying down with his leg in a machine that moved his knee slowly through a range of motions. That was followed by six months of physical therapy, which was often painful and always difficult, physically and emotionally, Mrs. Link said.

Now, a year after the operation, Collin is starting to play a nontackle form of football, worried about injury if he played regular football and got tackled again. And he is running track.

Having the operation "was a difficult decision to make," Mrs. Link said. "But if they can play sports, it's the only option."

From *The New York Times*, February 18, 2008. Copyright © 2008 by The New York Times Company. Reprinted by permission via PARS International.

The Skinny Sweepstakes

In the push for achievement, the perfect body is now part of the perfect résumé. Deprived of an internal compass, girls compete to be "hottest," turning colleges into incubators of eating disorders.

HARA ESTROFF MARANO

"I started starving myself when I was 12 or 13," Chloe, an absolute beauty, recalls. "I wasn't overweight, but I wasn't as thin as a lot of my friends. It was just something I noticed."

Around that time, "a lot of problems" erupted in her family. "Dieting made me feel like I was in control of something. It was the one thing I knew I could change on my own. I would diet and get positive feedback and feel really good. So I wouldn't eat for a few days at a time."

Dieting also bound her to her peers. "A lot of girls at school would skip meals. We'd do it together. We went on fad diets together, too." Her family never noticed her food fetishes. "I had trouble impressing my mother. I could never achieve enough for her. But she definitely noticed when I lost weight."

From the beginning, starving consumed her life. "You think about it everywhere you go. And you compare yourself to other people. Each of my friends was vying to be better than the others. I was in a restaurant with my boyfriend and a girl walked in who was really pretty and much thinner than me. I saw him glance at her. I went into the bathroom and cried."

She couldn't look at a picture of a celebrity without feeling bad, either. The boys at her public school didn't help. "They're constantly comparing women to each other: 'That girl is really hot; she's so much hotter than her friends.' So we compete to be the hotter friend. Some days it makes you feel fat. On particularly bad days, I can look at children and think that when I'm older, that little 3-year-old girl is going to steal my husband."

In a culture of plenty where the young are pressured to succeed even before birth, the achievement package has come to include, especially for girls, a "perfect" body. Starting at puberty, sometimes before, the mounting pressure launches girls into the stratosphere of fat fear, in part fueled by the ubiquity of food, in part by new sensitivities adolescence brings to the judgments of others.

But perhaps the greatest accelerant of fat fear and distorted eating is the peer culture to which adolescents have been consigned for the past few decades. Age segregation isn't new to America's schools. But since the middle of the 20th century, it

has gathered critical mass until it has also come to dominate the extracurricular life of the young in their insular march through middle school, high school, and beyond.

Between 1960 and 2000, the percentages of 20-, 25-, and 30-year-olds enrolled in school more than doubled, with females becoming an increasingly larger part of the total.

The extension of schooling for more young people, especially girls—now the majority of college attendees—requires them to be warehoused together for years with those deliberately selected to share many of the same attributes, constraining exposure to the broader range of humanity. Ongoing shifts in communication technology (think: MySpace, YouTube, and mp3 files) may employ up-to-the-nanosecond science, but they turn out to be extraordinarily conservative social and developmental forces, keeping the young tightly tethered to each other, cloistered among those like themselves, and sharing sights, sounds, and other cultural effusions targeted exclusively at them, further age-stratifying their souls.

Superimpose on that nature's compulsory contribution, the mating sweepstakes, and each cohort of girls seems forced to make ever more minute distinctions between themselves—just as they compete to distinguish themselves on their college application essays. Thus does dieting become a competitive sport with the gold medal going to the thinnest, a triumph of the cultural ideal for appearance that almost every American girl will unwittingly internalize by middle school.

The strongest predictor of eating disorders among middle-school girls today is the importance that peers place on weight and eating, researchers report in the *International Journal of Eating Disorders*. The perceptions of peers outweighs, as it were, such traditional factors as confidence level, actual body mass, trying to look like the girls and women appearing on television and in magazines, even being teased by family and others about weight.

In highly age-stratified education, particularly for females, whose attractiveness depends so heavily on youth, "all the most attractive females of a cohort are competing with each other" for the attention of males, explains Geoffrey Miller. "They are seeing only rivals who are quite similar to themselves," says the University of New Mexico psychologist. "They're not seeing the mating market as a whole. Their frame of reference is artificially constricted."

The result is "extreme intensification of sexual competition." And with increasing numbers of young women not merely going to college but getting advanced degrees, age segregation and stratification continue much later in life than they did even a few decades ago.

> **On bad days, I can look at children and think that when I'm older, that little 3-year-old girl is going to steal my husband.**

Modern schools, Miller points out, are often so homogenous in terms of class and race as well as age that "kids have to invent ways to be different from each other that they never would have had to invent a hundred years ago." As they jockey intensely for skinny status, their very limited involvement with the outside world helps keep them highly focused on themselves.

Adrift Amid Peer Pressure

Richard Hersh calls it the culture of neglect: kids grow up overly dependent on their peers—"in essence, kids raising kids"—without developing a strong sense of self. A RAND scholar, former director of Harvard's Center for Moral Education, as well as former president of Trinity College and William Smith and Hobart Colleges, Hersh contends that adults—parents, neighbors, teachers, professors—have inadvertently done children and adolescents an injustice. They allow them to be socialized by television, the Internet, and by their peers rather than by caring, demanding, and mentoring adults. At the same time, the adults view kids as helpless, sheltering them from a wide range of experiences, "the risk of failure and being hurt being so great."

Both forms of deprivation weaken the young from within, so that kids go off to college socially and emotionally fragile, manifest in a rising tide of distress: anorexia and bulimia, along with depression, physical violence, alcohol and other drug abuse, and suicide attempts. Approximately 40 percent of females now experience an eating disorder at some point during their years of college, data show.

Missing in action is a rich internal life independent of peers. Hersh sees residential college life perpetuating and intensifying an adolescent pattern of overreliance on peer approval. It also, he says, elevates the body over the mind. And that combination subverts the developmental challenge of finding something far more durable: a stable identity.

The way New York psychotherapist Steven Levenkron sees it, the adults essentially outsource parenting. Levenkron has been treating young women with eating disorders for more than 30 years. He wrote one of the first books about anorexia, *The Best Little Girl in the World*, in 1978, and he has written textbooks on treatment of the disorder. Why is it, he asks, that some

girls succumb to the peer pressure and some don't? "Those who aren't mentored by parents are not inoculated against peer pressure. They wind up turning to their peers and to the media, to the outside society, for guidance on how to appeal to men." Without a strong, healthy attachment to parents, kids become fair game for what he sees as destructive messages about femininity from Hollywood.

But the damage goes especially deep because contemporary adolescents "have no language for reflection," he says. "They don't know how to think about hurts. That makes them feel alone in the world." Anorexics, he contends, have only a very primitive language. "They can talk your head off about body measurements and fats. It's all transacted with about 12 words."

From Comparison to Cutthroat Competition

It's bad enough that teens are swaddled in software and bound by a branch of consumer culture crafted exclusively for them. But there is something about herding them together 24/7 that actively distorts their thinking, specifically about bodies. As a result, America's universities have become incubators of eating disorders. Attending a residential college actually warps perception of self in relation to others, finds psychologist Catherine Sanderson. At a time and place where people should be getting smarter about everything, they are getting a lot less smart about themselves.

A professor of psychology at Amherst College, Sanderson looked at perceptions of the norms of thinness among women at Amherst, Princeton, and Smith colleges. When women arrive at college as freshmen, they believe that all the other women at their school are highly motivated to be thin—much thinner than they themselves want to be.

Mistakenly, they assume that other people's statements accurately reflect their behavior. They know that they themselves talk the talk in the dining hall and other public places—but privately slip out later for a bag of Doritos. They feel ashamed and isolated, without realizing that almost everyone else is wolfing down chips in private, too. Students develop a false impression of the norm.

But the damage is done. The feelings of shame and isolation lead almost directly to bingeing and purging and other forms of disordered eating. "The more women perceive themselves as different, the more symptoms they show of anorexia or bulimia," Sanderson finds.

"The problem with college is that the norms are in your face," she notes. You eat in a common dining hall, exercise in a common fitness center, shower together, and get dressed together. "The togetherness surrounds people at the key life period in which this stuff matters."

Norms matter especially at times of transition, such as going off to boarding school or starting college. In order to make it in their new environment, students look to others there to figure out what's normal. We all navigate the social universe by making comparisons to others, but researchers have long known that widespread insecurity (Will I get into Harvard? Is my family coming apart at the seams? Do I even have an identity of my own? Why do I feel so different from everyone?) exacerbates the process, turning comparison—with peers, with media figures—into cutthroat competition.

In such environments, misperception accelerates over time. Asked what they weigh, freshmen say "around 130," exactly what they believe other women weigh. But surveyed again the next year, after gaining about five pounds, the same women say—accurately—that they weigh 135. However, they think others weigh "around 125." "You're gaining weight and you know it, yet you believe that other women are losing weight," explains Sanderson. It's ironic, she notes, that this is a topic about which college actually makes people stupid: The more time they spend in school, the less accurate they become in their perceptions.

Puppets of Fear...

Columbia University psychologist Barbara Von Bulow co-runs a day-treatment program in Manhattan for eating disordered students who have been sent home on leave, asked by their out-of-town colleges to take time off for treatment. So competitive are the women about their weight-control strategies that the program has had to separate the bulimics from the anorexics.

"It's difficult to treat anorexics if they don't see themselves as unhealthy," Von Bulow observes. "Yet the bulimics look at the anorexics as successes because they are so thin." On the other hand, the anorexics "are terrified when they look at the bulimics, most of whom are normal weight. They see them as failed anorexics."

In reality, as in the dictionary, anorexia comes before bulimia; about 50 percent of the time, restrictive eating begets binge eating. Candice Sombrero, 19, a sophomore at Babson College outside Boston, endured six months of anorexia while a student at the prestigious Iolani School in Honolulu, where she grew up. "I'd grab coffee at home and tell my parents I'd get breakfast at school, which I never did. For lunch I prided myself on sipping an extra-large Diet Coke." The endless hunger made her preoccupied with food. "Once you get your hands on food, you stuff yourself. Then you feel physically uncomfortable and guilty for eating, so you start to purge." For the next year and a half, she was "stuck in the bulimic cycle, throwing up eight to 10 times a day."

Bulimia testifies to the difficulty of the restrictive eating that defines anorexia. On the other hand, not every girl can make herself throw up. Katy Palmer is one of the latter.

At 17, she was at the top of her high school class in Atlanta, looking at colleges and locked into competition with another girl for class valedictorian. "We knew each other's GPA down to the hundredth of a point," she recalls. The academic pressure was intense. That year her grandfather died, and suddenly family life was dominated by grieving. "I didn't have control over the college application process and I couldn't make any school accept me; I knew it was an arbitrary process. I didn't have control over what was happening in my family. Eating became the least complicated thing I could do that was under my control. I read an article in *Self* magazine all about calories. Cause and effect were clear: Fewer calories equal less weight."

Pressure Control

Just as there is no single cause of eating disorders among the young—they are rooted in conditions set long before college—there is no one solution. But many contributing elements can be addressed by schools, parents, and the culture at large.

- Attenuate the competitive pressure on kids; dispute the idea that the only path to success runs through Harvard Yard.
- Combat the pursuit of perfection: Discuss the impossibility of being perfect, the self-preoccupation that dogs perfectionists, and perfectionism's ultimately self-defeating nature.
- Allow the young meaningful engagement in a broad range of experiences beyond their usual routines.
- Encourage kids to experiment by giving them permission to fail, so they can claim their own experience and construct a strong sense of self.
- Discard helicopter parenting for real parenting, because authentic connection inoculates kids against the excesses of peer culture.
- Expose kids to alternatives to the pseudo culture mass manufactured for their consumption.
- Lobby upper schools to dampen the college-entrance sweepstakes. This in turn could force colleges to revamp admissions policies predicated on excess selectivity favoring ultracompetitive overachievers.

Today, kids have to invent ways to be different from each other that they never would have had to invent years ago.

Gradually, she shriveled into her five-foot-10-inch frame, until she weighed 115 pounds. "I was always in a bad mood. I stopped having a personality. I stopped thinking about boys. All I thought about was food. Everything had to be carefully portioned. Any spread of food, any open box, was dangerous waters. I was always hungry. My dreams were nightmares about eating too much."

But people told her she looked great. And her parents never picked up on her calorie restriction. In fact, she became locked into competition with her mother, a true peer in weight obsession. "She'd say, 'Your thighs are skinnier than mine; let's get out the tape measure.' We never actually did, but we did feed off each other. We talked about how good it feels to be hungry. She told me she wouldn't be attracted to my father if he were overweight.

"Initially it's a choice," she says now. "You start dieting to be in control. But then it veers out of control. Anorexia is so dictated by fear. You're just a puppet of fear." That sleight of slight is likely accomplished through an array of cognitive changes, purely the effects of starvation on the brain.

. . . But Perfect on Paper

Fear is the dark heart of contemporary girl culture. Courtney Martin, an instructor at Barnard College and author of *Perfect Girls, Starving Daughters: The Frightening New Normalcy of Hating Your Body,* contends that a whole generation of young women was told that they could be anything. What they heard was slightly different: "We have to be everything." And that's terrifying. The pre-college emphasis on achievement leads them "to compose the self as perfect, with a perfect résumé and a perfect body," since they were socialized to believe they can look any way they want if they just try hard enough. Unfortunately, it's hard to create a sustainable self-image without a sense of self.

The pursuit of perfection is always self-consuming, and it locks young women into a vicious cycle. The struggle to achieve so much in so many different areas overwhelms them with anxiety, and anxiety generates constant comparison, which only makes them see themselves more negatively, which pressures them to try harder.

Martin regards the rising rate of suicide among girls 10 to 14 as alarming proof that girls today increasingly lack the inner resources to disarm the anxiety of achievement pressure and fat fear. "Neither parents nor schools are nurturing kids' well-being," she says, "because they themselves are caught up in the anxiety dance."

Psychologist Janell Mensinger views it as fallout of the Superwoman Syndrome. Head of health research at Reading Hospital in Pennsylvania, Mensinger has been looking at eating disorders among girls for over a decade. In a recent study reported in the journal *Sex Roles,* she and her colleagues found that the more adolescent girls perceived behavioral commands for excellence in academics, appearance, and dating, the more they subscribed to the superwoman ideal and the more disordered their eating became.

What's more, in surveying 1,200 students in 11 schools in New York City and Philadelphia, she found that the all-girls schools fostered greater competitiveness on appearance-related issues than did the coed schools. "Girls at single-sex schools appear to be at a disadvantage in that they are more dissatisfied with their bodies," she reports.

That body competition is worse among students at all-girls schools makes perfect sense to Geoffrey Miller. The psyche reads the environment as a scarcity of males. And that only ups the mate competition among females. "It's a supply-and-demand effect," he suggests. Candice Sombrero would agree. A transfer student, she finds that eating disorders are much less prevalent at Babson than at most other schools. "This is a business college, and the ratio of males to females is 60:40 or 70:30."

If it is indeed a supply-and-demand effect, then America's campuses ought to be bracing for a near epidemic of eating disorders. The ratio of males to females is shrinking dramatically at most colleges; even Babson, able to draw from a larger pool of women, aims to add more female students.

It is a particularly cruel irony that, through unforeseen shifts in gender balance, higher education as it's now constituted winds up lowering the threshold for one of the most mentally and physically disabling disorders of our time.

From *Psychology Today,* January/February 2008. Copyright © 2008 by Sussex Publishers, LLC. Reprinted by permission.

Dieting on a Budget

Plus the secrets of thin people, based on our survey of 21,000 readers.

With jobs being cut and retirement accounts seemingly shrinking by the day, it's too bad our waistlines aren't dwindling, too. We can't rectify that cosmic injustice, but in this issue we aim to help you figure out the most effective, least expensive ways to stay trim and fit.

Though most Americans find themselves overweight by middle age, an enviable minority stay slim throughout their lives. Are those people just genetically gifted? Or do they, too, have to work at keeping down their weight?

To find out, the Consumer Reports National Research Center asked subscribers to *Consumer Reports* about their lifetime weight history and their eating, dieting, and exercising habits. And now we have our answer:

People who have never become overweight aren't sitting in recliners with a bowl of corn chips in their laps. In our group of always-slim respondents, a mere 3 percent reported that they never exercised and that they ate whatever they pleased. The eating and exercise habits of the vast majority of the always-slim group look surprisingly like those of people who have successfully lost weight and kept it off.

Both groups eat healthful foods such as fruits, vegetables, and whole grains and eschew excessive dietary fat; practice portion control; and exercise vigorously and regularly. The only advantage the always-slim have over the successful dieters is that those habits seem to come a bit more naturally to them.

"When we've compared people maintaining a weight loss with controls who've always had a normal weight, we've found that both groups are working hard at it; the maintainers are just working a little harder," says Suzanne Phelan, Ph.D., an assistant professor of kinesiology at California Polytechnic State University and co-investigator of the National Weight Control Registry, which tracks people who have successfully maintained a weight loss over time. For our respondents, that meant exercising a little more and eating with a bit more restraint than an always-thin person—plus using more monitoring strategies such as weighing themselves or keeping a food diary.

A total of 21,632 readers completed the 2007 survey. The always thin, who had never been overweight, comprised 16 percent of our sample. Successful losers made up an additional 15 percent. We defined that group as people who, at the time of the survey, weighed at least 10 percent less than they did at their heaviest, and had been at that lower weight for at least three years. Failed dieters, who said they would like to slim down yet

Price vs. Nutrition: Making Smart Choices

Although healthful foods often cost more than high-calorie junk such as cookies and soda, we unearthed some encouraging exceptions. As illustrated below, two rich sources of nutrients, black beans and eggs, cost mere pennies per serving—and less than plain noodles, which supply fewer nutrients. And for the same price as a doughnut, packed with empty calories, you can buy a serving of broccoli.

- **Cooked black beans**
  - Serving size 1/2 cup
  - Calories per serving 114
  - Cost per serving 74¢
- **Hard-boiled egg**
  - Serving size one medium
  - Calories per serving 78
  - Cost per serving 94¢
- **Cooked noodles**
  - Serving size 3/4 cup
  - Calories per serving 166
  - Cost per serving 134¢
- **Glazed doughnut**
  - Serving size 1 medium
  - Calories per serving 239
  - Cost per serving 324¢
- **Cooked broccoli**
  - Serving size 1/2 cup chopped
  - Calories per serving 27
  - Cost per serving 334¢
- **Chicken breast**
  - Serving size 4 oz.
  - Calories per serving 142
  - Cost per serving 364¢

Sources: Adam Drewnowski, Ph.D., director of the Center for Public Health Nutrition, University of Washington: USDA Nutrient Database for Standard Reference.

still weighed at or near their lifetime high, were, sad to say, the largest group: 42 percent. (The remaining 27 percent of respondents, such as people who had lost weight more recently, didn't fit into any of the categories.)

Stay-Thin Strategies

Successful losers and the always thin do a lot of the same things—and they do them more frequently than failed dieters do. For the dietary strategies below, numbers reflect those who said they are that way at least five days a week, a key tipping point, our analysis found. (Differences of less than 4 percentage points are not statistically meaningful.)

Lifetime Weight History

Failed dieters: overweight and have tried to lose, but still close to highest weight. **Always thin:** never overweight. **Successful losers:** once overweight but now at least 10 percent lighter and have kept pounds off for at least three years.

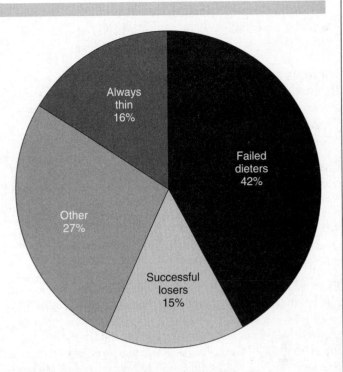

Strength Train at Least Once a Week

Always thin	31%
Successful loser	32%
Failed dieter	23%

Do Vigorous Exercise at Least Four Days a Week

Always thin	35%
Successful loser	41%
Failed dieter	27%

Eat Fruit and Vegetables at Least Five Times a Day

Always thin	49%
Successful loser	49%
Failed dieter	38%

Eat Whole Grains, Not Refined

Always thin	56%
Successful loser	61%
Failed dieter	49%

Eat Less Than 1/3 Calories from Fat

Always thin	47%
Successful loser	53%
Failed dieter	35%

Observe Portion Control at Every Meal

Always thin	57%
Successful loser	62%
Failed dieter	42%

Count Calories

Always thin	9%
Successful loser	47%
Failed dieter	9%

An encouraging note: More than half of our successful losers reported shedding the weight themselves, without aid of a commercial diet program, a medical treatment, a book, or diet pills. That confirms what we found in our last large diet survey, in 2002, in which 83 percent of "superlosers"—people who'd lost at least 10 percent of their starting weight and kept it off for five years or more—had done it entirely on their own.

6 Secrets of the Slim

Through statistical analyses, we were able to identify six key behaviors that correlated the most strongly with having a healthy body mass index (BMI), a measure of weight that takes height into account. Always thin people were only slightly less likely than successful losers to embrace each of the behaviors—and significantly more likely to do so than failed dieters. By following the behaviors, you can, quite literally, live like a thin person.

Watch portions. Of all the eating behaviors we asked about, carefully controlling portion size at each meal correlated most strongly with having a lower BMI. Successful losers—even those who were still overweight—were especially likely (**62 percent) to report practicing portion control at least five days per week. So did** 57 percent of the always thin, but only 42 percent of failed dieters.

Portion control is strongly linked to a lower BMI.

Limit fat. Specifically, that means restricting fat to less than one-third of daily calorie intake. Fifty-three percent of successful losers and 47 percent of the always thin said they did that five or more days a week, compared with just 35 percent of failed dieters.

Eat fruits and vegetables. The more days that respondents are five or more servings of fruits or vegetables, the lower their average BMI score. Forty-nine percent of successful losers and the always thin said they ate that way at least five days a week, while 38 percent of failed dieters did so.

Choose whole grains over refined. People with lower body weights consistently opted for whole-wheat breads, cereals, and other grains over refined (white) grains.

Eat at home. As the number of days per week respondents are restaurant or takeout meals for dinner increased, so did their weight. Eating at home can save a lot of money, too.

Exercise, exercise, exercise. Regular **vigorous exercise— the type that increases breathing and heart rate for 30 minutes** or longer—was strongly linked to a lower BMI. Although only about one quarter of **respondents said they did strength training at least once a week, that practice was significantly more prevalent among successful losers (32 percent) and always thin** respondents (31 percent) than it was among failed dieters (23 percent).

What Didn't Matter

One weight-loss strategy is conspicuously absent from the list: going low-carb. Of course we asked about it, and it turned out that limiting carbohydrates was linked to higher BMIs in our survey. That doesn't necessarily mean low-carb plans such as the Atkins or South Beach diets don't work. "If you go to the hospital and everyone there is sick, that doesn't mean the hospital made them sick," says Eric C. Westman, M.D., associate professor of medicine and director of the Lifestyle Medicine Clinic at Duke University Medical School. "just as people go to hospitals because they're ill, people may go to carb restriction because they have a higher BMI, not the other way around." At the same time, the findings do suggest that cutting carbs alone, without other healthful behaviors such as exercise and portion control, might not lead to great results.

Eating many small meals, or never eating between meals, didn't seem to make much difference one way or another. Including lean protein with most meals also didn't by itself predict a healthier weight.

Realistic Expectations

Sixty-six percent of our respondents, all subscribers to *Consumer Reports,* were overweight as assessed by their body mass index; that's the same percentage as the population as a whole. One third of the overweight group, or 22 percent of the overall sample, qualified as obese.

Are You Overweight?

A body mass index under 25 is considered normal weight: from 25 to 29, overweight; and 30 or above, obese. To calculate your BMI, multiply your weight in pounds by 703, then divide by your height squared in inches.

Although that might seem discouraging, the survey actually contains good news for would-be dieters. Our respondents did much better at losing weight than published clinical studies would predict. Though such studies are deemed successful if participants are 5 percent lighter after a year, our successful losers had managed to shed an average of 16 percent of their peak weight, an average of almost 34 pounds. They had an impressive average BMI of 25.7, meaning they were just barely overweight.

One key to weight loss success is having realistic goals and our subscribers responses proved encouraging. A staggering 70 percent of them said they currently wanted to lose weight. But when we asked how many pounds they hoped to take off, we found that their goals were modest: The vast majority reported wanting to lose 15 percent or less of their overall body weight; 65 percent sought to lose between 1 and 10 percent. Keeping expectations in check might help dieters from becoming discouraged when they don't achieve, say, a 70-pound weight loss or drop from a size 20 to a size 6—a common problem in behavioral weight loss studies.

Realistic goals are one key to weight loss.

What You Can Do

Weight loss is a highly individual process, and what matters most is finding the combination of habits that work for you. But our findings suggest that there are key behaviors common to people who have successfully lost weight and to those who have never gained it in the first place. By embracing some or all of those behaviors, you can probably increase your chances of weight-loss success, and live a healthier life in the process. In addition to following the steps above, consider these tips:

Don't get discouraged. Studies show that prospective dieters often have unrealistic ideas about how much weight they can lose. A 10 percent loss might not sound like much, but it significantly improves overall health and reduces risk of disease.

Ask for support. Though only a small minority of respondents overall reported that a spouse or family member interfered with their healthful eating efforts, that problem was much more likely among failed dieters, 31 percent of whom reported some form of spousal sabotage in the month prior to the survey. Ask housemates to help you stay on track by, for example, not pestering you to eat foods you're trying to avoid, or not eating those foods in front of you.

Get up and move. While regular vigorous exercise correlated most strongly with healthy body weight, our findings suggest that any physical activity is helpful, including activities you might not even consider exercise. Everyday activities such as housework, yard work, and playing with kids were modestly tied to lower weight. By contrast, hours spent sitting each day, whether at an office desk or at home watching television, correlated with higher weight.

Copyright © 2009 by Consumers Union of U.S., Inc. Yonkers, NY 10703-1057, a nonprofit organization. Reprinted with permission from the February 2009 issue of CONSUMER REPORTS® for educational purposes only. No commercial use or reproduction permitted. www.ConsumerReports.org.

"Fat Chance"

Doesn't "everyone know" that serving supersize meals to a young couch potato with plus-size parents is a sure recipe for an obese child? So why is the current epidemic of childhood obesity such a mystery to science?

SUSAN OKIE

Rudolph L. Leibel's genes may have predisposed him to become a scientist, but his decision to spend his life trying to discover the causes of obesity was environmental happenstance, the result of a chance encounter. In the spring of 1977, Randall, a severely overweight child, and Randall's mother showed up at the pediatric clinic of Cambridge Hospital in Massachusetts, where Leibel was a specialist in hormone disorders. Leibel could find no evidence that hormone deficiency or, indeed, any other known medical condition, was the cause of Randall's obesity. But what struck the young doctor was the response of Randall's mother when Leibel told her there was little he or anyone else could do for her son: "Let's get out of here, Randall," she snapped. "This doctor doesn't know s--t."

Chastened by her words, Leibel soon traded his hospital post for the low-paying toil of a rookie laboratory scientist. At the Rockefeller University laboratory of Jules Hirsch, a leading figure in research on obesity, Leibel and Hirsch conducted extensive studies of weight homeostasis: how the body responds both to weight gain and weight loss by fighting to restore the status quo ante.

In one of the studies, volunteers were induced to overeat to gain weight—a task that proved remarkably difficult. Whether they were fat or lean at the outset, the volunteers' bodies responded by turning up the metabolic rate, boosting the levels of certain hormones, reducing hunger, and burning up more calories as heat—all in a coordinated effort by the autonomic nervous system to restore the body's original weight. By contrast, when volunteers' food intake was restricted in order to promote weight loss, their bodies fought back even more fiercely: metabolisms slowed; the volunteers moved around less often and, even when they were exercising, their muscles burned fewer calories; and everyone felt constantly and uncomfortably hungry. A host of physiological defense mechanisms had swung into play, all aimed at regaining the lost pounds.

Such tight physiological regulation of body weight persuaded Leibel that a chemical signal from the body's stores of fat was being sent to the brain. Leibel's hypothesis led to the discovery of a gene that coded for the hormone leptin, which is produced by fat cells. Animal studies soon proved that leptin does indeed pass through the circulatory system to the brain. Could leptin be the key player in the signaling system Leibel had envisioned? If the brain detected enough leptin, would it decide that enough fat cells were storing energy, and so conclude that it was safe to stop eating? Sure enough, mice that could not produce leptin ate nonstop and grew enormously obese. Treating such mice with leptin normalized their body weight.

The gene for leptin was identified and sequenced as the result of an intensive collaborative effort between Leibel and his Rockefeller colleague Jeffrey M. Friedman. When the announcement was made in 1994, it was greeted with much fanfare. Many people (along with some drug companies) predicted that the newly identified gene would enable the hormone to become a miracle cure for obesity. It has not turned out that way.

Some evidence suggests body weight reaches a "set point" during puberty. So untreated childhood obesity can lead to the medical risks of adult obesity.

Today, instead, the United States and many other countries are faced with an epidemic. Most people tend to think of an epidemic as an outbreak of a contagious illness. But to public health officials, obesity rates since the mid 1980s have exploded dramatically and unexpectedly, just as if they reflected the outbreak of a new infectious disease. Noting that obesity and physical inactivity, along with tobacco smoking, are the major causes of "noncommunicable diseases," the World Health Organization estimated that 60 percent of the 56 million deaths worldwide in 2001 were caused by such obesity-related illnesses as heart disease and type 2 diabetes. Among children, obesity can have adverse effects that persist for life, just as surely as a virus can.

For example, there is evidence suggesting that a person's general body weight reaches a "set point" sometime during puberty, and so extreme obesity in childhood, left untreated, carries with it all the health risks of obesity for the rest of one's life: substantial increases in the risks of diabetes, heart disease, and other adverse medical consequences. Some officials have even begun to respond with the kind of alarm that might greet the global resurgence of polio. As David L. Katz of the Yale School of Public Health puts it:

> Children growing up in the United States today will suffer more chronic disease and premature death because of the way they eat and [because of] their lack of physical activity than [they will] from exposure to tobacco, drugs, and alcohol combined.

Even though the discovery of leptin has not led to a cure for childhood obesity, it has helped to show that the condition is largely biological, and not simply the result of faulty parenting or lack of willpower. And the years since the discovery have been hailed as a golden age for obesity research. In little more than a decade, investigators have sketched, in broad outlines, the biological system that regulates body weight. They have also learned a great deal about genetic vulnerability to obesity.

The control centers for tracking energy balance and regulating body weight are situated primarily in the hypothalamus, a small part of the brain that specializes in integrating messages from many parts of the body and orchestrating the organism's response to its environment. The hypothalamus communicates via nerve pathways and chemical signals with many other areas of the brain, as well as with the organs of the cardiovascular, digestive, reproductive, and endocrine systems (the latter encompasses the glands that secrete the hormones circulating in the blood).

The output of the hypothalamus can fine-tune a number of unconscious processes that affect a person's weight, such as the rate at which the body burns calories in carrying out certain cellular processes or through spontaneous muscle activity, such as fidgeting. Conceptually, at least, understanding how the body controls such unconscious processes is fairly straightforward. What is surprising for some people is that signals from the hypothalamus also affect the cerebral cortex, the "thinking" part of the brain. The hypothalamus can modify such conscious, purposeful behaviors as food-seeking, simply by increasing or decreasing the appetite. As Leibel puts it, those unconscious signals contribute to such conscious actions as ordering a pizza or having a second piece of pie. Just because a behavior is conscious, he adds, doesn't mean that all aspects of it are voluntary.

To exert its control, the hypothalamus needs reliable, relevant information about the body's current need for food. But where does that information come from? Leptin and, to a lesser extent, insulin carry information about long-term energy depots. The level of leptin in the blood reflects how much fat is stored in the body. Its chief function seems to be to protect energy stores and prevent starvation. When a human or other mammal's food intake is severely restricted, leptin levels drop within twenty-four hours—well before fat stores have been materially depleted by being burned for energy. The fall in leptin immediately prompts the hypothalamus to lower the metabolic rate, increase the appetite, and, to some extent, suppress the reproductive and immune systems so as to focus the body's resources on gaining food.

Insulin, the hormone produced by the beta cells of the pancreas, is released into the bloodstream in response to glucose from food. It helps the body maintain a balance between storing glucose and fat and burning them. Insulin also serves as another signal to certain nerve cells in the brain, informing them about the body's overall nutritional status. The brain also receives messages from the digestive tract. Constant updates about food availability and the timing of meals are relayed to the hypothalamus by various messenger molecules released by cells in the stomach and intestinal tract.

What about the genetics? If Randall were Leibel's young patient today, the boy might undergo testing for a genetic cause of his obesity. A few unlucky people are born with a single genetic mutation that stacks the deck against them so overwhelmingly that they become severely overweight almost no matter what the environment. At least five distinct "obesity genes" have been identified so far. Each of them is so critical to the regulation of appetite and food intake that certain mutations in any of them can lead to extreme obesity.

The mutations that cause such "monogenic," or single-gene, obesity are quite rare. Moreover, even if a physician can diagnose such a condition, there is still no guarantee that it can be treated successfully. Nevertheless, monogenic cases of severe obesity have helped investigators understand how the body regulates food intake and fat stores in people without such debilitating mutations. And even though monogenic obesity is rare, Leibel notes, it does reinforce the idea that specific molecules are highly potent in determining energy balance and body weight in humans.

What about the vast majority of overweight children and adults, whose obesity is not the result of a single defective gene? The scientific consensus is that such people may have multiple genes whose net effect predisposes them to eat a few extra calories, burn up a bit less energy than they take in, or store the excess as fat. Like the members of a band, the genes in each person's personal collection play together, along with various factors in the environment, to determine the person's specific vulnerability to becoming overweight.

How many genes might be at play? Investigators don't yet know. At first, just after leptin was discovered, many people thought there must be a single obesity gene, and some believed it had been found. Now at least sixty genes are being investigated, and some workers fear that as many as a hundred genes could be contributing to the obesity risk.

Leibel's own suspicion, after examining patterns of obesity inheritance in families drawn from various populations and ethnic groups, is that the number of important players is much smaller. He suggests that each person may have as many as a dozen genes that combine to determine the individual risk of obesity. Some genes—perhaps six or seven of them—are probably major players that help determine the likelihood of obesity in people all over the planet. The rest of the dozen or so genes may have arisen from gene variants more common in one ethnic population than in another. That, says Leibel, is what makes the genetics so complicated. No one knows which genes are major players, and which genes are minor ones. And so the geneticists have no way of knowing how to apportion their efforts.

Most people, of course, do not become severely obese, even in today's calorie-rich environment. The average person consumes between 7.5 million and 10 million calories per decade, yet Americans and people in other developed countries typically gain only half a pound to a pound a year throughout their adult lives. To gain any weight at all, they must eat more calories than they burn—but the amount needed to account for the typical weight gain is only about ten to twenty calories a day. That's about the equivalent of one Ritz cracker, or less than 1 percent of the average adult's daily intake.

A calorie imbalance that small can't be reliably measured by studying people in their normal habitat. To study how weight gain and loss quantitatively affect people's appetite and metabolism, Leibel and his associates had to confine volunteers to hospital research wards and measure every mouthful. They found, surprisingly, that obese people do not eat more than lean people in proportion to their body size. Nor do obese people have slower metabolisms than lean ones, as long as they remain at what is their own "normal" weight. They still balance their calorie intake and output very precisely to maintain a constant weight, just as lean people do. It's just that the weight they maintain is higher.

To gain half a pound to a pound a year, an adult needs to eat just ten to twenty calories a day more than she burns. That's about the equivalent of one Ritz cracker.

Yet the laws of thermodynamics dictate that people who are overweight must, at some point, have taken in more energy than they spent in order to gain the extra pounds. "There's no way around it," Leibel says. "You cannot eat like a canary and become the size of a pterodactyl." But in most cases, once obese people have reached a personal set point determined by their own physiology, their weight stabilizes. Their food intake and their metabolic rates, when adjusted for their body size, are similar to those of lean people.

When a person loses weight, however, the circumstances shift dramatically. Whether people start out lean or obese, when they lose 10 to 20 percent of their body weight, their bodies respond by becoming more efficient and using less energy, in an effort to conserve calories and replenish lost reserves of fat. The reduction in energy expenditure is about 15 percent larger than would be expected for the amount of weight lost. That almost certainly accounts for some of the tremendous recidivism among dieters, Leibel says. Studies suggest that some 95 percent of people who lose weight by dieting gain it back within five years.

So though genes determine individual vulnerability to weight gain, environmental factors help dictate the outcome—the weight that a person reaches during childhood or adulthood. Imagine, Leibel says, that you can rank a hundred people, on the basis of their genetic endowment, from 1 to 100 according to their tendency to store excess calories as body fat. Then that same genetic ranking will tell you how they'll line up relative to one another in most environments. What it won't tell you, though, is what those hundred people will look like in any particular environment. For example, if a hundred people were exposed to famine and had to subsist on a starvation diet, they would all become thin—but some would lose less weight than others, according to their genetic endowments.

In spite of the scientific progress made in disentangling the body's complex systems for regulating food intake, energy use, and energy storage, no one really knows how to treat most cases of obesity. Meanwhile, most of the developed world is facing an expanding public health crisis that clearly has not arisen because of newly mutated genes. Obesity is increasing at an unprecedented rate in the United States, and in many other countries as well. For example: in a study conducted in Europe between 1983 and 1986, more than half of the adults between the ages of thirty-five and sixty-five were either overweight or obese; and even in Japan and China, and throughout Southeast Asia, obesity rates have risen sharply during the past two decades. Recent shifts in the modern environment are undoubtedly at the root of the epidemic. People eat more and move around less. Most of us in the developed world enjoy an abundance of cheap, tasty, high-calorie foods, rely on cars, elevators, and other forms of motorized transportation, and lead sedentary lifestyles, in part because of the difficulty of incorporating walking and other kinds of activity into our daily routines.

Such a "toxic environment," in the words of Kelly D. Brownell, a health psychologist at Yale University, is playing on individual genetic vulnerability, thereby causing unhealthy weight gain in increasing numbers of people. And if environmental factors are at fault, then by changing the environment—or by learning ways whereby we can consciously change our responses to it—it may be possible to slow down or even reverse the trend. Nevertheless, one must sound a cautionary note on what may be too sanguine an assessment: obesity experts who are studying the epidemic think that a comprehensive solution to the rise in obesity will require broad environmental and social changes—a daunting task.

eibel is proud that his genetic research has helped put a stop to "blaming the victim," shifting the blame for fatness away from the people who suffer from it. The continuing discovery of obesity genes is proof that biological variation in vulnerability to weight gain is the main reason some people are fat and others are lean. That's why Leibel views much of the current national debate about measures to prevent obesity with some concern. He points out that no one yet knows precisely what actions will be most effective. "On some level this is a disease that everybody thinks they understand, and yet in fact nobody understands," he says. "We really don't know what has happened, other than on a very macro, thermodynamic level. Food intake is greater than energy expenditure. Period."

This article was adapted from **SUSAN OKIE**'s forthcoming book, *Fed Up! Winning the War Against Childhood Obesity,* which is being published by Joseph Henry Press (http://www.jhpress.org) in September 2006.

From *Fed Up! Winning the War Against Childhood Obesity* by Susan Okie. Copyright © 2005 by National Academies Press. Reprinted by permission.

UNIT 5

Drugs and Health

Unit Selections

Key Points to Consider

- What are the risks associated with college students' drinking?

- What are the risks versus benefits of statin drugs?

- Do you think America has a drug problem? Defend your answer.

- Why do teenagers use drugs despite the messages they've heard from DARE and "Just Say No"?

- What are the risks of taking over-the-counter pain medications?

- Why have certain over-the-counter medicines been moved behind the counter of drugstores?

- What can companies do to help workers quit smoking?

- Is it safe to buy drugs on the Internet?

Student Website
www.mhcls.com

Internet References

Food and Drug Administration (FDA)
   http://www.fda.gov/
National Institute on Drug Abuse (NIDA)
   http://www.nida.nih.gov/

As a culture, Americans have come to rely on drugs not only as a treatment for disease but also as an aid for living normal, productive lives. This view of drugs has fostered a casual attitude regarding their use and resulted in a tremendous drug abuse problem. Drug use and abuse has become so widespread that there is no way to describe the typical drug abuser.

There is no simple explanation for why America has become a drug-taking culture, but there certainly is evidence to suggest some of the factors that have contributed to this development.

From the time that we are children, we are constantly bombarded by advertisements about how certain drugs can make us feel and look better. While most of these ads deal with proprietary drugs, the belief created is that drugs are a legitimate and effective way to help us cope with everyday problems. Certainly drugs can have a profound effect on how we feel and act, but research has also demonstrated that our mind plays a major role in the healing process. For many people, it's easier to take a drug than to adopt a healthier lifestyle. They are more willing to take statin drugs to lower their cholesterol than to change their diet, exercise, and lose weight. Tara Parker-Pope addresses this issue related to usage of one of the most commonly prescribed medicines in the United States.

Growing up, most of us probably had a medicine cabinet full of over-the-counter (OTC) drugs, freely dispensed to family members to treat a variety of ailments. This familiarity with OTC drugs, coupled with rising health care costs, has prompted many people to diagnose and medicate themselves with OTC medications without sufficient knowledge of the possible side effects.

Though most of these preparations have little potential for abuse, it does not mean that they are innocuous. Generally speaking, OTC drugs are relatively safe if taken at the recommended dosage by healthy people, but the risk of dangerous side effects rises sharply when people exceed the recommended dosage. Another potential danger associated with the use of OTC drugs is the drug interactions that can occur when they are taken in conjunction with prescription medications. The gravest danger associated with the use of OTC drugs is that an individual may use them to control symptoms of an underlying disease and thus prevent its early diagnosis and treatment. In "Some Cold Medicines Move Behind Counter," Linda Bren discusses why certain OTC cold and allergy medicines are being taken off the shelves and stored behind the counter. Many of these non-prescription drugs contain ingredients of illegally produced methamphetamine.

Another category of over-the-counter medications, herbal preparations, has become extremely popular. They include approximately 750 substances such as herbal teas and other products of botanical origin that are believed to have medicinal properties. Many have been used for centuries with no ill effects, but others have questionable safety records. One drug with a checkered history is the herb *ephedra,* used in over-the-counter weight control products sold in pharmacies, mall kiosks, and via the Internet. The death of 23 year old Baltimore Orioles

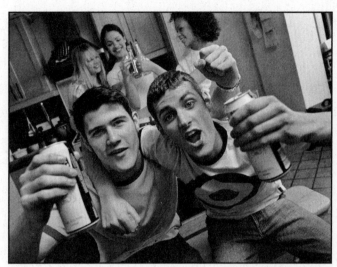

© BananaStock/PunchStock

pitcher Steve Bechler in February 2003, attributed to the use of *ephedra,* brought attention to the risks of the herb. Soon after Bechler's death, the minor league baseball board banned the herb, joining other sports organizations that had already banned its use. Health officials caution consumers against the use of the drug, especially if it's combined with other stimulants such as caffeine, or if strenuous exercise is involved. Many of these drugs and herbs are available online and many are legal. In "Online Drugs: Most Legal, Maybe Lethal," Tom Spring addresses the availability of drugs online.

As a culture, we have grown up believing that there is, or should be, a drug to treat any malady or discomfort that befalls us. Would we have a drug problem if there was no demand for drugs? One drug which is used widely in the United States is alcohol, especially on college campuses. Every year, over 1,000 students die from alcohol-related causes, mostly drinking and driving. In "Drinking Too Much, Too Young," author Garry Boulard, discusses other risks associated with students drinking including missed classes, falling behind in school work, damage to property, and injuries which occur while under the influence of alcohol. In addition to alcohol, teenagers are also abusing drugs such as prescription pain relievers. In "The Changing Face of Teenage Drug Abuse," Richard Friedman addresses the careless monitoring and regulation of addictive narcotics.

In addition to alcohol, another widely used legal drug is tobacco. Millions still smoke despite all the well publicized health effects linked to smoking. Many Americans have quit and many others would like to quit. To facilitate this process, some companies have developed programs to help employees quit the habit. Because smoking and its related diseases cost approximately $150 billion dollars each year, the stakes are enormous. Pamela Babcock addresses this issue in "Helping Workers Kick the Habit."

Great Drug, but Does It Prolong Life?

TARA PARKER-POPE

Statins are among the most prescribed drugs in the world, and there is no doubt that they work as advertised—that they lower not only cholesterol but also the risk for heart attack.

But in the fallout from the headline-making trial of Vytorin, a combination drug that was found to be no more effective than a simple statin in reducing arterial plaque, many people are asking a more fundamental question about statins in general: Do they prolong your life?

And for many users, the surprising answer appears to be no.

Some patients do receive significant benefits from statins, like Lipitor (from Pfizer), Crestor (AstraZeneca) and Pravachol (Bristol-Myers Squibb). In studies of middle-aged men with cardiovascular disease, statin users were less likely to die than those who were given a placebo.

But many statin users don't have established heart disease; they simply have high cholesterol. For healthy men, for women with or without heart disease and for people over 70, there is little evidence, if any, that taking a statin will make a meaningful difference in how long they live.

"High-risk groups have a lot to gain," said Dr. Mark H. Ebell, a professor at the University of Georgia who is deputy editor of the journal American Family Physician. "But patients at low risk benefit very little if at all. We end up overtreating a lot of patients." (Like the other doctors quoted in this column, Dr. Ebell has no ties to drug makers.)

How is this possible, if statins lower the risk of heart attack? Because preventing a heart attack is not the same thing as saving a life. In many statin studies that show lower heart attack risk, the same number of patients end up dying, whether they are taking statins or not.

"You may have helped the heart, but you haven't helped the patient," said Dr. Beatrice Golomb, an associate professor of medicine at the University of California, San Diego, and a co-author of a 2004 editorial in *The Journal of the American College of Cardiology* questioning the data on statins. "You still have to look at the impact on the patient over all."

A 2006 study in The Archives of Internal Medicine looked at seven trials of statin use in nearly 43,000 patients, mostly middle-aged men without heart disease. In that review, statins didn't lower mortality.

Nor did they in a study called Prosper, published in The Lancet in 2002, which studied statin use in people 70 and older. Nor did they in a 2004 review in The Journal of the American Medical Association, which looked at 13 studies of nearly 20,000 women, both healthy and with established heart disease.

Indications that statins aren't all they're cracked up to be.

A Pfizer spokeswoman notes that a decline in heart disease death rates reported recently by the American Heart Association suggests that medications like statins are having an impact. But to consistently show a mortality benefit from statins in a research setting would take years of study. "We've concentrated on whether Lipitor reduces risk of heart attacks and strokes," says Halit Bander, medical team leader for Lipitor. "We've proven that again and again."

This month, *The Journal of the American College of Cardiology* published a report combining data from several studies of people 65 and older who had a prior heart attack or established heart disease. This "meta-analysis" showed that 18.7 percent of the placebo users died during the studies, compared with 15.6 percent of the statin users.

This translates into a 22 percent lower mortality risk for high-risk patients over 65. A co-author of the study, Dr. Jonathan Afilalo, a cardiology fellow at McGill University in Montreal, says that for every 28 patients over 65 with heart disease who take statins, one life will be saved.

"If a patient has had a heart attack," Dr. Afilalo said, "they generally should be on a statin."

Of course, prolonging life is not the only measure that matters. If preventing a heart attack improved the quality of life, that would be an argument for taking statins even if it didn't reduce mortality. But critics say there's no evidence that statin users have a better quality of life than other people.

"If you can show me one study that people who have a disability from their heart are worse off than people who have a disability from other causes, I would find that a compelling argument," Dr. Golomb said. "There's not a shred of evidence that you've mitigated suffering in the groups where there is not a mortality benefit."

One big concern is that the side effects of statins haven't been well studied. Reported side effects include muscle pain, cognitive problems and impotence.

"Statins have side effects that are underrated," said Dr. Uffe Ravnskov, a retired Swedish physician and a vocal critic of statins. "It's much more frequent and serious than has been reported."

Dr. Ebell acknowledges that there are probably patients with heart disease who could benefit from a statin but who aren't taking it.

But he added, "There are probably more of the opposite—patients who are taking a statin when they probably don't need one."

From *The New York Times,* January 29, 2008. Copyright © 2008 by The New York Times Company. Reprinted by permission via PARS International.

Some Cold Medicines Move Behind Counter

Some over-the-counter (OTC) cold and allergy medicines are being moved behind the counter at pharmacies nationwide as part of the fight against illegal drug production.

Linda Bren

Under the Patriot Act signed by President Bush on March 9, 2006, all drug products that contain the ingredient pseudoephedrine must be kept behind the pharmacy counter and must be sold in limited quantities to consumers after they show identification and sign a logbook.

Pseudoephedrine is a drug found in both OTC and prescription products used to relieve nasal or sinus congestion caused by the common cold, sinusitis, hay fever, and other respiratory allergies. The drug is also a key ingredient in making methamphetamine—a powerful, highly addictive stimulant often produced illegally by "meth cooks" in home laboratories.

The new legal provisions for selling and purchasing pseudoephedrine-containing products are part of the Combat Methamphetamine Epidemic Act of 2005, which was incorporated into the Patriot Act. These "anti-meth" provisions introduce safeguards to make certain ingredients used in methamphetamine manufacturing more difficult to obtain in bulk and easier for law enforcement to track.

According to the National Institute on Drug Abuse, methamphetamine use and abuse is associated with serious health conditions including memory loss, aggression, violence, paranoia, hallucinations, and potential heart and brain damage. The Drug Enforcement Administration says there is a direct relationship between methamphetamine abuse and increased incidents of domestic violence and child abuse.

Meth users ingest the substance by swallowing, inhaling, injecting, or smoking it. There are currently no safe and tested medications for treating methamphetamine addiction.

The new law affects several hundred OTC products for children and adults, such as Sudafed Nasal Decongestant Tablets, Advil Allergy Sinus Caplets, TheraFlu Daytime Severe Cold SoftGels, Tylenol Flu NightTime Gelcaps, and Children's Vicks NyQuil Cold/Cough Relief. "There are very few decongestants on the market that don't contain pseudoephedrine," says Charles Ganley, M.D., director of the Food and Drug Administration's Office of Nonprescription Products.

Ganley says that products containing pseudoephedrine are still available without a prescription and that they are packaged the same way as any OTC drug. "The only difference is that people will have to go to the pharmacist to buy them," he says. "They just need to ask for them and show ID, and know that there's a limit to the amount they can purchase."

Buyers must show a government-issued photo ID, such as a driver's license, and sign a logbook. Stores are required to keep a record about purchases, which includes the product name, quantity sold, name and address of purchaser, and date and time of the sale, for at least two years. Single-dose packages containing 60 milligrams or less of pseudoephedrine are excluded from the recordkeeping requirement, but must still be stored behind the counter.

The federal law limits the amount of pseudoephedrine an individual can purchase to 3.6 grams in a single day and 9 grams in a month at a retail store. For example, a person may buy Advil Allergy Sinus Caplets, which contain pseudoephedrine and other ingredients, in quantities of up to 146 tablets in one day and 366 tablets in one month. The number of pills or amount of liquid medicine allowable will vary depending on the type of product and its strength.

The limits on the amount an individual can purchase became effective April 8, 2006. The requirements to place products behind the counter and to keep a logbook take effect Sept. 30, 2006. Many drug stores are already complying voluntarily or because some state laws require similar controls.

Drug companies are reformulating some of their products to eliminate pseudoephedrine. Pfizer, for example, while still offering Sudafed nasal decongestants, which contain pseudoephedrine, also markets a line called Sudafed PE as an "on the shelf" alternative. Sudafed PE contains the active ingredient phenylephrine, which is not used to make methamphetamine, and so is not under the same restrictions as pseudoephedrine.

"Drugs that contain phenylephrine are also safe and effective," says Ganley. "The dosing is a little different—you have to take them a little more frequently than the pseudoephedrine-containing drugs because their effects are not as long-lasting."

The anti-meth provisions of the Patriot Act restrict the sale of two other drug ingredients, ephedrine and phenylpropanolamine, because of their potential to be used illegally to make methamphetamine. Like pseudoephedrine, drugs containing these ingredients must be placed behind the counter, and buyers must show identification to purchase a limited quantity.

Synthetic ephedrine is used in some topical drugs, such as nose drops, to temporarily relieve congestion due to colds, hay fever, sinusitis, or other upper respiratory allergies. It is also used orally for temporary relief of asthma symptoms.

Phenylpropanolamine was commonly used in OTC decongestants and weight-loss drugs. Today, it is unlikely that consumers will find phenylpropanolamine in their drug stores, says Ganley. In 2000, the FDA asked drug manufacturers to discontinue marketing products containing phenylpropanolamine because of an increased risk of bleeding in the brain (hemorrhagic stroke) associated with the ingredient. The FDA has taken regulatory actions to remove phenylpropanolamine from all drug products.

From *FDA Consumer,* July/August 2006, pp. 18–19.

Drinking Too Much, Too Young

Trying to find an answer to the persistent habit of binge drinking among young people vexes the nation's policymakers.

GARRY BOULARD

The stories have been shocking, abruptly reminding a nation of a problem that remains unsolved: in the last half of 2004, six college-age students in Colorado died as a result of binge drinking.

Although each fatality was different in its circumstance—Samantha Spady, 19, a sophomore at Colorado State University, died after drinking vanilla vodka and more than two dozen beers, while Benett Bertoli, 20, also a CSU student, was found dead on a couch at an off-campus party from a combination of alcohol, methadone and benzodiazepene—the events leading up to the deaths were maddeningly familiar.

In almost every case, the fatalities were the unexpected ending to a boisterous party almost always involving large gatherings of young people on weekend nights consuming prodigious amounts of alcohol, sometimes for two days straight.

The number of Colorado deaths from binge drinking in late 2004 was exceptionally large, but the state is not alone. It killed Thomas Ryan Hauser, 23, a student at Virginia Tech in September. Blake Hammontree, 19, died at his fraternity house at the University of Oklahoma, also in September. Bradley Kemp, 20, died in October at his home near the University of Arkansas, where he was a student. Steven Judd died celebrating his 21st birthday with fraternity friends at New Mexico State University in November.

Those deaths did not occur in a vacuum. According to statistics from the National Institute for Alcohol Abuse and Alcoholism, more than 1,400 college students die from alcohol-related deaths each year including motor vehicle crashes. Unfortunately, that number has remained constant even though both high school and college-age drinking has decreased.

"The numbers have been going in the right direction," says Peter Cressy, the president of the Distilled Spirits Council of the United States. "There is today less regular use of alcohol on college campuses than there was 20 years ago. There has been a drop in the number of college students both of age and not of age who drink at all during any given month. And the data for eighth, 10th, and 12th graders who consume alcohol has also shown a downward trend."

Bucking the Trend

But what hasn't changed, industry, health and alcohol experts all agree, is the stubborn number of young people who continue to engage in destructive behavior.

"The issue is not the 30,000 kids on the campus of the University of Colorado, or any other school, who drink legally or illegally, but somehow manage to do it without any great peril," says Ralph Blackman, the president of the Century Council, a not-for-profit organization dedicated to fighting drunk driving and underage drinking.

"The issue is binge drinking and the continuing large numbers of kids who insist on over consumption to a level that has a very decided risk for a dangerous result," continues Blackman. "That is a phenomenon that very much remains with us."

Trying to find a specific reason for the persistence of binge drinking among the young is a subject that both vexes and causes great debate among the nation's policymakers. Do younger people just naturally like to get drunk, or in some cases, very drunk? Is it a matter of upbringing or income? Is it a reflection of a troubled and anxious society?

"You could ask questions like that all day, and not really get any solid answers," says Paul Hanson, a professor emeritus of sociology at the State University of New York, Potsdam.

"The only thing you could be sure of is that no matter how many different ways we approach it with different solutions, binge drinking continues among the very young, generation after generation."

But some experts believe one thing that is different with those who are a part of what demographers call the Millennials—those born in 1980 or after—and their predecessors, is that binge drinking today is out of the closet and celebrated on almost a worldwide basis due to the Internet.

"There is a huge difference from when many of us went to school in the 1960s and '70s and today," says Stephen Bentley, a coordinator of substance abuse services at the Wardenberg Health Center at the University of Colorado.

"Back in our day we really did not want any attention of any kind, we did not want adults or the world to know that we were drinking and partying excessively," continues Bentley.

"But today young people who engage in this kind of behavior are actually very proud of what they are doing, they post their own websites about their parties so that everyone else can see what they did."

One of the websites, called shamings.com, features pictures of drunken young men, updated on a regular basis, sometimes sleeping in their own vomit, often half naked, and many times covered with magic marker salutations alluding to their drinking prowess or lack thereof.

One of the website creators, Ricky Van Veen, explained to the Washington Post the guidelines used by the website in determining whether or not to post a binge drinker's picture: "The standard rule is, if you fall asleep with your shoes on, you're fair game," he said.

Youth Targets

For Julia Sherman, field director with the Center on Alcohol Marketing and Youth, binge drinking self-promotion is almost a natural outgrowth of what she says is the alcohol industry's "preoccupation with the young."

"The ads that are being put out there today are not your Mom and Pop, 'Mabel, Black Label,' ads of another era, but ads that are very much geared toward an exceedingly young demographic," she says.

"The whole ad focus of the alcohol industry has changed both in tenor and in numbers," says Sherman. "Their Web site ads now feature computer games and premiums for downloading music. They run ads in what are called the 'laddie magazines,' that are edgier than anything adults are seeing in their magazines. It is all part of a non-stop, never-ending pitch for the youth market."

According to a study released by the Center on Alcohol Marketing and Youth last October, the number of alcohol ads on TV jumped by nearly 90,000 between 2001 and 2003, with some 23 percent of the ads "more likely to be seen by the average underage person for every four seen by the average adult."

Cressey of the Distilled Spirits Council, among other industry leaders, disputes that there has been any concerted targeting of young people, and notes that his group will not permit any member to advertise where the media is not at least a 70/30, adult to minor, demographic.

"We also require through our code that all models in our ads be at least 25 years old," adds Cressey, a requirement that is also generally followed by members of the Beer Institute.

But even working within those parameters, the impact of drinking ads, usually showing young people at a beach party, rap concert, or skate boarding, remains a matter of contention.

"The problem is that how we view television has changed greatly in the last generation," says Sherman. "It used to be that there was one TV and the entire family was watching it, which meant that there would probably be some sort of adult filtering or response to whatever the ad message was. But that is much harder today when over 30 percent of kids aged two to eight, and two-thirds over the age of eight, have their own TVs in their own rooms."

The end result may not only be a message received early on that drinking alcohol is attractive, but an actual inability

---

Binge Drinking—The Facts

- In 2001, 44% of U.S. college students engaged in binge drinking; this rate has not changed since 1993.
- 51% of the men drank five or more drinks in a row.
- 40% of the women drank four or more drinks in a row.
- Students more likely to binge drink are white, age 23 or younger, and are residents of a fraternity or sorority.
- 75.1% of fraternity residents and 62.4% of sorority residents report binge drinking.
- Binge drinkers in high school are three times more likely to binge in college.
- From 1993 to 2001, more students abstained from alcohol (16% to 19%), but more also frequently drank heavily (19.7% to 22.8%).
- Just as many freshman (those under 21) as seniors binge drink.
- Frequent binge drinkers are eight times more likely than others to miss a class, fall behind in schoolwork, get hurt or injured, and damage property.
- 91% of women and 78% of the men who are frequent binge drinkers consider themselves to be moderate or light drinkers.
- 1,400 college students every year die from alcohol-related causes; 1,100 of these deaths involve drinking and driving.

Sources: Harvard University's School of Public Health; Robert Wood Johnson Foundation.

---

at an age leading all the way up to college to discern alcohol's potential danger. "There is a lot of research out there showing that even up to the age of 21 and beyond a young body is not fully developed and it does not absorb alcohol as well as it might in an older person," says Blackman of the Century Council. "Just as important is the evidence that your brain is not fully developed at that point either, so that issues of risk-taking and behavior are assessed in a different way."

To make matters worse, State University of New York's Hanson says, zero tolerance alcohol programs or efforts to make campuses virtually alcohol-free have a funny way of backfiring. "Prohibition is a classic example of how the laws in these matters can end up being counterproductive by actually making the thing that is being prohibited more attractive. That remains especially true for young people who don't like to be told what not to do."

"And when that happens," says Hanson, "young people very often find themselves involved in these dangerous events centered around heavy episodic drinking, which is the very last thing we want to see happen."

Teaching Moderation

Hanson has also noticed in his own research that the percentage of students who drink tends to decrease as they go from being freshmen to seniors. He says policymakers would be wiser to focus on what he calls "harm reduction policies" that acknowledge young people are going to drink no matter what, but emphasize responsible drinking through education—even to minors.

Similarly Colorado University's Bentley has noticed the effectiveness of the restorative justice approach on many college campuses that require students who have engaged in binge drinking to face the people who suffered the consequences of their behavior when they were drunk.

"That means the neighbors who were trying to study when the party was blaring," says Bentley, "or friends who had to take care of them when they were throwing up all over themselves or were otherwise dead drunk."

Legislatively, some lawmakers are looking at keg-registration laws in order to keep better track of who buys what for whom, particularly when such kegs end up at parties heavily populated with minors. So far, 24 states and the District of Columbia have adopted keg registration laws of varying severity.

"It is only a tool that might possibly reduce binge drinking and underage drinking," says Arizona Representative Ted Downing, who has introduced legislation requiring the state to put tracking numbers on every keg of beer sold.

"The way my legislation reads is that if you want to buy a keg, you have to show identification, fill out a form, leave a deposit, and detail where the keg is going to go and for what purpose" says Downing.

Other lawmakers believe that by making underage consumption and distribution more legally challenging, they can, at the very least, chip away at the roughly 33 percent of the nation's college students who are below the age of 21.

"It's worth a try," says Colorado Representative Angie Paccione, who has introduced legislation making it a class one misdemeanor to distribute alcohol to someone under the age of 21, with jail time of up to 18 months and fines topping out at $5,000.

"We want to give the DAs a tool that they can use for prosecuting and that the police can use in order to effect behavior changes," Paccione says, adding that problem college drinking is very often proceeded by problem high school drinking.

"I was a dean in a high school and have seen more than my share of kids who have had liquid lunches," she says. "So I know that this is a problem that begins very early."

Education Works

And although a new look at both underage and binge drinking from the legislative perspective may be in order, Jeff Becker, president of the Beer Institute, says lawmakers should not lose sight of the progress that has already been made in reducing both high school and college drinking.

"The education and awareness programs have really worked, whether it is at the college or high school level; and I think lawmakers should take credit for any support they have given to those efforts and continue those programs," says Becker.

"Maybe these most recent deaths will serve as a wake-up call and get all of us to look once more at what works and what doesn't work," he adds. "But from the community, family and school level it is very clear that making kids aware of the dangers has also made them smarter. And I don't think we should stop doing that."

In Connecticut, Senator Biagio "Billy" Ciotto, a long-time advocate of programs that educate high school students on the harmful effects of both drinking and driving and binge drinking, says he remains convinced that lawmakers should concentrate on what he calls the "realistic goal of reduction" vs. the "impossible idea," of elimination.

"You are never going to get rid of this kind of drinking completely," Ciotto says. "But I have no doubt in my mind that you can reduce the abuse simply by staying with it, never giving up, always trying to let kids know, without lecturing them, about the harmful effects of alcohol abuse."

Ciotto's efforts have even won the support of the Connecticut Coalition to Stop Underage Drinking, which named him "Outstanding Legislator in Reducing Underage Drinking" in 2004.

"I think they and just about everyone else recognize that we have to work on the big majority of kids who will not abuse alcohol if they know the dangers, and just figure that there is always going to be a minority that will do what they want to do no matter what," he says.

Arizona's Downing agrees: "It would be very foolish for any state representative or senator to feel that you can propose a bill that will somehow magically get rid of the problems of binge drinking or underage drinking."

"You can't," says Downing. "And we have to admit that. All you can really do is nudge things in a certain direction, which is what so many of our laws do anyway. If people are going to behave in the wrong way no matter what, there is only so much we can do. But we can help those who want to do the right thing, or don't want to break any laws just to have a little fun. That is the group we need to appeal to."

Freelancer **GARRY BOULARD** is a frequent contributor to State Legislatures.

From *State Legislatures*, April 2005, pp. 12–15. Copyright © 2005 by National Conference of State Legislatures. Reprinted by permission.

The Changing Face of Teenage Drug Abuse
The Trend toward Prescription Drugs

RICHARD A. FRIEDMAN, MD

When Eric, an 18-year-old who lives in San Francisco, wants to get some Vicodin (hydrocodone–acetaminophen), it's a simple matter. "I can get prescription drugs from different places and don't ever have to see a doctor," he explained. "I have friends whose parents are pill addicts, and we 'borrow' from them. Other times I have friends who have ailments who get lots of pills and sell them for cheap. As long as prescription pills are taken right, they're much safer than street drugs."

Eric's habits reflect an emerging pattern in drug use by teenagers: illicit street drugs such as "ecstasy" (3,4-methylenedioxymethamphetamine) and cocaine are decreasing in popularity, whereas the nonmedical use of certain prescription drugs is on the rise. These findings were reported in the Monitoring the Future survey, which is sponsored by the National Institute on Drug Abuse and designed and conducted by researchers at the University of Michigan.[1] The study, which began in 1975, annually surveys a nationally representative sample of about 50,000 students in 400 public and private secondary schools in the United States.

We're living in a time that seems decidedly more apocalyptic. . . . Maybe we need something to slow down.

Overall, the proportion of teens who reported having used any illicit drug during the previous year has dropped by more than a third among 8th graders and by about 10 percent among 12th graders since the peaks reported in the mid-to-late 1990s, according to the 2005 survey. Alcohol use and cigarette smoking among teens are now at historic lows. In contrast, the number of high-school students who are abusing prescription pain relievers such as oxycodone (OxyContin), a potent and highly addictive opiate, or sedatives is on the rise. A total of 7.2 percent of high-school seniors reported nonmedical use of sedatives in 2005, up

from a low of 2.8 percent in 1992 (see graph). Reported use of oxycodone in this group increased from 4.0 percent in 2002 to 5.5 percent in 2005.

The survey did not ask teenagers how they obtained their prescription drugs, but there is little doubt that the medications are easy to get from a variety of sources. "Prescription drugs are a lot easier to get than street drugs," said John, a high-school sophomore in Austin, Texas. "Kids can get them on the street, from parents and friends, or on the Internet."

They can also get them all too easily from physicians, according to recent data from the National Center on Addiction and Substance Abuse at Columbia University.[2] A 2004 survey of physicians found that 43 percent did not ask about prescription-drug abuse when taking a patient's history, and one third did not regularly call or obtain records from the patient's previous physician before prescribing potentially addictive drugs. These alarming data suggest that physicians are much too lax in prescribing controlled drugs. Claire, an 18-year-old who lives in Maine, told me, "You can always find a doctor who you can convince that you have a sleeping problem to get Ambien [zolpidem] or that you have ADD [attention-deficit disorder] and get Adderall." And even if most teenagers do not seek controlled prescription drugs directly from doctors, physicians are surely the original source of much of the medication that teens use, which has been diverted from its intended recipients.

In explaining the increase in the recreational use of prescription drugs, many teenagers draw key distinctions between these drugs and illicit street drugs. Teenagers whom I interviewed said that whereas they used illicit drugs only for recreation, they often used prescription drugs for "practical" effects: hypnotic drugs for sleep, stimulants to enhance their school performance, and tranquilizers such as benzodiazepines to decrease stress. They often characterized their use of prescription drugs as "responsible," "controlled," or "safe." The growing popularity of prescription drugs also reflects the perception that these drugs are safer than street drugs. According to the Monitoring the Future survey, for example, the use of sedatives among

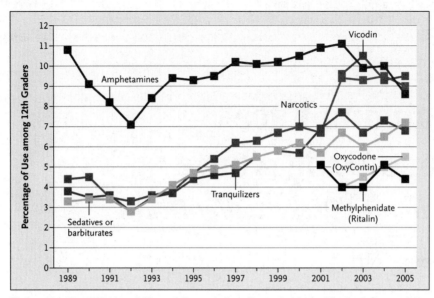

Figure 1 Prevalence of Use of Prescription Drugs without Medical Supervision among 12th Graders.

Data are from the Monitoring the Future survey. In 2001, the text of the question regarding tranquilizers was changed in half the questionnaire forms: Miltown (meprobamate) was replaced by Xanax (alprazolam) in the list of examples. This resulted in a slight increase in the reported prevalence. In 2002, the remaining questionnaire forms were changed. Also in 2002, the text of the question about narcotics other than heroin was changed in half the questionnaire forms: Talwin (pentazocine–naloxone), laudanum, and paregoric (which all reportedly had negligible rates of use by 2001) were replaced with Vicodin (hydrocodone–acetaminophen), OxyContin (oxycodone), and Percocet (oxycodone–acetaminophen). This resulted in an increase in reported prevalence, and in 2003, the remaining questionnaire forms were changed.

high-school seniors has increased in tandem with a decrease in the perceived risk and an increase in peer-group approval of the use of sedatives, whereas amphetamine use has steadily dropped as the perceived risk and societal disapproval have increased.

What might explain the growing confidence in the safety of prescription drugs? Negative media attention is frequently cited as a factor in the decreasing popularity of cocaine and stimulants among teenagers. The converse appears to be true regarding prescription medications. Nowadays, it is nearly impossible to open a newspaper, turn on the television, or search the Internet without encountering an advertisement for a prescription medication. Expenditures by the pharmaceutical industry for direct-to-consumer advertising increased from $1.8 billion in 1999 to $4.2 billion in 2004.[3,4] One effect has been to foster an image of prescription drugs as an integral and routine aspect of everyday life. Any adverse effects are relegated to the fine print of an advertisement or dispatched in a few seconds of rapid-fire speech.

Not all prescription drugs, however, have equal appeal among teenagers. According to the Monitoring the Future study, calming prescription drugs have become more popular, whereas the use of stimulants is decreasing. Whether this trend reflects the differential availability of sedative drugs, the selective effects of advertising, or other social factors is anyone's guess. Asked to speculate about it, teenagers said more or less what John,

the teen from Austin, expressed in an e-mail message: "We're living in a time that seems decidedly more apocalyptic, especially since 9/11 and all the recent natural disasters. Maybe we need something to slow down."

The perception that prescription drugs are largely safe seems to justify the attitude that occasional use poses little risk. And indeed, there is little doubt that many more people try drugs than become serious drug abusers. For example, in the 2004 National Household Survey on Drug Abuse, 19 percent of persons between 12 and 17 years of age reported ever having used marijuana, whereas 14.5 percent reported use during the previous year, and only 7.6 percent reported use during the previous month.[5]

Still, the fact that 50 percent of students have tried an illicit drug by the time they finish high school—another finding of the Monitoring the Future survey—is nothing to be happy about, not to mention the 5.5 percent of 12th graders who have tried the highly addictive oxycodone. For a substantial number of teenagers with risk factors, such as a psychiatric illness or a family history of drug abuse, crossing the line from abstinence to exposure will be the first step toward serious substance abuse.

Moreover, even in small doses, sedatives, hypnotics, and opiates have subtle effects on cognition and motor skills that may increase the risk of injury, particularly during sports activities or driving. From a longer-term perspective, the brains of teenagers are still developing, and the effects of drug abuse may be harmful in ways that are not yet understood. Do we really want teenagers to think nothing of popping a pill to relax, get through the tedium of a long homework assignment, or relieve normal anxieties?

Clearly, physicians play an important role in this problem, given their apparent laxness in prescribing controlled drugs. Physicians should routinely assess their patients for substance use and psychiatric illness before they put pen to a prescription pad. They should also discuss with their adult patients who have teenage children the risks associated with controlled drugs and the need to restrict the availability of such drugs at home.

In order to address these problems appropriately, physicians need adequate education in substance abuse. The survey by the National Center on Addiction and Substance Abuse reveals that physicians do not feel they are well trained to spot signs of substance abuse or addiction—a skill that should be taught in all medical schools and residency programs.

Finally, educators and parents must address the potential dangers of prescription-drug abuse with teenagers. As Claire put it, "In a way, prescription drugs are more dangerous than street drugs, because we don't recognize their dangers."

(The names of the teenagers who were interviewed have been changed to protect their privacy.)

References

Johnston LD, O'Malley PM, Bachman JG, Schulenberg JE. Monitoring the future: national results on adolescent drug use: overview of key findings, 2005. Bethesda, Md.: National Institute on Drug Abuse (in press).

Doe J. Under the counter: the diversion and abuse of controlled prescription drugs in the U.S. New York: National Center on Addiction and Substance Abuse of Columbia University, 2005.

R&D spending. In: PhRMA annual membership survey. Washington, D.C.: Pharmaceutical Research and Manufacturers of America, 2004.

Promotional data. In: Integrated Promotional Services and CMR. Fairfield, Conn.: IMS Health, June 2004.

Office of Applied Studies. Results from the 2004 National Survey on Drug Use & Health: national findings. NSDUH series H-28. Rockville, Md.: Substance Abuse and Mental Health Services Administration, 2005. (DHHS publication no. SMA 05-4062.)

DR. FRIEDMAN is a psychiatrist and the director of the Psychopharmacology Clinic at Weill Cornell Medical College, New York.

From *The New England Journal of Medicine,* April 6, 2006, pp. 1448–1450. Copyright © 2006 by Massachusetts Medical Society. All rights reserved. Reprinted by permission.

Helping Workers Kick the Habit

Programs aimed at helping employees give up tobacco can pay off in lower health care costs.

PAMELA BABCOCK

Smoking is more than a health threat for the 45 million Americans who use tobacco. It's also an employers' problem because it raises health cost issues and productivity concerns.

Smoking and the illnesses that link to it, such as cancer and heart disease, account for annual medical costs of $150 billion or more, by some estimates. In turn, those costs affect the premiums for employer-sponsored health care. As employers try to exert control over their fast-rising health costs through wellness programs and other efforts to improve employees' health, some are adopting smoking-cessation programs as one of their tools.

Smoking-cessation approaches range from reminding employees of the health effects of smoking, to offering them multifaceted assistance programs, to requiring them to quit smoking if they want to keep their jobs.

In that middle ground between encouragement and ultimatum reside a number of generally affordable programs that typically offer counseling—sometimes one-on-one—and various types of drugs formulated to help smokers quit. Health coverage companies, behavioral health organizations, stand-alone wellness companies, hospitals and others number among the providers.

As the availability of smoking-cessation programs increases and as new drugs arrive in the market, it's important for benefits specialists to know how to choose a cessation approach that will work best for their employees, and where to turn when looking for a program.

The Will to Quit

Although about 47 million Americans say they have quit smoking, almost as many still smoke. About 70 percent of those who smoke say they want to quit, but only 5 percent

succeed long term, the U.S. Centers for Disease Control and Prevention reports.

Indeed, quitting is difficult. Less than 7 percent of smokers who try to quit on their own abstain for longer than a year; most light up within a few days of attempting to quit, according to pharmaceutical manufacturer Pfizer Inc. It takes about 10 attempts, with or without treatment, before the average smoker kicks the habit for good, says Pfizer. The company recently introduced a smoking-cessation drug.

"Although we have made significant progress, tobacco use is still the leading cause of preventable illness and death," says Susan Butterworth, director of Health Management Services within the School of Nursing at Oregon Health & Science University (OHSU), based in Portland. "Nicotine dependency is more than a lifestyle choice. It's an addiction, and employees need assistance in addressing it," she says.

How Programs Work

Butterworth and many other smoking-cessation experts recommend a strategic approach that includes "quit medications" and health counseling.

Medications available over the counter include nicotine patches and nicotine gum; prescription drugs include nasal sprays, inhalers and pills. An article on the U.S. Food and Drug Administration's website describes how these medications work: "Most medical aids to smoking cessation are nicotine replacement products. They deliver small, steady doses of nicotine into the body to relieve some of the withdrawal symptoms, without the 'buzz' that keeps smokers hooked. . . . Like cigarettes, the products deliver nicotine into the blood, but they don't contain the tar and carbon monoxide that are largely responsible for cigarettes' dangerous health consequences."

Nicotine dependency is . . . an addiction, and employees need assistance in addressing it.

Many programs that operate under an employer-sponsored wellness initiative include a personal health assessment that identifies smoking as a health risk. Follow-up efforts often involve counseling—increasingly delivered by the Internet with threaded discussion, chat or e-mail. The vast majority, Butterworth says, deliver counseling by phone, while others deliver it in person.

One of the largest cessation companies, Free & Clear Inc., a coaching-based provider in Seattle, has been named the official quit-smoking program for 16 states and more than 100 large employers and health plans. Last year, the company registered more than 115,000 people into tobacco-cessation programs and completed nearly 700,000 intervention calls, says Dr. Tim McAfee, senior vice president for clinical and behavioral sciences at Free & Clear.

The company offers a personal Internet application, called Web Coach, in its Quit For Life Program. It also offers Vital Signs, a real-time, online reporting tool for clients. OHSU's Health Management Services competes in the field, offering smoking cessation as one of its health-coaching services for outside clients.

Other major providers of smoking-cessation programs include QuitNet, WebMD and the Mayo Clinic. For more

Online Resources

For additional information about helping employees to quit smoking, see the online version of this article at www.shrm.org/hrmagazine/07September for links to:

- A SHRM article on employers who want to help employees quit smoking.
- An *HR Magazine* article on the legal issues in providing smoking-cessation programs.
- An *HR News* article on tobacco's drain on employee productivity.
- A SHRM article about a Rhode Island law mandating employer health plan coverage of smoking-cessation treatment programs.
- Information from the Centers for Disease Control and Prevention on helping employees who smoke to quit.
- The American Legacy Foundation's survey on smoking cessation as an employer-sponsored health benefit.

on those organizations, including their smoking-cessation approaches, see the online version of this article at www.shrm.org/hrmagazine/07September.

Employers should avoid "going with a canned or low-cost program that doesn't embrace best practice in nicotine dependence treatment," says Butterworth, also an associate professor in OHSU's School of Nursing. Look for programs that use best practices—a combination of quit medications and coaching—and that demonstrate measurable outcomes, she says.

Measurable outcomes are determined by quit rates at one year compared with the rates in a control group in a random controlled study, Butterworth says. When the quit rate significantly exceeds the rate in the control group, the treatment is considered effective.

The combined use of coaching and quit medications—she calls it "the gold standard"— seems to work equally well across demographic and cultural differences within workplaces, but she adds that it's important for health coaches "to understand the culture, to be sensitive to employee norms, and to be acquainted with their benefits and other resources."

Employees may prefer accessing information in different ways, for example. Office workers who have desktops may prefer Internet products, while those on a manufacturing line may do better with telephone coaching or printed handouts.

Costs and Savings

Employers can provide programs such as a telephone "quit line"—generally the lowest-price approach—for under 5 cents per employee per month, a figure based on the total population of employees and their covered dependents, not on the number of employees using the service. The figure is in the results of research commissioned by the American Legacy Foundation, a Washington, D.C., organization that focuses on smoking prevention and cessation, and carried out by Milliman, a global consulting organization based in Seattle.

The research report, *Covering Smoking Cessation as a Health Benefit: A Case for Employers*, released last December, found that more-comprehensive coverage that includes therapy and selected pharmaceuticals costs 28 cents to 45 cents per health plan member per month.

The annual savings for each smoker who quits, according to the report, is about $210 through reductions in costs for smoking-related conditions such as stroke, coronary heart disease, pneumonia, childhood respiratory disease and low birth weight. The dollar savings alone may not fully offset an employer's annual cost for a cessation program, but they can make a difference over time, since they accrue each year the employee remains a nonsmoker.

In addition, smoking cessation reduces annual medical and life insurance costs almost immediately, says the study's author, Bruce Pyenson, a principal and consulting actuary with Milliman in New York.

Among the approaches compared in the study, telephonic quit lines, with no face-to-face contact with employees, had quit rates of 4.5 percent, Pyenson says. Programs with more features, such as counseling and a range of medications, cost more but had higher quit rates, up to about 30 percent.

Noting that the costs of cessation programs vary according to the type of service provided and the vendor providing it, Butterworth says one-time fees for each health-coaching participant range from $100 to $250.

Building the Base

Before settling on a particular program, benefits specialists should determine the incidence of smoking among the company's employees, experts suggest, and start their searches by tapping their trusted sources of information, such as brokers and health plan providers.

Christopher J. Mathews, a Washington, D.C.-based senior health consultant and vice president of the Segal Co., a benefits consulting organization headquartered in New York, recommends working with your health plan or advisor to find out whether smoking is a real problem in your employee population. Employee surveys can be used to determine how many smokers you have and whether any are really interested in quitting.

If your CEO is a cigar smoker and there's no way he's going to quit, there's a problem.

If your organization's smoker population is made up of those who have been smoking for 30 years, you might not get a lot of traction. "But if the smoker population is comprised of those who sincerely wish to quit, then the prospects for success are greatly improved," Mathews explains.

Karen Roberts, a senior vice president in Aon Consulting's Health and Benefits Practice in Las Vegas, recommends making sure that the program has support from the top. "If your CEO is a cigar smoker and there's no way he's going to quit, there's a problem," she says. "You really have to walk the talk with these programs."

Take inventory of your physical premises to determine how committed you are to the cessation program. Are you going to push cessation but still have designated smoking areas on your property or allow smoking in company cars?

Also, take inventory of provisions in your health benefits plan to determine if there are barriers to a program's success, such as lack of coverage for smoking-cessation drugs or for coaching or counseling, Mathews says. If such coverage isn't provided, he says, and your plan, in effect, becomes "a barrier to providing the necessary support needed for smokers to quit, it will need to be modified."

As sponsor of your health plan, you should decide how many attempts to quit smoking by an individual will be covered by your plan and whether there would be a maximum on the benefit per employee, Mathews says.

For OHSU's own tobacco-cessation program, provided by Health Management Services, the university has structured its employee health plan so that over-the-counter quit medications such as patches and gum are free, and there are no co-payments for prescription-only quit medicines approved by the U.S. Food and Drug Administration. Employees who sign up also receive an individual quit plan.

Butterworth and her staff acknowledge that some smokers may want to try alternative cessation approaches such as acupuncture and hypnosis; they are not included in any OHSU plan, however.

Butterworth recommends motivational interviewing, an approach "used by many reputable vendors" to help tobacco users develop the self-confidence necessary to quit. It's important, she says, to "engage smokers who aren't ready to quit" to "help them consider their options, draw out their ambivalence and help them weigh the pros and cons of quitting."

OHSU's smoking-cessation campaign expands this month to its entire Portland campus—12,000 employees, thousands of patients and students. All smoking will be banned, even on streets and sidewalks.

Try a Little Tenderness

Roger Reed, a nurse practitioner and executive vice president of Gordian Health Solutions, a health management provider based in Franklin, Tenn., says a positive and benevolent approach can go a long way in a smoking-cessation initiative. "The biggest mistake," he says, "is to start taking a list of smokers and singling them out with some kind of punitive action, such as saying you have 12 months to quit or you won't work here anymore."

Gordian provides one-on-one coaching, online information and health materials via mail to large employers, health plans and government entities. Last year, the company had 6,755 people enrolled in tobacco-cessation programs.

"Most people try to stop smoking multiple times, and it's just that one time when they make that one more attempt that it actually works," Reed says, adding, "You never know." It could be that when their employer provides that extra opportunity, it just might be the employee's time to quit for good.

PAMELA BABCOCK is a freelance writer based in the New York City area.

From *HR Magazine*, September 2007. Copyright © 2007 by Society for Human Resource Management. Reprinted by permission via the Copyright Clearance Center.

UNIT 6

Sexuality and Relationships

Unit Selections

Key Points to Consider

- Do you feel at risk of contracting AIDS or other STDs? If not, why not? If you do, what are you doing to reduce your risk?

- What specific issues do nontraditional couples face in our society?

- Should parents be permitted to choose the sex of their baby before birth?

- What role does scent play in sexual attraction?

- What role does pornography play in relationships?

Student Website

www.mhcls.com

Internet References

Planned Parenthood
  http://www.plannedparenthood.org/
Sexuality Information and Education Council of the United States (SIECUS)
  http://www.siecus.org/

Sexuality is an important part of both self awareness and intimate relationships. How important is physical attraction in establishing and maintaining intimate relationships? Researchers in the area of evolutionary psychology have proposed numerous theories that attempt to explain the mutual attraction that occurs between the sexes. The most controversial of these theories postulates that our perception of beauty or physical attractiveness is not subjective but rather a biological component hardwired into our brains. It is generally assumed that perceptions of beauty vary from era to era and culture to culture, but evidence is mounting that suggests that people all over share a common sense of beauty that is based on physical symmetry. In addition to a sense of physical beauty, researchers believe that scent is an important component of who we end up with. Physical attraction may be based on smell, which may be a significant component of what we think of as "chemistry" between partners.

While physical attraction is clearly an important issue when it comes to dating, how important is it in long-term, loving relationships? For many Americans the answer may be very important, because we tend to be a "Love Culture," a culture that places a premium on passion in the selection of our mates. Is passion an essential ingredient in love, and can passion serve to sustain a long-term, meaningful relationship? Because most people can't imagine marrying someone that they don't love, we must assume that most marriages are based on this feeling we call love. That being the case, why is it that so few marriages survive the rigors of day-to-day living? Perhaps the answer has more to do with our limited definition of love rather than love itself. An interesting look at love can be found in "Love at the Margins," which discusses nontraditional couples, and the demands they face. These relationships can demand, or may require, extreme commitments along with the coping with social disapproval. A related topic is one that argues that sex is good for health. Studies are showing that an active sex life may lead to a longer life, better ability to withstand pain, a healthy immune system, lesser risk of heart diseases and cancer, and lower rates of depression.

An important topic of interest and controversy in the area of human sexuality is sex education. While most states mandate some type of school-based sex education, many parents believe that they should be the source of their children's sex education and not the schools. A somewhat unrelated topic addresses the questions of parents choosing the sex of their unborn children. In "Girl or Boy?," Denise Grady questions whether couples should have the option of choosing the gender of their baby. Currently, some doctors are willing to accommodate parents, while others question the ethics of choosing the sex before birth.

Perhaps no topic in the area of human sexuality has garnered more publicity and public concern than the dangers associated with unprotected sex. Although the concept of "safe sex" is nothing new, the degree of open and public discussion regarding sexual behaviors is. With the emergence of AIDS as a disease of epidemic proportions and the rapid spreading of other sexually transmitted diseases (STDs), the surgeon general of the United States initiated an aggressive educational campaign, based on the assumption that knowledge would change behavior. If STD rates among teens are any indication of the effectiveness of this approach, then we must conclude that our educational efforts are failing. Conservatives believe that while education may play a role in curbing the spread of STDs, the root of the problem is promiscuity, and that promiscuity rises when a society is undergoing a moral decline. The solution, according to conservatives, is a joint effort between parents and educators to teach students the importance of values such as respect, responsibility, and integrity. Liberals, on the other hand, think that preventing promiscuity is unrealistic, and instead the focus should be on establishing open and frank discussions between the sexes. Their premise is that we are all sexual

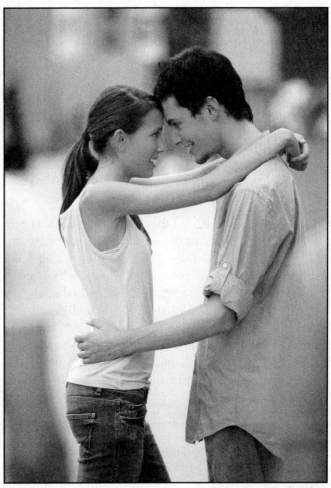

© 2008 Jupiterimages

beings, and the best way to combat STDs is to establish open discussions between sexual partners, so that condoms will be used correctly when couples engage in intercourse.

While education undoubtedly has had a positive impact on slowing the spread of STDs, perhaps it was unrealistic to think that education alone was the solution, given the magnitude and the nature of the problem. Most experts agree that for education to succeed in changing personal behaviors, the following conditions must be met: (1) The recipients of the information must first perceive themselves as vulnerable and, thus, be motivated to explore replacement behaviors, and (2) the replacement behaviors must satisfy the needs that were the basis of the problem behaviors. To date, most education programs have failed to meet these criteria. Given all the information that we now have on the dangers associated with AIDS and STDs, why is it that people do not perceive themselves at risk? It is not so much the denial of risks as it is the notion of most people that they use good judgment when it comes to choosing sex partners. Unfortunately, most decisions regarding sexual behavior are based on subjective criteria that bear little or no relationship to one's actual risk. Even when individuals do view themselves as vulnerable to AIDS and STDs, there are currently only two viable options for reducing the risk of contracting these diseases. The first is the use of a condom and the second is sexual abstinence, neither of which is an ideal solution to the problem.

Scents and Sensibility

"Sexual chemistry" is more than just a way of talking about heated attraction. Subtle chemical keys actually help determine who we fall for. But here comes news that our lifestyles may unwittingly undermine our natural sex appeal.

ELIZABETH SVOBODA

Psychologists Rachel Herz and Estelle Campenni were just getting to know each other, swapping stories about their lives over coffee, when Campenni confided something unexpected: She was living proof, she said, of love at first smell. "I knew I would marry my husband the minute I smelled him," she told Herz. "I've always been into smell, but this was different; he really smelled good to me. His scent made me feel safe and at the same time turned on—and I'm talking about his real body smell, not cologne or soap. I'd never felt like that from a man's smell before. We've been married for eight years now and have three kids, and his smell is always very sexy to me."

Everyone knows what it's like to be powerfully affected by a partner's smell—witness men who bury their noses in their wives' hair and women who can't stop sniffing their boyfriends' T-shirts. And couples have long testified to the ways scent-based chemistry affects their relationships. "One of the most common things women tell marriage counselors is, 'I can't stand his smell,'" says Herz, the author of *The Scent of Desire*.

Sexual attraction remains one of life's biggest mysteries. We might say we go for partners who are tall and thin, love to cook, or have a mania for exercise, but when push comes to shove, studies show, the people we actually end up with possess few of the traits we claim to want. Some researchers think scent could be the hidden cosmological constant in the sexual universe, the missing factor that explains who we end up with. It may even explain why we feel "chemistry"—or "sparks" or "electricity"—with one person and not with another.

Physical attraction itself may literally be based on smell. We discount the importance of scent-centric communication only because it operates on such a subtle level. "This is not something that jumps out at you, like smelling a good steak cooking on the grill," says Randy Thornhill, an evolutionary psychologist at the University of New Mexico. "But the scent capability is there, and it's not surprising to find smell capacity in the context of sexual behavior." As a result, we may find ourselves drawn to the counter attendant at the local drugstore, but have no idea why—or, conversely, find ourselves put off by potential dating partners even though they seem perfect on paper.

Though we may remain partially oblivious to scent signals we're sending and receiving, new research suggests that we not only come equipped to choose a romantic partner who smells good to us, but that this choice has profound biological implications. As we act out the complex rituals of courtship, many of them inscribed deep in our brain, scent-based cues help us zero in on optimal partners—the ones most likely to stay faithful to us and to create healthy children with us.

At first blush, the idea of scent-based attraction might seem hypothetical and ephemeral, but when we unknowingly interfere with the transmission of subtle olfactory messages operating below the level of conscious awareness, the results can be both concrete and devastating. When we disregard what our noses tell us, we can find ourselves mired in partnerships that breed sexual discontent, infertility, and even—in extreme cases—unhealthy offspring.

The Scent of Desire

When you're turned on by your partner's scent, taking a deep whiff of his chest or the back of her neck feels like taking a powerful drug—it's an instant flume ride to bliss, however momentary. Research has shown that we use scent-based signaling mechanisms to suss out compatibility. Claus Wedekind, a biologist at the University of Lausanne in Switzerland, created Exhibit A of this evidence by giving 44 men new T-shirts and instructing them to wear the shirts for two straight nights. To ensure that the sweat collecting on the shirts would remain "odor-neutral," he supplied the men with scent-free soap and aftershave.

After the men were allowed to change, 49 women sniffed the shirts and specified which odors they found most attractive. Far more often than chance would predict, the women preferred the smell of T-shirts worn by men who were immunologically dissimilar to them. The difference lay in the sequence of more than 100 immune system genes known as the MHC, or major histocompatibility complex. These genes code for proteins that help the immune system recognize pathogens. The smell of their favorite shirts also reminded the women of their past and current boyfriends, suggesting that MHC does indeed influence women's dating decisions in real life.

I knew I would marry my husband the minute I first smelled him. His body scent made me feel safe and turned on.

Women's preference for MHC-distinct mates makes perfect sense from a biological point of view. Ever since ancestral times, partners whose immune systems are different have produced offspring who are more disease-resistant. With more immune genes expressed, kids are buffered against a wider variety of pathogens and toxins.

But that doesn't mean women prefer men whose MHC genes are most different from theirs, as University of Chicago evolutionary biologist Martha McClintock found when she performed a T-shirt study similar to Wedekind's. Women are not attracted to the smell of men with whom they had no MHC genes in common. "This might be a case where you're protecting yourself against a mate who's too similar or too dissimilar, but there's a middle range where you're OK," McClintock says.

Women consistently outperform men in smell sensitivity tests, and they also make greater time and energy sacrifices on their children's behalf than men do—in addition to bearing off-spring, they look after them most of the time. These factors may explain why women are more discriminating in sniffing out MHC compatibility.

Men are sensitive to smell as well, but because women shoulder a greater reproductive burden, and are therefore choosier about potential mates, researchers are not surprised to find that women are also more discriminating in sniffing out MHC compatibility.

Unlike, say, blood types, MHC gene complements differ so much from one person to the next that there's no obvious way to reliably predict who's MHC-compatible with whom. Skin color, for instance, isn't much help,

Follow Your Nose

How to Put Your Nose to Work in Choosing a Partner—or Evaluating an Existing One

Think twice about opting for the pill if you're seeking a long-term partner. The first few weeks of a relationship are critical to assessing compatibility, so make sure your nose is up to the task.

Try a fragrance-free week. Eliminate factors that could throw your nostrils off. Have your partner set aside scented shower gels in favor of fragrance-free soap, nix the cologne, and use only unscented deodorant.

Keep smell's importance in context. If you sometimes find your partner's scent off-putting, don't panic; it doesn't necessarily mean fertility issues are in your future. Connections between MHC compatibility and conception problems have yet to be confirmed in large-scale population studies, so don't plunk down big bucks for MHC testing at this point.

since groups of people living in different areas of the world might happen to evolve genetic resistance to some of the same germs. "People of different ethnicities can have similar profiles, so race is not a good predictor of MHC dissimilarity," Thornhill says.

And because people's MHC profiles are as distinct as fingerprints—there are thousands of possible gene combinations—a potential sex partner who smells good to one woman may completely repel another. "There's no Brad Pitt of smell," Herz says. "Body odor is an external manifestation of the immune system, and the smells we think are attractive come from the people who are most genetically compatible with us." Much of what we vaguely call "sexual chemistry," she adds, is likely a direct result of this scent-based compatibility.

Typically, our noses steer us in the right direction when it comes to picking a reproductively compatible partner. But what if they fail us and we wind up with a mate whose MHC profile is too similar to our own? Carol Ober, a geneticist at the University of Chicago, explored this question in her studies of members of the Hutterite religious clan, an Amish-like closed society that consists of some 40,000 members and extends through the rural Midwest. Hutterites marry only other members of their clan, so the variety in their gene pool is relatively low. Within these imposed limits, Hutterite women nevertheless manage to find partners who are MHC-distinct from them most of the time.

The few couples with a high degree of MHC similarity, however, suffered higher rates of miscarriage and experienced longer intervals between pregnancies, indicating more difficulty conceiving. Some scientists speculate that miscarriages may be the body's way of curtailing investment in a child who isn't likely to have a strong immune system anyway.

What's more, among heterosexual couples, similar MHC profiles spell relational difficulty, Christine Garver-Apgar, a psychologist at the University of New Mexico, has found. "As the proportion of MHC alleles increased, women's sexual responsiveness to their partners decreased, and their number of sex partners outside the relationship increased," Garver-Apgar reports. The number of MHC genes couples shared corresponded directly with the likelihood that they would cheat on one another; if a man and woman had 50 percent of their MHC alleles in common, the woman had a 50 percent chance of sleeping with another man behind her partner's back.

The Divorce Pill?

Women generally prefer the smell of men whose MHC gene complements are different from theirs, setting the stage for the best biological match. But Wedekind's T-shirt study revealed one notable exception to this rule: women on the birth-control pill. When the pill users among his subjects sniffed the array of pre-worn T-shirts, they preferred the scent of men whose MHC profiles were similar to theirs—the opposite of their pill-free counterparts.

This dramatic reversal of smell preferences may reflect the pill's mechanism of action: It prevents the ovaries from releasing an egg, fooling the body into thinking it's pregnant. And since pregnancy is such a vulnerable state, it seems to activate a preference for kin, who are genetically similar to us and likely to serve as protectors. "When pregnant rodent females are exposed to strange males, they can spontaneously abort," Herz says. "The same may be true for human females." What's more, some women report a deficit in sex drive when they take the pill, a possible consequence of its pregnancy-mimicking function.

The tendency to favor mates with similar MHC genes could potentially hamper the durability of pill users' relationships in the long term. While Herz shies away from dubbing hormonal birth control "the divorce pill," as a few media outlets have done in response to her theories, she does think the pill jumbles women's smell preferences. "It's like picking your cousins as marriage partners," Herz says. "It constitutes a biological error." As a result, explains Charles Wysocki, a psychobiologist at Florida State University, when such a couple decides to have children and the woman stops taking birth control, she may find herself less attracted to her mate for reasons she doesn't quite understand. "On a subconscious level, her brain is realizing a mistake was made—she married the wrong guy," he says.

"Some couples' fertility problems may be related to the pill-induced flip-flop in MHC preferences," Garver-Apgar adds. No one has yet collected data to indicate whether the pill has created a large-scale problem in compatibility. Still, Herz recommends that women seeking a long-term partner consider alternative birth control methods, at least until they get to know their potential significant other well and are sure they like the way he smells. "If you're looking for a man to be the father of your child," she says, "go off the pill before you start your search."

If you were on the pill when you met your current partner, the situation is more complicated. Once a relationship has progressed to long-term commitment, says Herz, a woman's perception of her partner's smell is so intertwined with her emotional reaction to him that it could be difficult for her to assess his scent as if he were a stranger. "If she's in love, he could smell like a garbage can and she'd still be attracted to him."

Crossed Signals

The pill subverts a woman's ability to sniff out a compatible mate by causing her to misinterpret the scent messages she receives. But it may warp olfactory communication channels in the other direction as well, distorting the signals she sends—and making her seem less appealing to men, an irony given that women typically take the pill to boost their appeal in a partner's eyes.

Geoffrey Miller, an evolutionary psychologist at the University of New Mexico and author of *The Mating Mind*, noticed the pill's connection to waning male desire while studying a group of exotic dancers—women whose livelihoods depend on how sexually appealing they are to male customers. Non-pill-using dancers made about 50 percent more in tips than dancers on oral contraceptives. In other words, women who were on the pill were only about two-thirds as sexy as women who weren't.

Why were the pill-takers in the study so much less attractive to men? "Women are probably doing something unconsciously, and men are responding to it unconsciously," says Miller. "We just don't know whether it has to do with a shift in their psychology, their tone of voice, or if it's more physical, as in the kind of pheromones they're putting out."

The biggest earners in Miller's study were non-pill-using dancers at the time of ovulation. Other studies have shown that men rate women as smelling best when they are at the most fertile point of their menstrual cycles, suggesting that women give offscent-based signals that broadcast their level of fecundity. "The pill might be producing cues that a woman is in the early stage of pregnancy, which would not tend to elicit a lot of male sexual

Solving the Mystery of Gaydar

The Ability to Discern Sexual Orientation May Be Based on Scent

Everyone knows someone with impeccable "gaydar," the seemingly telepathic ability to tell whether someone is gay or straight. New research is robbing gaydar of its sixth-sense mystique, revealing that some people literally have the power to sniff out another person's sexual orientation—and that the ability is strongly rooted in biology.

When Charles Wysocki, a geneticist at the University of Pennsylvania's Monell Chemical Senses Center, asked volunteers to sniff underarm sweat from donors of a variety of genders and sexual orientations, some clear patterns began to emerge. Gay men strongly preferred the odor of other gay men, lesbians gravitated toward the smell of other lesbians, and straight women rated the odor of straight men higher than that of gay men. Each group, in short, preferred the smell of their first-choice mates, indicating a scent-based ability to assess sexual orientation. Another study confirmed that gay men and lesbians can recognize and identify the odor of others who share their sexual preference. This kind of scent-based gaydar enables gays to pinpoint potential partners instantly.

Researchers at Karolinska University in Sweden have added to Wysocki's findings, identifying a potential reason why gay men find the smell of other males so enticing. They found that androstenone, a steroid compound men secrete in their sweat, excited brain areas that control sexual behavior in gay men but left the brains of straight men unaffected. This suggests the chemical may be an integral part of the scent-driven signaling mechanism that attracts gay men to each other.

interest," Miller says. "It makes sense for men to be sensitive to that and for them not to feel the same chemistry with the woman."

Drowning in Fragrance

The pill isn't the only way we might confound sexual chemistry. Every day, far more people may be subverting their quest for love with soap and bottled fragrances. In ancestral times, smelling ripe was just a fact of life, absent hot showers and shampoo. This held true well into the 19th century, when the miasma of body odor in Parisian streets grew so thick that it was dubbed "The Great Stink of 1880." Back when a person's scent could waft across a room, a mere handshake could provide valuable information about attraction.

The need to smell our mates—and the difficulty in doing so over the sensory din of modern perfumes and colognes—may drive the sexual disinhibition of modern society.

Since the 20th-century hygiene revolution and the rise of the personal-care industry, however, companies have pitched deodorants, perfumes, and colognes to consumers as the epitome of sex appeal. But instead of furthering our quest to find the perfect mate, such products may actually derail it, say researchers, by masking our true scent and making it difficult for prospects to assess compatibility. "Humans abuse body smell signals by hiding them, masking them, putting on deodorant," says Devendra Singh, a psychologist at the University of Texas. "The noise-to-signal ratio was much better in primitive society."

Miller argues that modern hygiene may be such an impediment to sexual signaling that it could explain why so many people in our culture get so physical so fast. "Hunter-gatherers didn't have to do a lot of kissing, because they could smell each other pretty clearly from a few feet away," Miller says. "With all the showering, scents, and soap, we have to get our noses and mouths really up close to people to get a good idea of their biochemistry. People are more motivated to do a lot more kissing and petting, to do that assessment before they have sex." In other words, the need to smell our mates—and the comparative difficulty of doing so in today's environment of perfumes and colognes—may actually be driving the sexual disinhibition of modern society.

Other scientists counter that odor detection is a bit subtler. For one thing, it's possible we select store-bought scents to complement our natural odorprints, rather than mask them entirely: One study found that people with similar MHC profiles tend to go for the same colognes. And Garver-Apgar points out that in spending hours together each day, partners have ample opportunity to experience each other sans artificial scents. "Once you're in a close enough relationship," she says, "you're going to get a real whiff at some point."

Scents and Sensibility

There's no way to know whether couples who shell out thousands of dollars to fertility clinics—and those who struggle to make a relationship work because "the chemistry just isn't there"—suffer MHC incompatibility. We might never know, since a multitude of factors contributes to every reproductive and romantic outcome. But we can, at least, be cognizant of the importance of natural scent.

"Scent can be a deal breaker if it's not right, just like someone being too stupid or unkind or short," says Miller. Nevertheless, smell isn't the be-all and end-all of attraction, but one of a constellation of important factors. Armed with knowledge of how scent-based attraction operates, we have some power to decide how much priority we want to accord it. Is it more important to be with the partner who smells amazing and with whom you have great chemistry, or with the one who may not attract you quite as much on a physical level but is honest and reliable?

"People tend to treat this as an either-or situation: Either we're completely driven by pheromones, like moths, or we're completely in charge of our own destiny," University of Chicago psychologist McClintock says. "But it's not a wild idea that both factors are involved." While people like Estelle Campenni have reaped untold benefits by trusting their scent impressions, it's ultimately up to us how highly we value what our noses tell us.

ELIZABETH SVOBODA contributes regularly to the *New York Times*, *Discover*, and *Popular Science*. She lives in San Jose, California.

From *Psychology Today*, January/February 2008. Copyright © 2008 by Sussex Publishers, LLC. Reprinted by permission.

Love at the Margins

Extreme Relationships Demand Extreme Commitment

Nontraditional couples may be seen as weird, discomfiting or even sinful by others, but if they survive the crucible of social censure and self-doubt they can forge powerful bonds—and teach others about enduring love.

MARK TEICH

It's not easy being a lesbian couple in a suburban New Jersey community. "We're surrounded by married couples and families, and we stand out," says Allison. Madeleine adds, "By now I'm sure the neighbors can guess our situation. I feel comfortable with a few, but I'd rather keep things secret from the rest."

When they first dated, Allison, an artist, was in her element in Manhattan. Madeleine spent weekends at Allison's place. "In the city, no one noticed us," Allison says. "I never felt we were marginalized until I moved to New Jersey." Ultimately she'd felt she had to make the commitment to move in with Madeleine, because her girlfriend was the major breadwinner then, with a stable job as a computer software engineer 20 minutes from home.

"I love my work," notes Madeleine. "But there's a lot of prejudice in this field, so I don't mention Allison. I'd never bring her to an office party."

Sustaining a relationship is a challenge for anyone, but couples deemed inappropriate or abnormal by traditional social norms must forge their unions in the face of both internal and external pressures. Walking down the street or dining out, a gay or interracial couple or, say, a 50-year-old man embracing a 27-year-old woman (or vice versa) may be stared at, or viewed as suspect or even unnatural. More important, they may often face the wrath and rejection of their families, colleagues and friends. Couples considered marginal can encounter impediments from the law or organized religion—any institution built on traditional belief. No wonder they often hesitate to invest emotionally in one another, balking at moving in together or taking their partners to Christmas gatherings with their friends or families.

Nonetheless, many nontraditional couples end up thriving for decades. How do they move past the stigmas, ridicule and rejection to build some of the most enduring unions?

The answer lies in a kind of emotional trifecta. First, somewhere amid the prejudice, resentment and doubt they face, they find a support system that sustains them and confirms their relationship; second, like Romeo and Juliet, they discover an us-against-them inner strength that defies all naysayers; third, they simply stand the test of time, until both they and those who doubted them come to be believers.

The Glue That Binds

The question is: Why do it—especially with all the extra stress from such disapproval? Why begin a romance with so many strikes against you?

Certainly, physical attraction can override social concerns. Floridians Ken and Sara Benjamin were immediately drawn to one another at a computer conference 18 years ago, even though she had just turned 40 (a blond, young-looking 40) and he was only 24. "I thought she was an attractive female with great legs," he remembers. "But I also felt something deeper almost immediately. I wanted something much more than a one-night stand."

For some nontraditional couples, friendship comes first. Steven and Joyce Boro, a Jewish-American married to a black emigrant from Dominica, were roommates and buddies at Brooklyn College in New York well before they became involved. "We knew one another a full year first," says Steven. "We hung out, hitchhiked around together

Steven and Joyce Boro, Portland, Oregon

Couples on the margins of society may discover that a relationship frowned on in one locale is encouraged elsewhere. For Steven and Joyce Boro, a white Jewish man and a black Caribbean woman, that meant moving their show west—far from the disapproving eyes of family and friends in New York—to a commune. "I'd mainly dated white guys, but I never brought them to meet my mother," says Joyce. "It was probably intentional, because I wanted to avoid the racial issue with her. And Steven's mother thought blacks were the scum of the earth." By moving to the commune, they simultaneously limited their contact with their parents and gained a network of supportive friends. Ultimately they moved to Portland, where they raised their two children and have remained happily married for more than 30 years. Of course, like all interracial couples, they have been subject to some negative scrutiny. "Just the other day, I got angry looks from a black guy when we were walking together in Seattle," says Steven. "We've had our share of looks from whites, too. But none of that means anything to me. I've never really seen Joyce's color. It looks good on her, though."

Steven Pearl and Gino Grenek, Brooklyn, New York

Steven, a 40-year-old editor, and Gino, a 33-year-old dancer, finish each other's sentences with an edgy intimacy. They met at a party six years ago, felt an instant simpatico and attraction, and soon became a pair. Today they share an apartment in Brooklyn and consider themselves official domestic partners even if New York rejects same-sex marriage. This barrier notwithstanding, Steven and Gino find New York City especially accepting ("It's not Brokeback Mountain out here," Gino says)—so much so that their greatest relationship challenges come not from their same-sex status but from religion and involvement with work. Steven is Jewish, while Gino is Russian Orthodox. Both come from observant families. "We have learned to celebrate these differences and participate in each other's rituals," Steven explains. Gino travels with his troupe, while Steven works regular hours as an editor. "I told him that dance comes first and he comes second, but I've softened a bit on that," Gino states. According to Steven, the one complexity that may rear its head in the future involves having a family. "A lot of gay men and women don't often think of themselves as having children," he comments, "and to some degree I've internalized that." Yet, growing their family is something they consider. Says Gino, "If we decide to have a family I think we'll both be fantastic fathers and role models for our kids."

and became good friends before anything romantic happened. I always felt good being with her."

While relatives usually react badly at first to these unions, in some cases family acceptance launches the relationship. Stephanie, a young Chinese-American from California, who planned a career in medicine, met Juan, a poor construction worker, in a little town in Honduras when she was serving as a Peace Corps health worker. His family was the initial glue; Stephanie actually met them first, when Juan was working out of town. His mother, a coworker, kept inviting her home. "He has a big family, with 10 brothers and sisters, and lots of cousins, and they interact every day. They were all so nice, and kind of adopted me."

By the time Juan arrived on the scene, she was already a fixture. "We never really dated, we just spent a lot of time together," she recalls.

Vive La Difference

Marginalized couples come together for many of the same reasons as other couples. But the very extremity of their differences may give their relationship an extra dimension. "The primary thing people look for in relationships is to expand themselves," asserts Arthur Aron, psychologist at the State University of New York at Stony Brook. "Those we grow close to become part of who we are, widening our social resources and our perspective. We want someone different from ourselves to increase our efficacy and range of influence. If you're black and they're white, if you're older and they're younger, if you're one nationality and they're another, you've expanded your knowledge and opportunities."

The more you and your partner differ, the better—until the stress exceeds the thrill.

As a same-sex couple fairly close in age, Allison and Madeleine clearly don't have these kinds of disparities. But their personalities couldn't be more different. Allison is a free-spirited artist, Madeleine a meticulous software expert. Allison is comfortable living hand to mouth, while Madeleine thrives on the security of a lucrative career; Allison is assertive and public about being gay, displaying her pictures online with other lesbian artists; Madeleine likes to keep her sexual orientation off the radar. "When I met Allison, she would blatantly flirt with me so that everyone knew she had a crush on me, and I was horrified," Madeleine says.

The more radical your choices in a partner, the better—until the stress exceeds the thrill. "The key to a successful relationship is the tension between similar and opposite," says Aron. "Difference increases excitement and resources, but similarity ups the chance of maintaining the relationship long-term."

Allison's free-spiritedness and openness (as well as a slinky black dress) helped win Madeleine over, while Madeleine's intelligence, seriousness and solidity did the trick for Allison. Ultimately they learned that despite major personality differences, they had lots in common.

Coming to the Crossroads

The tension between commonality and difference eventually brings most nontraditional couples to a crossroads. Families' and communities' initial reactions reflect age-old cultural fears of letting the invaders in, of polluting and depleting the race. That's why, for example, Hasidic Jewish families traditionally hold funerals when a family member marries outside the faith.

Faced with such strong disapproval, even the happiest partners experience serious reservations early on, which can lead to moments of reckoning. Purdue University social psychologists Justin Lehmiller and Christopher Agnew have shown that at the start, nontraditional couples invest less of themselves in their relationships and are less committed than traditional couples, probably for this very reason.

Differences increase excitement, but similarity ups the chance of maintaining the relationship long-term.

Steven Boro, whose father (a Holocaust survivor) and mother were appalled that he was dating a black woman, simply set off without Joyce, hitching around the U.S. and Canada the moment he graduated from college, though Joyce and he had been involved for months. He had no plans of coming back. "I was committed not to her but to what I saw as my 'spiritual journey,'" Steven recalls. "Really I was floating like a leaf on a stream. On my 22nd birthday, I vowed that I wouldn't marry until I was 30 and that I'd never have kids.'"

It took Joyce to save the relationship. When she received a letter from Steven that he had settled on a commune in the Washington wilderness—and was involved with another woman there—she sought out his brother

Ken and Sara Benjamin, Taverna, Florida

When Ken and Sara were dating 18 years ago, they faced problems: Ken wanted to marry, but Sara was twice divorced. Ken, then 24, was interested in having children, but Sara, then 40, already had two going off to college, "I liked marriage, but I was at the end of child-rearing and wanted to stretch my wings," Sara recalls. Adding insult to injury, people kept mistaking Sara for Ken's mother.

They found a unique way to solve their dilemmas: They backpacked around the world for two years. "I wouldn't say we went on the trip to escape the problems," says Sara. "We just needed to get into a neutral area to work things out." They went to India and Nepal, stayed in hostels and hiked mountains. "In these places, where people's life spans were very contracted, we would tell people we were a couple, and they would respond flat out: 'That's not possible; she's too old," remembers Ken.

There was no escaping the issues, but the longer they were together, the more they loved one another. So they compromised: On their return, Sara agreed to marry Ken and he passed up having children. "I didn't want children as a concept, I just wanted her children," says Ken. In fact, it all worked out. "Even though I'm only five years older than Sara's daughter, she needed support and I was glad to fill that role."

Fred to help her go after her boyfriend. "I hadn't been in this country that long, and I was still very naive. I didn't even know what a commune was, and I almost headed for Washington, D.C.,'" says Joyce. "Fred put me on the right bus. I was still in school, and I thought I was going for the weekend, but it took me four days just to cross the country."

"Halfway there, in Nebraska, she called to tell me she was coming," says Steven. "I was really happy. I told her the other relationship was over."

Neither of them ever came back. They settled, along with 30 other people, on 120 acres of rolling hills and forests. Within a few weeks, their commune friends began suggesting they get married. "'You look so good together. You're such a great couple,' they kept telling us," says Steven. "I thought about it, and I realized they were right. Joyce was wonderful. So I said sure." Two months later, they were married. Three decades later, their two grown children are now out on their own, and the couple no longer live on the commune.

"Despite investing less in their relationship at first, marginalized partners ultimately tend to be significantly more committed than nonmarginalized couples," Lehmiller notes.

Tracie and Leo Auguste, Miami, Florida

Tracie Auguste, 30, is Chinese, and her husband, Leo, 31, is Haitian—but cultural and racial differences have never stood in their way. One reason: At North Miami Senior High, where they met when she was a junior and he a senior, they were simply fellow minority students in the multicultural melting pot that was their school. "People might have noticed if Tracie were white," comments Leo, "but we were both minorities and no one batted an eye." Even their families were accepting. "Leo's family wouldn't have cared if I was purple, they loved me like a daughter," says Tracie. Though Tracie's parents were more standoffish, they have heartily embraced Leo since the arrival of the couple's two children, ages four and one. By living and working in Miami (he's a carpenter and she's an assistant policy director for the mayor of Miami Dade) Leo and Tracie have continued to escape stigma. Leo is mindful, however, of the judgments his children may face. "America still teaches us to view people based on appearance," he says. "The best thing we can do for our children is to teach them to be proud of who they are."

Stephanie and Juan Carlos Valderramos, Bronx, New York

Serving as a Peace Corps volunteer in Honduras in 1998, Stephanie, an educated Chinese-American, was "adopted" by the family of a friendly coworker who happened to have a son named Juan. "I didn't have a TV, so I'd go to their house after work and watch it there. I had most of my meals there, "Stephanie recalls. Meeting Juan in the bosom of his nurturing family showed her just what she was getting, and their relationship took off.

To outsiders, they seemed mismatched: Stephanie had already applied to medical school, while Juan, who needed to work to pay the bills, was still in high school. But the differences didn't bother them. "Juan is really smart. We talk about everything—at first in Spanish, now more in English—and he always has an opinion," says Stephanie, who notes that Juan served as her cultural guide during their time in Honduras. Juan concurs: "I'm proud of who I am, and I liked her the way she was. If she wanted to be with me, it made no difference that she had more money or education."

Stephanie now works as a physician and Juan is studying at Bronx Community College and plans to become an environmental engineer.

Family Feuds

Often it takes every bit of that commitment for these couples to survive the extreme pressures their families impose on them; no other stressor is typically as great.

Like Steven and Joyce, Stephanie and Juan came to a crossroads relatively early in their relationship, in their case because of issues with *both* families. It started when Stephanie's Peace Corps stint was ending. She had to return home, and though she and Juan had been together a year and a half, he wasn't ready to go with her.

"Stephanie meant a lot to me, but I didn't want to leave my family," he says. They weren't dying to lose him either, even though they loved Stephanie. His parents were divorced. As the oldest brother, Juan was seen as "Papi" at home. So Stephanie headed back to the States thinking the relationship was over.

They kept communicating, though, and soon realized they missed each other too badly to stay apart. Juan applied for a fiance visa, and that's when the trouble with Stephanie's father began.

When he learned she was planning to marry Juan, he felt disrespected. He pointed to all the egregious differences between her and Juan: She was Chinese-American, he was Hispanic; she had been raised Buddhist, he was Catholic; she was a well-off medical school candidate, and he hadn't completed high school. What's more, Juan didn't speak English. "He's just using you to get a green card," her father said. When Stephanie married Juan and moved with him to the Bronx, New York, her father didn't talk to her for years.

Stephanie lived with a pang in her heart for her lost family. "I was with Juan for three and a half years before my family met him, and I'd never spoken to my father in all that time. I've always been close to my family, so it was awful," she says. "Juan is such a good, honest man, such a gentle soul, that I knew they would love him if they ever met him."

Marginalized partners ultimately tend to be significantly more committed than mainstream couples.

Finally, the couple was invited home one Christmas, and the response to Juan was everything Stephanie had hoped for: Her father was nice to him from the moment he met him. And after five years of marriage, Juan, now preparing to become an environmental engineer, has shown that he deserved the trust Stephanie always placed in him.

The advent of children typically brings a whole new level of familial turmoil to marginalized couples, as the in-laws are now involved. For the Boros, for instance,

Advice for the Rest of Us

Nontraditional couples who make it have a lot to teach us. Here's what we can learn from their success.

- The more you trust your gut instinct and the more comfortable you feel in your own skin, the less outsiders will be able to interfere.
- When partners bring different skills to a relationship, they enhance each other's positions in the world.
- You may be attracted to your opposite, but if you want the relationship to last, you need lots in common as well.
- Don't let outside disapproval of your partner determine the way you feel about him or her.
- Extended family or a close circle of friends can nurture your relationship.
- Friends and family who initially disapprove may change their minds as your relationship stands the test of time. But accept the possibility that they may not. Be prepared to reduce contact and forge new ties with others.
- If in-laws interfere in your relationship or take a strong stance on how you must raise your children, it may be time to limit their role.
- If you can deal with it together as a team, adversity will strengthen the relationship.
- Traditional couples can enhance their bonds by introducing exciting challenges. Climbing a mountain or building a company together can spice up the love.

Steven's mother was a continual irritant whenever she visited, "as much because Joyce wasn't Jewish as because she was black," Steven explains. "She was concerned about what faith the children would be raised in." Joyce recalls, "She'd tell my friends how disappointed she was that Steven was married to me, and though she grew to love the kids very much she felt embarrassed to be seen with them because they were dark."

When the World Rushes In

While families cause the most havoc, the censure of the world contributes its own share of trouble. The mixed-race Boro children, for instance, received some of the same rejection in school that they got from their grandmother. Trying to give the kids an ethnic identity and please Steven's parents, Joyce had converted to Judaism and enrolled the children in Jewish schools, but the schools never fully accepted them. Feeling rejected by Jewish people, they've committed themselves to black culture and are exclusively dating African-Americans. "But the black community tends to see them as white and hasn't embraced them either," Joyce says.

Partners with wide age differences experience a subtler form of marginalization, but social pressures can still be great. While they're not discriminated against in housing or social services, and not barred from marrying as gays are, they may make their families, friends and neighbors uneasy, and are often the butt of insulting misunderstandings or jokes.

"It's so nice that you brought your mother with you" is a typical comment that Ken, now 42, hears about his 58-year-old wife Sara. In the early days of their relationship it bothered them, but they had larger hurdles to worry about: Sara was reluctant to marry for a third time, and Ken had to accept that they might never have a biological child. (Sara was already the mother of teenagers.) Three years ago, Sara had a stroke that left her weak on her left side, in need of a cane and prone to epilepsy-related blackout seizures. "I can't imagine any physical infirmity that would test my commitment. The stroke is a life challenge, not a relationship challenge," says Ken.

Ever since, they have remained so secure in their relationship that rude comments roll off their backs. "We always understood we were abnormal in society's eyes," Sara says, "but what anybody else thinks about our relationship is far less important to us than the relationship itself."

"She's the love of my life," Ken says.

Staying the Course

In their research, Lehmiller and Agnew found that the key reason most marginal couples stayed together was not deep satisfaction in their relationships, but a sense of limited alternatives. In other words, they didn't think they could do better, so they settled for what they had.

But when told about these findings, the couples we interviewed couldn't have disagreed more.

"Joyce and I have been blessed to be as close as we are, and I can't imagine any couple being closer," asserts Steven Boro. "That sounds conceited," chides Joyce. "But we are extremely close."

"I liked and learned from my first two husbands, but neither was my soulmate," says Sara.

Having settled for less is the furthest thing from these couples' minds.

"Lehmiller and Agnew argue that people who stay in marginalized relationships feel they have worse options, but I'm not fully convinced," says Douglas T. Kenrick, Ph.D., professor of evolutionary psychology at Arizona State University. "We all make trade-offs. Maybe these couples just happened to land on partners who were well worth the trade-offs." You might not automatically put a poor construction worker from Honduras on your checklist of potential partners, but then you run into him and he has a wealth of other characteristics that are wonderful to you. If you have confidence in your feelings, you see that instinct through.

In fact, the chance to be true to yourself may be one of the greatest surprises—and rewards—of these relationships.

"You find a lot of freedom at the margins," says Joshua Gamson, a Jew married to a biracial man. "When you're at the center of society, you feel forced to obey the norms.

Marginalized couples have a lot of disadvantages, but since they're already outcasts in a sense, they're far freer to do what they really want, to put on their own show and be purely themselves."

MARK TEICH, a freelance writer living in Connecticut, has written for *Sports Illustrated, Redbook* and other magazines.

From *Psychology Today,* September/October 2006, pp. 88–95. Copyright © 2006 by Sussex Publishers, LLC. Reprinted by permission.

Girl or Boy?

As Fertility Technology Advances, So Does an Ethical Debate

DENISE GRADY

If people want to choose their baby's sex before pregnancy, should doctors help?

Some parents would love the chance to decide, while others wouldn't dream of meddling with nature. The medical world is also divided. Professional groups say sex selection is allowable in certain situations, but differ as to which ones. Meanwhile, it's not illegal, and some doctors are already cashing in on the demand.

There are several ways to pick a baby's sex before a woman becomes pregnant, or at least to shift the odds. Most of the procedures were originally developed to treat infertility or prevent genetic diseases.

The most reliable method is not easy or cheap. It requires in vitro fertilization, in which doctors prescribe drugs to stimulate the mother's ovaries, perform surgery to collect her eggs, fertilize them in the laboratory and then insert the embryos into her uterus.

Before the embryos are placed in the womb, some doctors will test for sex and, if there are enough embryos, let the parents decide whether to insert exclusively male or female ones. Pregnancy is not guaranteed, and the combined procedures can cost $20,000 or more, often not covered by insurance. Many doctors refuse to perform these invasive procedures just for sex selection, and some people are troubled by what eventually becomes of the embryos of the unwanted sex, which may be frozen or discarded.

Another method, used before the eggs are fertilized, involves sorting sperm, because it is the sperm and not the egg that determines a baby's sex. Semen normally has equal numbers of male- and female-producing sperm cells, but a technology called MicroSort can shift the ratio to either 88 percent female or 73 percent male. The "enriched" specimen can then be used for insemination or in vitro fertilization. It can cost $4,000 to $6,000, not including in vitro fertilization.

MicroSort is still experimental and available only as part of a study being done to apply for approval from the Food and Drug Administration. The technology was originally developed by the Agriculture Department for use in farm animals, and it was adapted for people by scientists at the Genetics and IVF Institute, a fertility clinic in Virginia. The technique has been used in more than 1,000 pregnancies, with more than 900 births so far, a spokesman for the clinic said. As of January 2006 (the most recent figures released), the success rate among parents who wanted girls was 91 percent, and for those who wanted boys, it was 76 percent.

Regardless of the method, the American College of Obstetricians and Gynecologists opposes sex selection except in people who carry a genetic disease that primarily affects one sex. But allowing sex selection just because the parents want it, with no medical reason, may support "sexist practices," the college said in an opinion paper published this month in its journal, Obstetrics and Gynecology.

Some people say sex selection is ethical if parents already have one or more boys and now want a girl, or vice versa. In that case, it's "family balancing," not sex discrimination. The MicroSort study accepts only people who have genetic disorders or request family balancing (they are asked for birth records), and a company spokesman said that even if the technique was approved, it would not be used for first babies.

The obstetricians group doesn't buy the family-balance argument, noting that some parents will say whatever they think the doctor wants to hear. The group also says that even if people are sincere about family balance, the very act of choosing a baby's sex "may be interpreted as condoning sexist values."

Much of the worry about this issue derives from what has happened in China and India, where preferences for boys led to widespread aborting of female fetuses when ultrasound and other tests made it possible to identify them. China's one-child policy is thought to have made matters worse. Last month, Chinese officials said that 118 boys were born for every 100 girls in 2005, and some reports have projected an excess of 30 million males in less than 15 years. The United Nations opposes sex selection for nonmedical reasons, and a number of countries have outlawed it, including Australia, Canada and Britain, and other nations in Asia, South America and Europe. Left unanswered is the question of whether societies, and families, that favor boys should just be allowed to have them, since attitudes are hard to change, and girls born into such environments may be abused.

The American Society for Reproductive Medicine, a group for infertility doctors, takes a somewhat more relaxed view of sex selection than does the college of obstetricians. Instead of opposing sex selection outright, it says that in people who already need in vitro fertilization and want to test the embryos' sex without a medical reason, the testing should "not be encouraged." And those who don't need in vitro fertilization but want it just for sex selection "should be discouraged," the group says.

But sperm sorting is another matter, the society says. It is noninvasive and does not involve discarding embryos of the "wrong" sex. The society concludes that "sex selection aimed at increasing gender variety in families may not so greatly increase the risk of harm to children, women or society that its use should be prohibited or condemned as unethical in all cases." The group also says it may eventually be reasonable to use sperm sorting for a first or only child.

Dr. Jamie Grifo, the program director of New York University's Fertility Center, said that he opposed using embryo testing just for sex selection, but that it was reasonable to honor the request in patients who were already having embryos screened for medical reasons, had a child and wanted one of the opposite sex. In those cases, he said, the information is already available and doesn't require an extra procedure.

"It's the patient's information, their desire," he said. "Who are we to decide, to play God? I've got news for you, it's not going to change the gender balance in the world. We get a handful of requests per year, and we're doing it. It's always been a controversy, but I don't think it's a big problem. We should preserve the autonomy of patients to make these very personal decisions."

Dr. Jeffrey M. Steinberg, from Encino, Calif., who has three clinics that offer sex selection and plans to open a fourth, in Manhattan, said: "We prefer to do it for family balancing, but we've never turned away someone who came in and said, 'I want my first to be a boy or a girl.' If they all said a boy first, we'd probably shy away, but it's 50-50."

"Reproductive choice, as far as I'm concerned, is a very personal issue," Dr. Steinberg said. "If it's not going to hurt anyone, we go ahead and give them what they want."

Many patients come from other countries, he said. John A. Robertson, a professor of law and bioethics at the University of Texas, said: "The distinction between doing it for so-called family balancing or gender variety would be a useful line to draw at this stage of the debate, just as maybe a practice guideline, and let's just see how it works out."

In the long run, Mr. Robertson said, he doubted that enough Americans would use genetic tests to skew the sex balance in the population, and he pointed out that so far, sperm sorting was more successful at producing girls than boys.

He concluded, "I think this will slowly get clarified, and people will see it's not as big a deal as they think."

From *The New York Times*, February 6, 2007. Copyright © 2007 by The New York Times Company. Reprinted by permission via PARS International.

Is Pornography Adultery?

Ross Douthat

The marriage of Christie Brinkley and Peter Cook collapsed the old-fashioned way in 2006, when she discovered that he was sleeping with his 18-year-old assistant. But their divorce trial this summer was a distinctly Internet-age affair. Having insisted on keeping the proceedings open to the media, Brinkley and her lawyers served up a long list of juicy allegations about Cook's taste in online porn: the $3,000 a month he dropped on adult Web sites, the nude photos he posted online, the user names he favored ("happyladdie2002," for instance, and "wannasee-all") while surfing swinger sites, even the videos he supposedly made of himself masturbating.

Perhaps the most interesting thing about the porn-related revelations, though, was the ambiguity about what line, precisely, Cook was accused of having crossed. Was the porn habit a betrayal in and of itself? Was it the financial irresponsibility that mattered most, or the addictive behavior it suggested? Was it the way his habit had segued into other online activities? Or was it about Cook's fitness as a parent, and the possibility that their son had stumbled upon his porn cache? Clearly, the court and the public were supposed to think that Cook was an even lousier husband than his affair with a teenager might have indicated. But it was considerably less clear whether the porn habit itself was supposed to prove this, or whether it was the particulars—the monthly bill, the swinger sites, the webcam, the danger to the kids—that made the difference.

The notion that pornography, and especially hard-core pornography, has *something* to do with marital infidelity has been floating around the edges of the American conversation for a while now, even as the porn industry, by some estimates, has swollen to rival professional sports and the major broadcast networks as a revenue-generating source of entertainment. A 2002 survey of the American Academy of Matrimonial Lawyers suggests that Internet porn plays a part in an increasing number of divorce cases, and the Brinkley-Cook divorce wasn't the first celebrity split to feature porn-related revelations. In 2005, at the start of their messy divorce, Denise Richards accused Charlie Sheen of posting shots of his genitalia online and cultivating a taste for "barely legal" porn sites. Two years later, Anne Heche,

Ellen DeGeneres's ex, accused her non-celeb husband of surfing porn sites when he was supposed to be taking care of their 5-year-old son. The country singer Sara Evans's 2006 divorce involved similar allegations, including the claim that her husband had collected 100 nude photographs of himself and solicited sex online.

But the attention paid to the connection between porn and infidelity doesn't translate into anything like a consensus on what that connection is. Polls show that Americans are almost evenly divided on questions like whether porn is bad for relationships, whether it's an inevitable feature of male existence, and whether it's demeaning to women. This divide tends to cut along gender lines, inevitably: women are more likely to look at pornography than in the past, but they remain considerably more hostile to porn than men are, and considerably less likely to make use of it. (Even among the Internet generation, the split between the sexes remains stark. A survey of American college students last year found that 70 percent of the women in the sample never looked at pornography, compared with just 14 percent of their male peers; almost half of the men surveyed looked at porn at least once a week, versus just 3 percent of the women.)

One perspective, broadly construed, treats porn as a harmless habit, near-universal among men, and at worst a little silly. This is the viewpoint that's transformed adult-industry icons like Jenna Jameson and Ron Jeremy from targets of opprobrium into C-list celebrities. It's what inspires fledgling stars to gin up sex tapes in the hope of boosting their careers. And it's made smut a staple of gross-out comedy: rising star funnyman Seth Rogen has gone from headlining Judd Apatow's *Knocked Up,* in which his character's aspiration to run a pornographic website was somewhat incidental to the plot, to starring in Kevin Smith's forthcoming *Zack and Miri Make* a Porno, in which the porn business promises to be rather more central.

A second perspective treats porn as a kind of gateway drug—a vice that paves the way for more-serious betrayals. A 2004 study found that married individuals who cheated on their spouses were three times as likely to have used Internet pornography as married people who hadn't committed adultery. In Tom Perrotta's bestselling *Little Children,* the female protagonist's husband—who is himself being cuckolded—progresses from obsessing over an online porn star named "Slurry Kay" to sending away for her panties to joining a club of fans who pay to vacation with her in person. Brinkley's husband may have followed a similar trajectory, along with many of the other porn-happy celebrity spouses who've featured in the gossip pages and divorce courts lately.

Maybe it's worth sharpening the debate. Over the past three decades, the VCR, on-demand cable service, and the Internet have completely overhauled the ways in which people interact with porn. Innovation has piled on innovation, making modern pornography a more immediate, visceral, and personalized experience. Nothing in the long history of erotica compares with the way millions of Americans experience porn today, and our moral intuitions are struggling to catch up. As we try to make sense of the brave new world that VHS and streaming video have built, we might start by asking a radical question: Is pornography use a form of adultery?

Nothing in the history of erotica compares with the way Americans experience porn today, and our moral intuitions are struggling to catch up.

The most stringent take on this matter comes, of course, from Jesus of Nazareth: "I tell you that anyone who looks at a woman lustfully has already committed adultery with her in his heart." But even among Christians, this teaching tends to be grouped with the Gospel injunctions about turning the other cheek and giving would-be robbers your possessions—as a guideline for saintliness, useful to Francis of Assisi and the Desert Fathers but less helpful to ordinary sinners trying to figure out what counts as a breach of marital trust. Jimmy Carter's confession to *Playboy* that he had "lusted in [his] heart" still inspires giggles three decades later. Most Americans, devout or secular, are inclined to distinguish lustful thoughts from lustful actions, and hew to the *Merriam-Webster* definition of adultery as "voluntary sexual intercourse between a married man and someone other than his wife or between a married woman and someone other than her husband."

On the face of things, this definition would seem to let porn users off the hook. Intercourse, after all, involves physicality, a flesh-and-blood encounter that Internet Explorer and the DVD player can't provide, no matter what sort of adultery the user happens to be committing in his heart.

But there's another way to look at it. During the long, latewinter week that transformed the governor of New York, Eliot Spitzer, into an alleged john, a late-night punch line, and finally an ex-governor, there was a lively debate on blogs and radio shows and op-ed pages about whether prostitution ought to be illegal at all. Yet amid all the chatter about whether the FBI should have cared about Spitzer's habit of paying for extramarital sex, next to nobody suggested, publicly at least, that *his wife* ought not to care—that Silda Spitzer ought to have been grateful he was seeking only sexual gratification elsewhere, and that so long as he was loyal to her in his mind and heart, it shouldn't matter what he did with his penis.

Start with the near-universal assumption that what Spitzer did in his hotel room constituted adultery, and then ponder whether Silda Spitzer would have had cause to feel betrayed if the FBI probe had revealed that her husband had paid merely to *watch* a prostitute perform sexual acts while he folded himself into a hotel armchair to masturbate. My suspicion is that an awful lot of people would say yes—not because there isn't some distinction between the two acts, but because the distinction isn't morally significant enough to prevent both from belonging to the zone, broadly defined, of cheating on your wife.

You can see where I'm going with this. If it's cheating on your wife to watch while another woman performs sexually in front of you, then why isn't it cheating to watch while the same sort of spectacle unfolds on your laptop or TV? Isn't the man who uses hard-core pornography already betraying his wife, whether or not the habit leads to anything worse? (The same goes, of course, for a wife betraying her husband—the arguments in this essay should be assumed to apply as well to the small minority of women who use porn.)

Fine, you might respond, but there are betrayals and then there are betrayals. The man who lets his eyes stray across the photo of Gisele Bündchen, bare-assed and beguiling on the cover of *GQ,* has betrayed his wife in some sense, but only a 21st-century Savonarola would describe that sort of thing as adultery. The line that matters is the one between fantasy and reality—between the call girl who's really there having sex with you, and the porn star who's selling the *image* of herself having sex to a host of men she'll never even meet. In this reading, porn is "a fictional, fantastical, even allegorical realm," as the cultural critic Laura Kipnis described it in the mid-1990s—"mythological and hyperbolic" rather than realistic, and experienced not as a form of intercourse but as a "popular-culture genre" like true crime or science fiction.

This seems like a potentially reasonable distinction to draw. But the fantasy-versus-reality, pixels-versus-flesh binary feels more appropriate to the pre-Internet landscape than to one where people spend hours every day in entirely virtual worlds, whether they're accumulating "friends" on Facebook, acting out Tolkienesque fantasies in World of Warcraft, or flirting with a sexy avatar in Second Life. And it feels much more appropriate to the tamer sorts of pornography, from the increasingly archaic (dirty playing cards and pinups, smutty books and the *Penthouse* letters section) to the of-the-moment (the topless photos and sex-scene stills in the more restrained precincts of the online pornosphere), than it does to the harder-core material at the heart of the porn economy. Masturbating to a *Sports Illustrated* swimsuit model (like Christie Brinkley, once upon a time) or a *Playboy* centerfold is a one-way street: the images are intended to provoke fantasies, not to embody reality, since the women pictured aren't having sex for the viewer's gratification. Even strippers, for all their flesh-and-blood appeal, are essentially fantasy objects-depending on how you respond to a lap dance, of course. But hard-core pornography is real sex by definition, and the two sexual acts involved—the on-camera copulation, and the masturbation it enables—are interdependent: neither would happen without the other. The whole point of a centerfold is her unattainability, but with hard-core porn, it's precisely the reverse: the star isn't just attainable, she's already being attained, and the user gets to be in on the action.

Moreover, the way the porn industry is evolving reflects the extent to which the Internet subverts the fantasy-reality dichotomy. After years of booming profits, the "mainstream" porn studios are increasingly losing ground to start-ups and freelancers—people making sex videos on their beds and sofas and shag carpeting and uploading them on the cheap. It turns out that, increasingly, Americans don't want porn as a "kind of science fiction," as Kipnis put it—they want realistic porn, porn that resembles the sex they might be having, and porn that at every moment holds out the promise that they can join in, like Peter Cook masturbating in front of his webcam.

So yes, there's an obvious line between leafing through a *Playboy* and pulling a Spitzer on your wife. But the line between Spitzer and the suburban husband who pays $29.95 a month to stream hard-core sex onto his laptop is considerably blurrier. The suburbanite with the hard-core porn hookup is masturbating to real sex, albeit at a DSL-enabled remove. He's experiencing it in an intimate setting, rather than in a grind house alongside other huddled masturbators in raincoats, and in a form that's customized to his tastes in a way that mass-market porn like *Deep Throat and Debbie Does Dallas* never was. There's no emotional connection, true—but there presumably wasn't one on Spitzer's part, either.

This isn't to say the distinction between hiring a prostitute and shelling out for online porn doesn't matter; in moral issues, every distinction matters. But if you approach infidelity as a continuum of betrayal rather than an either/or proposition, then the Internet era has ratcheted the experience of pornography much closer to adultery than I suspect most porn users would like to admit.

I t's possible, of course, to consider hard-core porn use a kind of infidelity and shrug it off even so. After all, human societies have frequently made sweeping accommodations for extramarital dalliances, usually on the assumption that the male libido simply can't be expected to submit to monogamy. When apologists for pornography aren't making Kipnis-style appeals to cultural transgression and sexual imagination, they tend to fall back on the defense that it's pointless to moralize about porn, because men are going to use it anyway.

Here's Dan Savage, the popular Seattle-based sex columnist, responding to a reader who fretted about her boyfriend's porn habit—"not because I'm jealous," she wrote, "but because I'm insecure. I'm sure many of those gifts are more attractive than me":

> All men look at porn . . . The handful of men who claim they don't look at porn are liars or castrates. Tearful discussions about your insecurities or your feminist principles will not stop a man from looking at porn. That's why the best advice for straight women is this: GET OVER IT. If you don't want to be with someone who looks at porn . . . get a woman, get a dog, or get a blind guy . . . While men shouldn't rub their female partners' noses in the fact that they look at porn—that's just inconsiderate—telling women that the porn "problem" can be resolved through good communication, couples counseling, or a chat with your pastor is neither helpful nor realistic.

Savage's perspective is hardly unique, and is found among women as well as men. In 2003, three psychology professors at Illinois State University surveyed a broad population of women who were, or had been, in a relationship with a man who they knew used pornography. About a third of the women described the porn habit as a form of betrayal and infidelity. But the majority were neutral or even positively disposed to their lover's taste for smut, responding slightly more favorably than not to prompts like "I do not mind my partner's pornography use" or "My partner's pornography use is perfectly normal."

This point of view—that looking at pornography is a "perfectly normal" activity, one that the more-judgmental third of women need to just stop whining about—has been strengthened by the erosion of the second-order arguments against the use of porn, especially the argument that it feeds misogyny and encourages rape. In the great porn debates of the 1980s, arguments linking porn to violence against women were advanced across the ideological spectrum.

Feminist crusaders like Andrea Dworkin and Catharine MacKinnon denounced smut as a weapon of the patriarchy; the Christian radio psychologist (and future religious-right fixture) James Dobson induced the serial killer Ted Bundy to confess on death row to a pornography addiction; the Meese Commission on Pornography declared, "In both clinical and experimental settings, exposure to sexually violent materials has indicated an increase in the likelihood of aggression." It all sounded plausible—but between 1980 and 2004, an era in which porn became more available, and in more varieties, the rate of reported sexual violence *dropped,* and by 85 percent. Correlation isn't necessarily causation, but the sharpness of the decline at least suggests that porn may reduce sexual violence, by providing an outlet for some potential sex offenders. (Indeed, the best way to deter a rapist might be to hook him up with a high-speed Internet connection: in a 2006 study, the Clemson economist Todd Kendall found that a 10 percent increase in Internet access is associated with a 7 percent decline in reported rapes.)

And what's true of rapists could be true of ordinary married men, a porn apologist might argue. For every Peter Cook, using porn *and* sleeping around, there might be countless men who use porn as a substitute for extramarital dalliances, satisfying their need for sexual variety without hiring a prostitute or kicking off a workplace romance.

Like Philip Weiss's friends, for instance. In the wake of the Spitzer affair, Weiss, a New York-based investigative journalist, came closer than any mainstream writer to endorsing not only the legalization of prostitution but the destigmatization of infidelity, in a rambling essay for *New York* magazine on the agonies that monogamy imposes on his buddies. Amid nostalgia for the days of courtesans and concubines and the usual plaints about how much more sophisticated things are in Europe, Weiss depicted porn as the modern man's "common answer" to the marital-sex deficit. Here's one of his pals dilating on his online outlets:

> "Porn captures these women [its performers] before they get smart," he said in a hot whisper as we sat in Schiller's Liquor Bar on the Lower East Side. Porn exploited the sexual desires, and naiveté, of women in their early twenties, he went on . . . He spoke of acts he observed online that his wife wouldn't do. "It's painful to say, but that's your boys' night out, and it takes an enlightened woman to say that."

The use of the term *enlightened* is telling, since the strongest argument for the acceptance of pornography—and the hard-core variety in particular—is precisely that it represents a form of sexual progress, a more civilized approach to the problem of the male libido than either the toleration of mass prostitution or the attempt, from the Victorian era onward, to simultaneously legislate prostitution away and hold married couples to an unreasonably high standard of fidelity. Porn may be an evil, this argument goes, but it's the least of several evils. The man who uses porn is cheating sexually, but he isn't involving himself in an emotional relationship. He's cheating in a way that carries none of the risks of intercourse, from pregnancy to venereal disease. And he's cheating with women who may be trading sex for money, but are doing so in vastly safer situations than streetwalkers or even high-end escorts.

Indeed, in a significant sense, the porn industry looks like what advocates of legalized prostitution hope to achieve for "sex workers." There are no bullying pimps and no police officers demanding sex in return for not putting the prostitutes in jail. There are regular tests for STDs, at least in the higher-end sectors of the industry. The performers are safely separated from their johns. And freelancers aren't wandering downtown intersections on their own; they're filming from the friendly confines of their homes.

If we would just accept Dan Savage's advice, then, and *get over it,* everyone would gain something. Weiss and his pals could have their "boys' night out" online and enjoy sexual experiences that their marriages deny them. The majority of wives could rest secure in the knowledge that worse forms of infidelity are being averted; some women could get into the act themselves, either solo or with their spouse, experiencing the thrill of a threesome or a '70s key party with fewer of the consequences. The porn industry's sex workers could earn a steady paycheck without worrying about pimps, police, or HIV. Every society lives with infidelity in one form or another, whether openly or hypocritically. Why shouldn't we learn to live with porn?

Live with it we almost, certainly will. But it's worth being clear about what were accepting. Yes, adultery is inevitable, but it s never been universal in the way that pornography has the potential to become—at least if we approach the use of hard-core porn as a normal outlet from the rigors of monogamy, and invest ourselves in a cultural paradigm that understands this as something all men do and all women need to live with. In the name of providing a low-risk alternative for males who would otherwise be tempted by "real" prostitutes and "real" affairs, we're ultimately universalizing, in a milder but not all that much milder form, the sort of degradation and betrayal that only a minority of men have traditionally been involved in.

Go back to Philip Weiss's pal and listen to him talk: *Porn captures these women before they get smart . . . It's painful to say, but that's your boys' night out.* This is the language of a man who has accepted, not as a temporary lapse but as a permanent and necessary aspect of his married life, a paid sexual relationship with women other than his wife. And it's the language of a man who has internalized a view of marriage as a sexual prison, rendered bearable only by frequent online furloughs with women more easily exploited than his spouse.

Calling porn a form of adultery isn't about pretending that we can make it disappear. The temptation will always be there, and of course people will give in to it. I've looked at porn; if you're male and breathing, chances are so have you. Rather, it's about what sort of people we aspire to be: how we define our ideals, how we draw the lines in our relationships, and how we feel about ourselves if we cross them. And it's about providing a way for everyone involved, men and women alike—whether they're using porn or merely tolerating it—to think about what, precisely, they're involving themselves in, and whether they should reconsider.

The extremes of anti-porn hysteria are unhelpful in this debate. If the turn toward an "everybody does it" approach to pornography and marriage is wrong, it's because that approach is wrong in and of itself, not because porn is going to wreck society, destroy the institution of marriage, and turn thousands of rapists loose to prey on unsuspecting women. Smut isn't going to bring down Western Civilization any more than Nero's orgies actually led to the fall of Rome, and a society that expects near-universal online infidelity may run just as smoothly as a society that doesn't.

Which is precisely why it's so easy to say that the spread of pornography means that we're just taking a turn, where sex and fidelity are concerned, toward realism, toward adulthood, toward sophistication. All we have to give up to get there is our sense of decency.

Ross Douthat, an Atlantic senior editor, blogs at rossdouthat .theatlantic.com

From *The Atlantic,* October 2008. Copyright © 2008 by Ross Douthat. Reprinted by permission of the author.

UNIT 7

Preventing and Fighting Disease

Unit Selections

Key Points to Consider

- What is the relationship between obesity and diabetes (Type 2)?

- What are the lifestyle changes that you can make to reduce your risk of developing cardiovascular disease, cancer, diabetes, and AIDS?

- Why are people still dying from AIDS?

- Should all young girls be vaccinated against HPV? What are the risks vs. the benefits of this vaccination?

Student Website
www.mhcls.com

Internet References

American Cancer Society
   http://www.cancer.org
American Diabetes Association Home Page
   http://www.diabetes.org
American Heart Association
   http://www.amhrt.org
National Institute of Allergy and Infectious Diseases (NIAID)
   http://www3.niaid.nih.gov/

Cardiovascular disease and cancer are the leading killers in this country. This is not altogether surprising given that the American population is growing increasingly older, and one's risk of developing both of these diseases is directly proportional to one's age. Another major risk factor, which has received considerable attention over the past 30 years, is one's genetic predisposition or family history. Historically, the significance of this risk factor has been emphasized as a basis for encouraging at-risk individuals to make prudent lifestyle choices, but this may be about to change as recent advances in genetic research, including mapping the human genome, may significantly improve the efficacy of both diagnostic and therapeutic procedures.

Just as cutting-edge genetic research is transforming the practice of medicine, startling new research findings in the health profession are transforming our views concerning adult health. This new research suggests that the primary determinants of our health as adults are the environmental conditions we experienced during our life in the womb. According to Dr. Peter Nathanielsz of Cornell University, conditions during gestation, ranging from hormones that flow from the mother to how well the placenta delivers nutrients to the tiny limbs and organs, program how our liver, heart, kidneys, and especially our brains function as adults. While it is too early to draw any firm conclusions regarding the significance of the "life in the womb factor," it appears that this avenue of research may yield important clues as to how we may best prevent or forestall chronic illness.

Of all the diseases in America, coronary heart disease is this nation's number one killer. Frequently, the first and only symptom of this disease is a sudden heart attack. Epidemiological studies have revealed a number of risk factors that increase one's likelihood of developing this disease. These include hypertension, a high serum cholesterol level, diabetes, cigarette smoking, obesity, a sedentary lifestyle, a family history of heart disease, age, sex, race, and stress. In addition to these well-established risk factors, scientists think they may have discovered several additional risk factors. These include the following: low birth weight, cytomegalovirus, *Chlamydia pneumoniae,* porphyromonasgingivalis, and c-reactive protein (CRP). CRP is a measure of inflammation somewhere in the body. In theory, a high CRP reading may be a good indicator of an impending heart attack. The article "The Battle Within" addresses research related to yet another possible link to heart disease.

One of the most startling and ominous health stories was the recent announcement by the Centers for Disease Control and Prevention (CDC) that the incidence of Type 2 adult onset diabetes increased significantly over the past 15 years. This sudden rise appears to cross all races and age groups, with the sharpest increase occurring among people aged 30 to 39 (about 70 percent). Health experts at the CDC believe that this startling rise in diabetes among 30- to 39-year-olds is linked to the rise in obesity observed among young adults (obesity rates rose from 12 to 20 percent nationally during this same time period). Experts at the CDC believe that there is a time lag of about 10–15 years between the deposition of body fat and the manifestation of Type 2 diabetes. This time lag could explain why individuals in their 30s are experiencing the greatest increase in developing Type 2 diabetes today. Current estimates suggest that 16 million Americans have

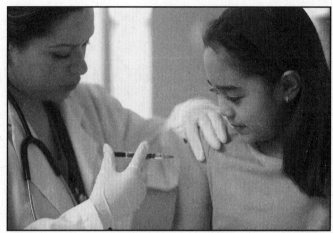

© Blend Images/Jupiterimages

diabetes; it kills approximately 180,000 Americans each year. Many experts now believe that our couch-potato culture is fueling the rising rates of both obesity and diabetes. Given what we know about the relationship between obesity and Type 2 diabetes, the only practical solution is for Americans to watch their total calorie intake and exercise regularly. "Diabesity, a Crisis in an Expanding Country" examines the rapid rise in the incidence of Type 2 diabetes among our youth and young adults, and suggests that the term "adult onset diabetes" may be a misnomer, given the growing number of young adults and teens with this form of diabetes.

Cardiovascular disease is America's number one killer, but cancer takes top billing in terms of the "fear factor." This fear of cancer stems from an awareness of the degenerative and disfiguring nature of the disease. Today, cancer specialists are employing a variety of complex agents and technologies, such as monoclonal antibodies, interferon, and immunotherapy, in their attempt to fight the disease. Progress has been slow, however, and the results, while promising, suggest that a cure may be several years away. A very disturbing aspect of this country's battle against cancer is the fact that millions of dollars are spent each year trying to advance the treatment of cancer, while the funding for the technologies used to detect cancer in its early stages is quite limited. A reallocation of funds would seem appropriate, given the medical community posits that early detection and treatment are the key elements in the successful cure of cancer. Until we have more effective methods for detecting cancer in the early stages our best hope for managing cancer is to prevent it through our lifestyle choices. The same lifestyle choices that may help prevent cancer can also help reduce the incidence of heart disease and diabetes.

Three articles address interesting issues: fighting disease among prison inmates, who still dies of AIDS, and the new vaccine to prevent cervical cancer. In the first, Susan Okie discusses the risky health behaviors that occur among inmates. These behaviors increase the risk of transmitting HIV. In the second article, Kate O'Beirne addresses the issue of the HPV vaccine and the questions that remain over who should be immunized. In the third piece, Gary Taubes discusses why the AIDS virus can still trump modern medicine and kill its victims.

'Diabesity,' a Crisis in an Expanding Country

Jane E. Brody

I can't understand why we still don't have a national initiative to control what is fast emerging as the most serious and costly health problem in America: excess weight. Are our schools, our parents, our national leaders blind to what is happening—a health crisis that looms even larger than our former and current smoking habits?

Just look at the numbers, so graphically described in an eye-opening new book, "Diabesity: The Obesity-Diabetes Epidemic That Threatens America—and What We Must Do to Stop It" (Bantam), by Dr. Francine R. Kaufman, a pediatric endocrinologist, the director of the diabetes clinic at Children's Hospital Los Angeles and a past president of the American Diabetes Association.

In just over a decade, she noted, the prevalence of diabetes nearly doubled in the American adult population: to 8.7 percent in 2002, from 4.9 percent in 1990. Furthermore, an estimated one-third of Americans with Type 2 diabetes don't even know they have it because the disease is hard to spot until it causes a medical crisis.

An estimated 18.2 million Americans now have diabetes, 90 percent of them the environmentally influenced type that used to be called adult-onset diabetes. But adults are no longer the only victims—a trend that prompted an official change in name in 1997 to Type 2 diabetes.

More and more children are developing this health-robbing disease or its precursor, prediabetes. Counting children and adults together, some 41 million Americans have a higher-than-normal blood sugar level that typically precedes the development of full-blown diabetes.

'Then Everything Changed'

And what is the reason for this runaway epidemic? Being overweight or obese, especially with the accumulation of large amounts of body fat around the abdomen. In Dr. Kaufman's first 15 years as a pediatric endocrinologist, 1978 to 1993, she wrote, "I never saw a young patient with Type 2 diabetes. But then everything changed."

Teenagers now come into her clinic weighing 200, 300, even nearly 400 pounds with blood sugar levels that are off the charts.

But, she adds, we cannot simply blame this problem on gluttony and laziness and "assume that the sole solution is individual change."

The major causes, Dr. Kaufman says, are "an economic structure that makes it cheaper to eat fries than fruit" and a food industry and mass media that lure children to eat the wrong foods and too much of them. "We have defined progress in terms of the quantity rather than the quality of our food," she wrote.

Her views are supported by a 15-year study published in January in The Lancet. A team headed by Dr. Mark A. Pereira of the University of Minnesota analyzed the eating habits of 3,031 young adults and found that weight gain and the development of prediabetes were directly related to unhealthful fast food.

Taking other factors into consideration, consuming fast food two or more times a week resulted, on average, in an extra weight gain of 10 pounds and doubled the risk of prediabetes over the 15-year period.

Other important factors in the diabesity epidemic, Dr. Kaufman explained, are the failure of schools to set good examples by providing only healthful fare, a loss of required physical activity in schools and the inability of many children these days to walk or bike safely to school or to play outside later.

Genes play a role as well. Some people are more prone to developing Type 2 diabetes than others. The risk is 1.6 times as great for blacks as for whites of similar age. It is 1.5 times as great for Hispanic-Americans, and 2 times as great for Mexican-Americans and Native Americans.

Unless we change our eating and exercise habits and pay greater attention to this disease, more than one-third of whites, two-fifths of blacks and half of Hispanic people in this country will develop diabetes.

It is also obvious from the disastrous patient histories recounted in Dr. Kaufman's book that the nation's medical structure is a factor as well. Many people do not have readily accessible medical care, and still many others have no coverage for preventive medicine. As a result, millions fall between the cracks until they are felled by heart attacks or strokes.

A Devastating Disease

There is a tendency in some older people to think of diabetes as "just a little sugar," a common family problem. They fail to take it seriously and make the connection between it and the costly, crippling and often fatal diseases that can ensue.

Diabetes, with its consequences of heart attack, stroke, kidney failure, amputations and blindness, among others, already ranks No. 1 in direct health care costs, consuming $1 of every $7 spent on health care.

Nor is this epidemic confined to American borders. Internationally, "we are witnessing an epidemic that is the scourge of the 21st century," Dr. Kaufman wrote.

Unlike some other killer diseases, Type 2 diabetes issues an easily detected wake-up call: the accumulation of excess weight, especially around the abdomen. When the average fasting level of blood sugar (glucose) rises above 100 milligrams per deciliter, diabetes is looming.

Abdominal fat is highly active. The chemical output of its cells increases blood levels of hormones like estrogen, providing the link between obesity and breast cancer, and decreases androgens, which can cause a decline in libido. As the cells in abdominal fat expand, they also release chemicals that increase fat accumulation, ensuring their own existence.

The result is an increasing cellular resistance to the effects of the hormone insulin, which enables cells to burn blood sugar for energy. As blood sugar rises with increasing insulin resistance, the pancreas puts out more and more insulin (promoting further fat storage) until this gland is exhausted. Then when your fasting blood sugar level reaches 126 milligrams, you have diabetes.

Two recent clinical trials showed that Type 2 diabetes could be prevented by changes in diet and exercise. The Diabetes Prevention Program Research Group involving 3,234 overweight adults showed that "intensive lifestyle intervention" was more effective than a drug that increases insulin sensitivity in preventing diabetes over three years.

The intervention, lasting 24 weeks, trains people to choose low-calorie, low-fat diets; increase activity; and change their habits. Likewise, the randomized, controlled Finnish Diabetes Prevention Study of 522 obese patients showed that introducing a moderate exercise program of at least 150 minutes a week and weight loss of at least 5 percent reduced the incidence of diabetes by 58 percent.

Many changes are needed to combat this epidemic, starting with schools and parents. Perhaps the quickest changes can be made in the workplace, where people can be encouraged to use stairs instead of elevators; vending machines can be removed or dispense only healthful snacks; and cafeterias can offer attractive healthful fare. Lunchrooms equipped with refrigerators and microwaves will allow workers to bring healthful meals to work.

Dr. Kaufman tells of a challenge to get fit and lose weight by Caesars Entertainment in which 4,600 workers who completed the program lost a total of 45,000 pounds in 90 days. Others could follow this example.

From *The New York Times,* March 29, 2005, 1 page. Copyright © 2005 by The New York Times Company. Reprinted by permission via PARS International.

Sex, Drugs, Prisons, and HIV

Susan Okie, MD

One recent morning at a medium-security compound at Rhode Island's state prison, Mr. M, a middle-aged black inmate, described some of the high-risk behavior he has witnessed while serving time. "I've seen it all," he said, smiling and rolling his eyes. "We have a lot of risky sexual activities. . . . Almost every second or minute, somebody's sneaking and doing something." Some participants are homosexual, he added; others are "curious, bisexual, bored, lonely, and . . . experimenting." As in all U.S. prisons, sex is illegal at the facility; as in nearly all, condoms are prohibited. Some inmates try to take precautions, fashioning makeshift condoms from latex gloves or sandwich bags. Most, however, "are so frustrated that they are not thinking of the consequences except for later," said Mr. M.

Drugs, and sometimes needles and syringes, find their way inside the walls. "I've seen the lifers that just don't care," Mr. M said. "They share needles and don't take a minute to rinse them." In the 1990s, he said, "needles were coming in by the handful," but prison officials have since stopped that traffic, and inmates who take illicit drugs usually snort or swallow them. Tattooing, although also prohibited, has been popular at times. "A lot of people I've known caught hepatitis from tattooing," Mr. M said. "They use staples, a nail . . . anything with a point."

Mr. M had just undergone a checkup performed by Dr. Josiah D. Rich, a professor of medicine at Brown University Medical School, who provides him with medical care as part of a long-standing arrangement between Brown and the Adult Correctional Institute in Cranston. Two years ago, Mr. M was hospitalized with pneumonia and meningitis. "I was scared and in denial," he said. Now, thanks to treatment with antiretroviral drugs, "I'm doing great, and I feel good," he reported. "I am HIV-positive and still healthy and still look fabulous."

U.S. public health experts consider the Rhode Island prison's human immunodeficiency virus (HIV) counseling and testing practices, medical care, and prerelease services to be among the best in the country. Yet according to international guidelines for reducing the risk of HIV transmission inside prisons, all U.S. prison systems fall short. Recognizing that sex occurs in prison despite prohibitions, the World Health Organization (WHO) and the Joint United Nations Program on HIV/AIDS (UNAIDS) have recommended for more than a decade that condoms be made available to prisoners. They also recommend that prisoners have access to bleach for cleaning injecting equipment, that drug-dependence treatment and methadone maintenance programs be offered in prisons if they are provided in the community, and that needle-exchange programs be considered.

Prisons in several Western European countries and in Australia, Canada, Kyrgyzstan, Belarus, Moldova, Indonesia, and Iran have adopted some or all of these approaches to "harm reduction," with largely favorable results. For example, programs providing sterile needles and syringes have been established in some 50 prisons in eight countries; evaluations of such programs in Switzerland, Spain, and Germany found no increase in drug use, a dramatic decrease in needle sharing, no new cases of infection with HIV or hepatitis B or C, and no reported instances of needles being used as weapons.[1] Nevertheless, in the United States, condoms are currently provided on a limited basis in only two state prison systems (Vermont and Mississippi) and five county jail systems (New York, Philadelphia, San Francisco, Los Angeles, and Washington, DC). Methadone maintenance programs are rarer still, and no U.S. prison has piloted a needle-exchange program.

The U.S. prison population has reached record numbers—at the end of 2005, more than 2.2 million American adults were incarcerated, according to the Justice Department. And drug-related offenses are a major reason for the population growth, accounting for 49% of the increase between 1995 and 2003. Moreover, in 2005, more than half of all inmates had a mental health problem, and doctors who treat prisoners say that many have used illicit drugs as self-medication for untreated mental disorders.

In the United States in 2004 (see table), 1.8% of prison inmates were HIV-positive, more than four times the estimated rate in the general population; the rate of confirmed AIDS cases is also substantially higher (see graph).[2] Some behaviors that increase the risk of contracting HIV and other bloodborne or sexually transmitted infections can also lead to incarceration, and the burden of infectious diseases in prisons is high. It has been estimated that each year, about 25% of all HIV-infected persons in the United States spend time in a correctional facility, as do 33% of persons with hepatitis C virus (HCV) infection and 40% of those with active tuberculosis.[3]

Critics in the public health community have been urging U.S. prison officials to do more to prevent HIV transmission, to improve diagnosis and treatment in prisons, and to expand programs for reducing high-risk behavior after release. The

HIV–AIDS among Prison Inmates at the End of 2004.*

Jurisdictions with the Most Prisoners Living with HIV–AIDS	No. of Inmates Living with HIV–AIDS	Prevalence of HIV–AIDS %
New York	4500	7.0
Florida	3250	3.9
Texas	2405	1.7
Federal system	1680	1.1
California	1212	0.7
Georgia	1109	2.2

*Data are from Maruschak.[2]

debate over such preventive strategies as providing condoms and needles reflects philosophical differences, as well as uncertainty about the frequency of HIV transmission inside prisons. The UNAIDS and WHO recommendations assume that sexual activity and injection of drugs by inmates cannot be entirely eliminated and aim to protect both prisoners and the public from HIV, HCV, and other diseases.

But many U.S. prison officials contend that providing needles or condoms would send a mixed message. By distributing condoms, "you're saying sex, whether consensual or not, is OK," said Lieutenant Gerald Ducharme, a guard at the Rhode Island prison. "It's a detriment to what we're trying to enforce." U.S. prison populations have higher rates of mental illness and violence than their European counterparts, which, some researchers argue, might make providing needles more dangerous. And some believe that whereas European prison officials tend to be pragmatic, many U.S. officials adopt a "just deserts" philosophy, viewing infections as the consequences of breaking prison rules.

Studies involving state-prison inmates suggest that the frequency of HIV transmission is low but not negligible. For example, between 1988—when the Georgia Department of Corrections began mandatory HIV testing of all inmates on entry to prison and voluntary testing thereafter—and 2005, HIV seroconversion occurred in 88 male inmates in Georgia state prisons. HIV transmission in prison was associated with men having sex with other men or receiving a tattoo.[4] In another study in a southeastern state, Christopher Krebs of RTI International documented that 33 of 5265 male prison inmates (0.63%) contracted HIV while in prison.[5] But Krebs points out that "when you have a large prison population, as our country does . . . you do start thinking about large numbers of people contracting HIV."

Studies of high-risk behavior in prisons yield widely varying frequency estimates: for example, estimates of the proportion of male inmates who have sex with other men range from 2 to 65%, and estimates of the proportion who are sexually assaulted range from 0 to 40%.[5] Such variations may reflect differences in research methods, inmate populations, and prison conditions that affect privacy and opportunity. Researchers emphasize that classifying prison sex as either consensual or forced is often overly simplistic: an inmate may provide sexual favors to another in

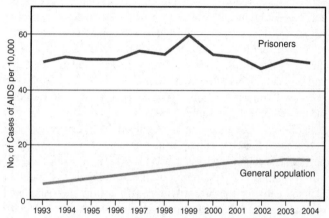

Rates of Confirmed AIDS Cases in the General Population and among State and Federal Prisoners, 1993–2004.

Data are from Maruschak.[2]

return for protection or for other reasons. Better information on sexual transmission of HIV in prisons may eventually become available as a result of the Prison Rape Elimination Act of 2003, which requires the Justice Department to collect statistics on prison rape and to provide funds for educating prison staff and inmates about the subject.

Theodore M. Hammett of the Domestic Health, Health Policy, and Clinical Research Division of Abt Associates, a Massachusetts-based policy research and consulting firm, acknowledged that for political reasons U.S. prisons are unlikely to accept needle-exchange programs, but he said adoption of other HIV-prevention measures is long overdue. "Condoms ought to be widely available in prisons," he said. "From a public health standpoint, I think there's little question that that should be done. Methadone, also—all kinds of drug [abuse] treatment should be much more widely available in correctional settings." Methadone maintenance programs for inmates have been established in a few jails and prisons, including those in New York City, Albuquerque, and San Juan, Puerto Rico. Brown University's Rich is currently conducting a randomized, controlled trial at the Rhode Island facility, sponsored by the National Institutes of Health, to determine whether starting methadone maintenance in heroin-addicted inmates a month before their release will lead to better health outcomes and reduced recidivism, as compared with providing either usual care or referral to community methadone programs at the time of release.

At the Rhode Island prison, the medical program focuses on identifying HIV-infected inmates, treating them, teaching them how to avoid transmitting the virus, addressing drug dependence, and when they're released, referring them to a program that arranges for HIV care and other assistance, including methadone maintenance treatment if needed. The prison offers routine HIV testing, and 90% of inmates accept it. One third of the state's HIV cases have been diagnosed at the prison. "These people are a target population and a captive one," noted Rich. "We should use this time" for health care and prevention. Nationally, 73% of state inmates and 77% of federal inmates surveyed in 2004 said they had been tested for HIV in prison. State policies vary, with 20 states reportedly testing all inmates and the rest offering tests for high-risk groups, at inmates' request, or in specific situations. Researchers said inmate acceptance rates also vary widely, depending on how the test is presented. Drugs for treating HIV-infected prisoners are not covered by federal programs, and prison budgets often contain inadequate funding for health services. "You can see how, in some cases, there could be a disincentive for really pushing testing," Hammett said.

Critics of U.S. penal policies contend that incarceration has exacerbated the HIV epidemic among blacks, who are disproportionately represented in the prison population, accounting for 40% of inmates. A new report by the National Minority AIDS Council calls for routine, voluntary HIV testing in prisons and on release, making condoms available, and expanding reentry programs that address HIV prevention, substance abuse, mental health, and housing needs as prisoners return to the community. "Any reservoir of infection that is as large as a prison would warrant, by simple public health logic, that we do our best . . . to reduce the risk of transmission" both inside and outside the walls, said Robert E. Fullilove of Columbia University's Mailman School of Public Health, who wrote the report. "The issue has never been, Do we understand what has to happen to reduce the risks? . . . It's always been, Do we have the political will necessary to put what we know is effective into operation?"

Notes

1. Dolan K, Rutter S, Wodak AD. Prison-based syringe exchange programmes: a review of international research and development. Addiction 2003;98:153–158.
2. Maruschak LM. HIV in prisons, 2004. Washington, DC: Bureau of Justice Statistics, November 2006.
3. Hammett TM, Harmon MP, Rhodes W. The burden of infectious disease among inmates of and releasees from US correctional facilities, 1997. Am J Public Health 2002;92:1789–1794.
4. HIV transmission among male inmates in a state prison system—Georgia, 1992–2005. MMWR Morb Mortal Wkly Rep 2006;55:421–6.
5. Krebs CP. Inmate factors associated with HIV transmission in prison. Criminology Public Policy 2006;5:113–36.

DR. OKIE is a contributing editor of the *Journal*.

From *The New England Journal of Medicine,* January 11, 2007, pp. 105–108. Copyright © 2007 by Massachusetts Medical Society. All rights reserved. Reprinted by permission.

The Battle Within
Our Anti-inflammation Diet

What do paper cuts, spicy foods, stubbed toes and intense workouts at the gym have to do with your odds of getting colon cancer, drifting into Alzheimer's or succumbing to a heart attack? A lot more than you might think.

The more scientists learn about these and other serious diseases, the more they are being linked with the long-term effects of inflammation on the body.

MICHAEL DOWNEY

The inflammation-disease connection has become a hot research topic. And it's about to explode.

Vital Nuisance

Inflammation is a vital immune response to infection, injury or irritation. It is the basis of humanity's earliest survival.

It's what causes the redness in that paper cut—the result of extra blood walling off the area and rushing macrophages, histamine and other bacteria-fighting immune factors to the wound.

The same inflammatory process is what makes your throat burn when you decide to impress your friends by chugging the extra-spicy suicide sauce—blood vessels leak fluid, proteins and cells to repair or remove damaged tissues. And fever is yet another form of that inflammatory burning.

Inflammation sparks the swelling in that stubbed toe—caused by fluid released into the banged-up cells to speed healing and cushion that toe against further injury.

It also causes that tenderness you feel after hours at the gym—because your immune system rushes fluids to the torn muscles to protect and repair them, compressing sensitive nerve endings in the process.

Inflammation isolates foreign invaders and rushes our strongest natural infection-fighters to the site deemed under attack. It cleans away debris from destroyed tissue; slows bleeding; starts clotting; and—if tissues cannot be restored—produces scar tissue. Without this sophisticated immune response, our species would have died out long ago.

Defensive Nutrition

- oily fish and fish oil supplements
- olive, walnut or flaxseed oil
- walnuts, flaxseeds and soy foods
- fruits and vegetables
- red wine
- antioxidant supplements
- garlic, ginger and turmeric (enreumin)
- sunflower seeds, eggs, herring, nuts or zinc tablets
- pineapple or bromelain supplements
- S-adenosyl-methionine (SAMe)

But it's a double-edged sword. In addition to its telltale redness, heat, swelling or pain, inflammation can cause serious dysfunction.

Problems begin when—for one reason or another—the inflammatory process becomes chronic, persisting long after it's needed.

Heart disease researchers were the first to notice that inflammation can play a role in cardiovascular disease.

Heart Mystery

Not long ago, doctors viewed heart disease as a plumbing problem. Cholesterol levels in the blood get too high, and, over the years, fatty deposits clog the pipes and cut off the blood supply.

There's just one problem with that explanation: Sometimes, it's dead wrong.

Half of all heart attacks occur in people with normal cholesterol levels and normal blood pressure. Something causes relatively minor deposits to burst, triggering massive clots that block the blood supply.

That something has turned out to be inflammation.

C-reactive protein (CRP)—a blood measure of inflammation—shoots up during an acute illness or infection. But CRP is also somewhat elevated among otherwise healthy people. And studies show that those with the highest CRP levels have three times the heart attack risk as those with the lowest levels. The inflammatory response, possibly reacting to cholesterol that has seeped into the lining of the artery, makes even normal fatty deposits unstable.

There are several causes of heart disease: smoking, high blood pressure and, yes, cholesterol. But we must now add inflammation to that list.

Runaway Reaction

Heart disease is just the tip of the inflammation iceberg. Studies over the past couple of years have suggested that higher CRP levels raise the risk of diabetes. It's too early to say whether lowering inflammation will keep diabetes from developing. But before insulin was isolated at the University of Toronto in the 1920s, doctors found that blood sugar levels could be decreased by using salicylates, a group of aspirin-like compounds known to reduce inflammation.

In the 1860s, German pathologist Rudolph Virchow speculated that cancerous tumors start at the site of chronic inflammation—basically, a wound that never heals. Then, in the middle of the 20th century, we came to understand the role of genetic mutations in cancerous tissue. Today, researchers are investigating the possibility that mutations and inflammation work together to turn normal cells into deadly tumors. Reducing chronic inflammation may yet become a prescription for keeping cancer at bay.

Researchers have found that people who take anti-inflammation medications—for arthritis, for example—succumb to Alzheimer's disease later in life more than those who don't. Plaque and tangles accumulate in the brains of Alzheimer's patients. Perhaps the immune system mistakenly sees these abnormalities as damaged tissue that should be eliminated. Early information suggests that low-dose aspirin and fish oil capsules—both known to reduce inflammation—lower the risk of Alzheimer's.

The cause of asthma is still unknown, but some suspect the inflammatory attack. The treatments that help relieve asthma work by reducing the inflammation involved.

Sometimes, for reasons that are not clear, perfectly healthy cells trigger the body's immune system. The inflammatory response is launched against normal cells in the joints, nerves, connective tissue or any part of the body. These autoimmune disorders include rheumatoid arthritis, multiple sclerosis, lupus, vitiligo, psoriasis and other versions of a body at war with itself. Even Crohn's disease and cystic fibrosis are associated with inflammation.

Some level of inflammatory immune reaction is usually present in our bodies, whether we're aware of it or not. And if inflammation really is the biological engine that drives many of our most feared illnesses, it suggests a new and possibly much simpler way of warding off disease. Instead of different treatments for all of these disorders, simply turning down the degree of our inflammatory attack might be a partial prevention for all of them.

Dampening the Fires

Many attributes of a Western lifestyle—such as a diet high in sugars and saturated fats, accompanied by little or no exercise—make it much easier for the body to become inflamed.

Losing weight helps because fat cells produce cytokines, which crank up inflammation. Thirty minutes a day of moderate exercise dampens the fire as well. Flossing your teeth combats gum disease, another source of chronic inflammation. And, of course, you should avoid excess alcohol intake and smoking.

Despite the injury they can do to the stomach, anti-inflammatory drugs such as aspirin and ibuprofen are often prescribed for treatment of inflammatory diseases, but they're not appropriate for prevention. Fish oil capsules have been shown to produce the same reduction in inflammatory cytokines.

Inflammation-promoting prostaglandins are made from the trans fats found in partially hydrogenated oils. So avoid margarines and vegetable shortenings that are made with them.

Getting a good supply of omega-3 fatty acids—and a minimum of omega-6 fats—is key to an immune system that's not overreactive. Opt for oily fish such as salmon, sardines, herring and mackerel; and on days that you don't have fish, take a fish oil supplement, eat walnuts, freshly ground flaxseeds or flaxseed oil and soy foods. Steer away from safflower, sunflower, corn and sesame oils, as well as polyunsaturated vegetable oils. Use walnut, flaxseed or extra virgin olive oils instead.

Fruits and vegetables are full of antioxidants that disable free radicals and minimize inflammation. All are good, but you should focus your diet on those that produce the highest antioxidant activity: blueberries and kiwi. Consider antioxidant supplements such as resveratrol, grape seed extract, quercetin, pycnogenol or citrus bioflavonoids, as well as beta-carotene and vitamins, C and E. And drink red wine in small quantities.

Garlic, ginger and turmeric are natural anti-inflammatory agents. Include them in your diet.

Zinc controls inflammation while promoting healing. It is found in sunflower seeds, eggs, nuts, wheat germ, herring and zinc supplements.

S-adenosyl-methionine (SAMe), alpha lipoic acid and coenzyme Q1O act as inflammation fighters. Also, bromelain—found in pineapple and supplements—may reduce inflammation.

So if you want to stop inflammation, get off that couch and head out to pick up oily fish, fresh produce, garlic and supplements. And try not to stub your toe on the way.

From *Better Nutrition*, February 2005, pp. 27–29. Copyright © 2005 by Michael Downey. Reprinted by permission of the author.

Who Still Dies of AIDS, and Why

In the age of HAART, the virus can still outwit modern medicine.

GARY TAUBES

In the video, filmed last November, Mel Cheren appears understandably dismayed. He's being interviewed by a reporter for CBS News on *Logo,* a gay-themed news program; he's sitting in a wheelchair, and he's talking about the indignity and the irony of dying from AIDS at a time when AIDS should be a chronic disease, not a fatal one. Cheren, a music producer and founder of West End Records, had been an AIDS activist since the earliest days of the epidemic. It was Cheren, in 1982, who gave the Gay Men's Health Crisis its first home, providing a floor of his brownstone on West 22nd Street. In the interview, Cheren talks about what it's like to lose more than 300 friends to the AIDS epidemic, outlive them all, and then get diagnosed yourself at age 74.

Indeed, the fact that Cheren had plenty of sex through the height of the epidemic, had been tested regularly, and had apparently emerged uninfected had led him to believe that testing was no longer necessary, or at least so one doctor had told him half a dozen years earlier. He's only learned the truth after he began losing weight, had trouble walking, and was finally referred to a specialist who didn't consider AIDS an unreasonable diagnosis for a man of Cheren's experience and advanced years and so ordered up the requisite blood test. "There was one guy," Cheren says in the interview, explaining how he might have been infected. A male escort. "We really hit it off, sexually . . ."

By the time Cheren learned he had AIDS, he was already suffering from a rare, drug-resistant pneumonia, what infectious-disease specialists refer to as an opportunistic infection, and he had lymphoma, an AIDS-related cancer that had spread to his bones.

Within a month of his diagnosis, Cheren was dead. The official cause was pneumonia, although, as his cousin Mark Cheren points out, cause of death in these cases is a moot point. "Infection from pneumonia was probably the culprit," he says, "but only because that acts quickest when you don't stop it."

Dying from AIDS, or dying with an HIV infection, which may not be the same thing, is a significantly less common event than it was a decade ago, but it's not nearly as uncommon as anyone would like. Bob Hattoy, for instance, died last year as well. Hattoy, 56, was "the first gay man with AIDS many Americans had knowingly laid eyes on," as *the New York Times* described

him after Hattoy announced his condition to the world in a speech at the 1992 Democratic National Convention. Hattoy went on the work in the Clinton White House as an advocate for gay and lesbian issues. In the summer of 1993, he told *the New York Times,* "I don't make real long-term plans." But the advent of an anti-retroviral drug known as a protease inhibitor, in 1995, and then, a year later multidrug cocktails called HAART—for highly active anti-retroviral therapy—gave Hattoy and a few hundred thousand HIV-infected Americans like him the opportunity to do just that.

If the pharmaceutical industry ever needed an icon for evidence of its good works, HAART would be it. Between 1995 and 1997, annual AIDS deaths in New York City dropped from 8,309 to 3,426, and that number has continued to decline ever since. The success of HAART has been so remarkable that it now tends to take us by surprise when anybody does succumb, although 2,076 New Yorkers died in 2006 (2007 figures are not yet available). Though many of the most prominent deaths, like Cheren's and Hattoy's, tend to be of gay men, the percentage of the dead who contracted the disease through gay sex is now reportedly as low as 15 percent (with a large proportion still reported as unknown). Intravenous-drug users make up the biggest group, 38.5 percent, and women account for almost one in three of total AIDS deaths.

One of the ironies of the success of HAART is that it has fostered the myth that the AIDS epidemic has come to an end, and that living with HIV is only marginally more problematic than living with herpes or genital warts. This is one obvious explanation for why HIV infection is once again on the rise among young men—specifically, MSMs, as they're now known in the public-health jargon, for men who have sex with men—increasing by a third between 2001 and 2006. Among those 30 and over, the infection rate is still decreasing, notes Thomas Frieden, commissioner of the city's Department of Health and Mental Hygiene, suggesting that the increased rate of infection among men under 30 is due in part to decreased awareness of the disease or the toll it can take.

"If you do the mathematics," Frieden says, "HAART became available in 1996. If you were of age before then, sexually active, and you saw a lot of people dying or sick or disfigured from AIDS, maybe you're more careful than if you came of age after 1996 and didn't see that. When we've done focus groups, what young men have told us is that the only thing they hear about HIV these days is that if you get it, you can climb mountains, like Magic Johnson. Certainly it's true that the treatment for HIV is very effective and it's possible to live a long and productive life with an HIV infection. It's also true that it remains an incurable infection. That the treatment is very arduous and sometimes unsuccessful. It remains a disease often fatal, and frequently disabling."

At the moment some 100,000 New Yorkers are infected with the HIV virus, and AIDS remains the third leading cause of death in men under 65, exceeded only by heart disease and cancer. The question of who will die from AIDS in the HAART era—or who dies with an HIV infection but not technically from AIDS—and what kills them is worth asking now that such deaths have become relatively infrequent.

Frieden's department of Health and Mental Hygiene tried to answer this question with a study it published in the summer of 2006. The newsworthy conclusions were that deaths among New Yorkers with AIDS were still dropping, thanks to HAART, and that one in four of these individuals was now living long enough to die of the same chronic diseases that are likely to kill the uninfected—particularly cancer or heart disease—although most of these non-HIV-related deaths were from the side effects of drug abuse. HIV-related illnesses were still responsible for the remaining three out of four deaths. Or at least "HIV disease," in these cases, was recorded as a cause of death on the death certificates.

What the Health Department study couldn't do is say precisely what these HIV-related deaths were. For the answer to this question, you have to go to physicians who specialize in treating HIV-infected patients. Michael Mullen, clinical director of infectious diseases at Mount Sinai School of Medicine, for instance, says the best way to think about AIDS deaths is to divide HIV-infected individuals into three groups.

The bulk of these deaths occur within the first group, those who either never started HAART to begin with or didn't stay on it once they did. For these patients, "it might as well still be the eighties," says Mullen, and they die from the same AIDS-defining illnesses that were the common causes of death twenty years ago-pneumocystis pneumonia, central-nervous system opportunistic infections (such as toxoplasmosis), lymphoma, Kaposi's sarcoma, etc.

A large proportion of these victims are indigent; many are intravenous-drug users—IVDUs, as they're known in the official jargon, accounted for 21 percent of HIV-positive New Yorkers in 2006, but, as noted above, 38.5 percent of the city's AIDS deaths. The virus is not more aggressive or virulent in these cases. Rather, these are the people who either don't or can't do what it takes to fight it. "These individuals are repeatedly admitted to the hospital," says Mullen, "sometimes for opportunistic infections, sometimes for drug-related issues, often for HIV-related lymphomas and malignancies. They will not take the medication, nine times out of ten, because of drug use." Often these individuals are co-infected with hepatitis, which increases the risk that the more toxic side effects of the antiretroviral drugs will lead to permanent liver or kidney damage.

By far the highest death rates in this group are in what the authorities now refer to as concurrent HIV/AIDS diagnoses. These patients never get diagnosed with HIV infection until they already have active AIDS. (Cheren, because of his age and his AIDS awareness, is an extreme case.) These constituted more than a quarter of the 3,745 new cases of HIV infections diagnosed in New York in 2006. "Those people have never been tested before," says Mullen. "Believe it or not, people like this still exist." Typically, they've had the infection for ten years—the average time between HIV infection and the emergence of AIDS—but won't know it or acknowledge it until admitted to the emergency room with pneumonia or some other opportunistic infection. These individuals are twice as likely to die in the three to four years after their diagnosis as someone who was just diagnosed with HIV alone. Half of these deaths will occur in the first four months after diagnosis, often from whatever AIDS-related ailment led them to the emergency room in the first place.

It's because of these concurrent HIV/AIDS diagnoses that the Centers for Disease Control and Prevention and the city's Department of Health and Mental Hygiene have been lobbying for HIV tests to be given routinely to anyone who visits an emergency room for any reason. In one recent study from South Carolina, almost three out of four of those people with concurrent HIV/AIDS diagnoses had visited a medical facility after their infection and prior to getting their blood tested for the virus—averaging six visits each before they were finally tested and diagnosed. "By remaining untested during their routine contacts with the health-care system," said Frieden, in testimony to the New York State Assembly Committee on Health, "they have missed the high-quality treatment that could improve their health and extend their lives. Many may have unknowingly infected their partners—and these partners may not learn that they are infected until they too are sick with AIDS. And so this cycle of death continues."

The second group of HIV-infected patients consists of those at the other extreme, the ones who are least likely to die from AIDS or its complications. These individuals were diagnosed with HIV after the advent of HAART and have taken their medications religiously ever since. In these cases, HAART is likely to suppress their virus for decades, and they're now significantly more likely to die of heart disease or cancer than of anything related to AIDS. To get an idea of the mortality rate among these patients, consider Alexander McMeeking's practice, on East 40th Street. McMeeking ran the HIV clinic at Bellevue from 1987 to 1989 and then left to start a private practice. To the best of his knowledge, only three of his 300-odd Bellevue patients survived long enough to get on HAART. They are still alive today. "Fortunately, thank God, all three are doing great," says McMeeking. "I tell them they will essentially die of old age."

McMeeking's practice now includes 600 HIV-infected patients, and last year he lost only two of those—one to lung cancer, another to liver cancer.

Now the question is whether these patients doing well with HAART are actually more susceptible to the kind of chronic diseases that kill the uninfected. Are they more likely to die from heart disease, cancers, liver and kidney failure, and other chronic diseases either because of the HIV itself or the anti-retroviral regimen keeping it under control? One observation made repeatedly in studies—including the 2006 report from the Department of Health and Mental Hygiene—is that these HIV-infected individuals appear to have higher rates of several different cancers, in particular lung cancer among smokers, non-Hodgkins lymphoma, and cancers of the rectal area. These cancers appear both more precocious and more aggressive in HIV-infected patients—they strike earlier and kill quicker. The reason is not yet clear, although a likely explanation is that the ability of the immune system to search out and destroy incipient malignancies is sufficiently compromised from either the anti-retroviral drugs, the virus, or the coexistence of several viruses—squamous-cell cancers of the rectal area are caused by the same human papilloma virus that causes cervical cancer in woman—that the cancers get a foothold they don't get in non-HIV-infected individuals.

One finding that's considered indisputable is that HAART, and particularly the protease inhibitors that are a critical part of the anti-retroviral cocktail, can play havoc with risk factors for heart disease. They raise cholesterol and triglyceride levels; they lower HDL, and they can cause increased resistance to the hormone insulin. These changes often accompany a condition known as HIV-related lipodystrophy, which afflicts maybe half of all individuals who go on HAART. Subcutaneous fat is lost on the face, arms, legs, and buttocks, while fat accumulates in the gut, upper back (a condition known as a buffalo hump), and breasts. The question is whether these metabolic disturbances actually increase the likelihood of having a heart attack. It's certainly reasonable to think they would, but it's remarkably difficult to demonstrate that the drugs or the virus itself is responsible: The fact that a relatively young man or woman with AIDS has a heart attack does not mean that the heart attack was caused by HIV or the disturbance in cholesterol and lipid levels induced by the therapy.

"If it's 1988, 1989," says one doctor, "and I have a patient with HIV disease and hypertension, he's not going to live long enough to die of hypertension. I want to treat the disease."

Any difference in disease incidence between HIV-infected and uninfected individuals, explains John Brooks, leader of the clinical-epidemiology team within the CDC's Division of HIV/AIDS Prevention, can be due to the infection itself, to the therapy—HAART—or to "the host, the person who has HIV infection, both physiologically and socioculturally." It's the last factor—the host—that complicates the science. Until recently, for instance, physicians saw little reason to worry about heart-disease risk factors in their HIV-infected patients and so didn't bother to aggressively treat risk factors in those patients, as they did the HIV-negative. "Think about it," says Brooks, "if it's

1988, 1989, and I have a patient with HIV disease and hypertension, he's not going to live long enough to die of hypertension. I want to treat the disease."

The rate of cigarette smoking among HIV-infected individuals is also twice as high as the national average. The rate of intravenous drug use is far higher, as is the rate of infection with hepatitis B or C, because intravenous drug use is a common route to getting both HIV and hepatitis. So the fact that an HIV-infected patient may seem to be suffering premature heart disease, diabetes, or liver or kidney disease earlier than seems normal for the population as a whole—or the fact that a study reports such a finding about a population of HIV-infected individuals—only raises the issue of whether the population as a whole is the relevant comparison group. "Since one of the major risk factors for HIV is intravenous drug use," says Brooks, "you have to ask, what's the contribution of heroin to somebody's kidney disease versus the HIV versus untreated high blood pressure versus smoking?"

"I still expect most of my patients to live a normal life expectancy," says an AIDS doctor, "but they may do so with a bit more nips and scrapes."

From his own clinical experience, McMeeking agrees that heart disease, certain cancers, and liver and kidney disease do seem to pose a greater threat to his HIV-infected patients than might otherwise be expected in a comparable uninfected population. "I still expect most of my patients to live a normal life expectancy," he says, "but they may do so with a bit more nips and scrapes."

The third group of HIV-infected individuals consists of those in the middle of the two extremes. HAART, in these cases, has literally been a life saver, but has not guaranteed a normal life expectancy. These are the patients, like Bob Hattoy, who were diagnosed with AIDS in the late eighties or early nineties, before the advent of HAART. They began on one drug (AZT, for instance) and then stayed alive long enough to get on protease inhibitors and the HAART cocktails. These patients were on the cusp of the HIV transformation from a deadly to a chronic-disease epidemic; they were infected late enough to survive but too early to derive all the benefits from HAART.

The anti-retroviral drugs of HAART work by attacking the life cycle of the virus. The earliest generation of HAART drugs attacked the enzymes that the virus virus uses to reproduce in the cells. (Protease inhibitors, for instance, go after an enzyme called HIV-1 protease, which the virus uses to assemble itself during reproduction.) The latest drugs go after the methods that the virus uses to enter cells in which it will replicate. The key to the effectiveness of HAART, as researchers discovered in the mid-nineties, was to include at least three drugs in the cocktail to which the patient's specific virus had no resistance. This would suppress viral replication sufficiently so that the virus wouldn't be able to mutate fast enough to evolve resistance to any of the drugs. But patients who began on one or two anti-AIDS drugs and only then moved to HAART already had time to evolve resistance to a few of the drugs in the cocktail. This made the entire package less effective and increased the likelihood that they would evolve resistance to the other drugs as well.

"We call it 'sins of the past,'" says Mullen. "We gave these patients sequential monotherapy; it was state-of-the-art at the time, and a lot of those people are alive today because of that. It got them through until HAART came along, but their HAART is not highly active, only fairly active. Their virus has baseline mutations that interfere with the response." This group of patients also includes those who were infected initially with a strain of HIV already resistant to one or several of the components of HAART, or those patients who were less than 99 percent faithful in taking the regimen of pills that constitute HAART. Anything less than that and the virus has the opportunity to evolve resistance.

Perhaps a quarter of all new cases, says Mullen, are infected with a strain of the virus resistant to one or more drugs in the HAART cocktail. "You can't use the frontline regimen, because the virus has already seen those drugs," he says. "You have to go to more complicated regimens. This is why we do resistance testing before we start a person on medication. We see what drugs the virus has seen or is resistant to and can take that into account."

Sins-of-the-past patients have to have faith that the pharmaceutical industry can stay one step ahead of their disease. The prognosis, at the moment, is promising. There are several entirely new classes of AIDS drugs, including one by Merck, called an integrase inhibitor, that was just approved by the FDA last October. A recent report of the discovery of 270 new human proteins employed by the AIDS virus to hijack cells and start replicating—the definition of a successful infection—means the pharmaceutical industry will not run out of new targets to block the infection in the near future.

Still, some sins-of-the-past patients simply do worse than others, and the occasional patient will lose the battle before new drugs come along or simply give up. "I had a friend who died last week," one sins-of-the-past patient told me recently. "He just lost faith. He would get sick a lot, would get better, then sick again. Finally he decided to try Eastern medicine, and stopped taking his [HAART] medications entirely. It killed him. It's not a good example, other than to show that people can reach their breaking point."

From *New York Magazine*, June 16, 2008. Copyright © 2008 by New York Magazine. Reprinted by permission.

A Mandate in Texas

The Story of a Compulsory Vaccination and What It Means

Kate O'Beirne

On February 2, Texas became the first state to require that young girls be vaccinated against some sexually transmitted viruses. This happened when Gov. Rick Perry issued an executive order requiring that students receive a new vaccine before entering the sixth grade. Perry's order has met with criticism from state legislators who object to his unilateral action, medical groups that welcome the breakthrough vaccine but oppose a mandate, and parents who believe that such coercion usurps their authority. The vaccine's manufacturer is aggressively lobbying other state legislatures to back mandates, and legislation to require the new vaccine is pending in over a dozen states.

Last June, the Food and Drug Administration approved Merck & Co.'s Gardasil vaccine for females aged 9 to 26. When administered to girls before they become sexually active, the vaccine can protect against two of the strains of the human papillomavirus (HPV) that cause about 70 percent of cervical cancers. Within a few weeks of the approval, the vaccine was added to the federal list of recommended routine immunizations for eleven- and twelve-year-old girls. The duration of immunity for the three-dose vaccine series, at a cost of about $360, is not yet known. The federal, means-tested Vaccines for Children program will now include the HPV vaccine, and insurance companies are expected to begin covering its costs.

There is little controversy over the recommendation that the vaccine be broadly used. HPV is the most common sexually transmitted infection, with about half of those who are sexually active carrying it at some point in their lives and about 6.2 million infected annually. The number of sexual partners is the most important risk factor for genital HPV infection. There are no treatments to cure HPV infections, but most are cleared by the immune system, with 90 percent disappearing within two years. Some infections do persist, causing genital warts, cancers of the cervix, and other types of cancer. Each year, over 9,000 new cases of cervical cancer are diagnosed, and the disease kills 3,700 women. Routine Pap tests have dramatically reduced the incidence of cervical cancers over the past 50 years, and it is recommended that even those immunized with the new vaccine continue to be tested, as the vaccine doesn't guard against eleven other high-risk strains of HPV that cause cancer.

Governor Perry recognized that "the newly approved HPV vaccine is a great advance in the protection of women's health" in a "whereas" clause on the way to his "therefore" order that rules be adopted to "mandate the age appropriate vaccination of all female children for HPV prior to admission to the sixth grade." In turning a federal recommendation into a state mandate, Perry has thrilled the vaccine manufacturer, while acting against the balance of medical opinion. And critics object to an opt-out provision that puts the onus on parents to file an affidavit seeking approval of their objection.

The American College of Pediatricians opposes requiring the vaccination for school attendance, saying that such a mandate would represent a "serious, precedent-setting action that trespasses on the rights of parents to make medical decisions for their children as well as on the rights of the children to attend school." The chairman of the American Academy of Pediatrics Committee on Infectious Diseases, Dr. Joseph A. Bocchini, believes a vaccine mandate is premature. "I think it's too early," he said. "This is a new vaccine. It would be wise to wait until we have additional information about the safety of the vaccine." The Texas Medical Association also opposes the mandate, expressing concerns over liability and costs.

Mandatory-education laws create a responsibility to make sure that children are vaccinated against contagious diseases they might be exposed to at school. Now states are considering compelling vaccination in the name of a broad public good, even though the disease in question would not be spread at schools.

Dr. Jon Abramson, the chairman of the Advisory Committee on Immunization Practices of the Centers for Disease Control, explains that protecting children against a virus that is spread by sexual activity is different from preventing the spread of measles. Abramson believes that mandating the HPV vaccine "is a much harder case to make, because you're not going to spread it in a school unless you're doing something you're not supposed to be doing in school." Non-vaccinated students would pose no risk to others while at school.

Texas state senator Glenn Hegar has introduced legislation to reverse Governor Perry's order on the grounds that research trials are still underway and "such mandates take away parents' rights to make medical decisions for their children and usurp parental authority." Twenty-six of 31 state senators believe the governor has usurped legislative authority too, and are calling on him to rescind the executive order. Perry stands by the order, but the rising controversy has discouraged other supporters of mandates.

The *Washington Post* recently reported that Virginia and 17 other states are considering the vaccine requirement "at the urging of New Jersey—based pharmaceutical giant Merck & Co. . . . [which] stands to earn hundreds of millions of dollars annually on Gardasil, according to Wall Street estimates." Public-health organizations have joined Merck in urging that the vaccine be made available in public clinics and encouraging its coverage by private insurers, but they don't support Merck's push for a school requirement.

There were 210 cases of cervical cancer in Maryland last year. Democratic state senator Delores Kelley introduced a bill to require the HPV vaccine for sixth-grade girls. Following complaints from parents and recent non-compliance problems with current mandated vaccinations, Kelley has withdrawn her bill (though she has spoken openly of reintroducing it next session). She explains that she was unaware of Merck & Co.'s lobbying efforts, and that she learned about the new HPV vaccine through a nonpartisan group of female legislators called Women in Government. More than half of its listed supporters are pharmaceutical manufacturers or other health-related companies. Women in Government is spearheading the campaign to mandate the HPV vaccine through school requirements, and some watchdog groups question the support it receives from Merck & Co. "It's not the vaccine community pushing for this," explains the director of the National Network for Immunization Information. Governor Perry's critics point to his own connection with Gardasil's manufacturer: His former chief of staff is a lobbyist for Merck & Co. in Texas.

The profit motive of a company can coincide with public-health interests, but the case for an HPV-vaccine mandate has not been made. The new vaccine does not prevent cervical cancer, but is a welcome protection against some strains of HPV. It is already available to parents who can decide whether it is appropriate for their young daughters. In substituting his judgment for theirs, Governor Perry has attempted to intrude upon their prerogatives and responsibilities. He has also substituted his own judgment for expert medical opinion. State officials who follow his lead won't enjoy immunity from the firestorm of criticism they will rightly earn.

From *The National Review,* March 5, 2007. Copyright © 2007 by National Review, Inc, 215 Lexington Avenue, New York, NY 10016. Reprinted by permission.

UNIT 8

Health Care and the Health Care System

Unit Selections

Key Points to Consider

- Is health care just another commodity? Should it be treated differently from other consumer services?

- Is quality health care a right or a privilege? Defend your answer.

- What can you as an individual do to help reduce health care costs? Give specific actions that can be taken.

- Should pharmacists be permitted to refuse to fill certain prescriptions?

- How does illiteracy affect the status of health?

- Why are more and more doctors banning drug sales representatives from pitching their products in the office?

- Should there be limits on health care provided to the terminally ill?

Student Website

www.mhcls.com

Internet References

American Medical Association (AMA)
   http://www.ama-assn.org
MedScape: The Online Resource for Better Patient Care
   http://www.medscape.com

Americans are healthier today than they have been at any time in this nation's history. Americans suffer more illness today than they have at any time in this nation's history. Which statement is true? They both are, depending on the statistics you quote. According to longevity statistics, Americans are living longer today and, therefore, must be healthier. Still, other statistics indicate that Americans today report twice as many acute illnesses as did our ancestors 60 years ago. They also report that their pain lasts longer. Unfortunately, this combination of living longer and feeling sicker places additional demands on a health care system that, according to experts, is already in a state of crisis.

Despite the clamor about the problems with our health care system, if you can afford it, then the American health care system is one of the best in the world. However, being the best does not mean that it is without problems. Each year, more than half a million Americans are injured or die due to preventable mistakes made by medical care professionals. In addition, countless unnecessary tests are preformed that not only add to the expense of health care, but may actually place the patient at risk. Reports such as these fuel the fire of public skepticism toward the quality of health care that Americans receive.

While these aspects of our health care system indicate a need for repair, they represent just the tip of the iceberg. Daniel Callahan, in "Curbing Medical Costs," discusses the number of Americans who are uninsured and the problems they face. As the number continues to rise, Callahan calls for the government to develop a universal system that covers all. He believes that universal coverage will not only insure all Americans, but it will also help to reduce the cost of health care. Callahan also believes that costs continue to rise due to the blockage of price controls by the pharmaceutical industry.

Some doctors, hospitals, and medical schools are trying to deal with the high cost of medications. They are banning drug sales representatives from pitching their products. The doctors and hospital-based professions believe that sales personnel promote new, expensive drugs that may cause serious side effects, as well as increase the costs of medications. An unrelated pharmaceutical issue is presented in "Pharmacist Refusals: A Threat to Women's Health." It relates to pharmacists who refuse to fill prescriptions for certain medications that violate their personal beliefs. These typically include oral contraceptives and morning after pills, which some pharmacists believe cause abortions.

While choices in health care providers are increasing, paying for services continues to be a challenge as medical costs continue to rise. Why have health care costs risen so much? The answer to this question is multifaceted, and includes such factors as physicians' fees, hospital costs, insurance costs, pharmaceutical costs, and health fraud. It could be argued that while these factors operate within any health care system, the lack of a meaningful form of outcomes assessment has permitted and encouraged waste and inefficiency within our system. Ironically, one of the major factors for the rise in the cost of health care is our rapidly expanding aging population—tangible evidence of an improving health care delivery system. This is obviously one factor that we hope will continue to rise. Another significant

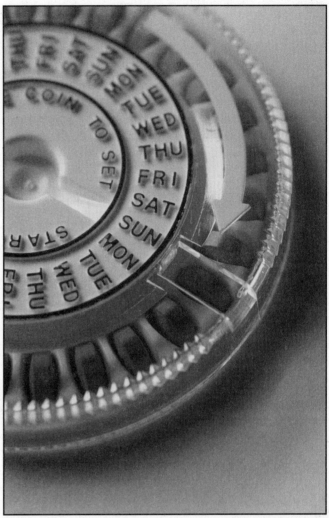

© Don Farrall/Getty Images

factor that is often overlooked is the constantly expanding boundaries of health care. It is somewhat ironic that as our success in treating various disorders has expanded, so has the domain of health care, and often into areas where previously health care had little or no involvement. "Incapacitated, Alone and Treated to Death" offers an interesting perspective of how the care and treatment of patients is often made independent of their wishes.

Traditionally, Americans have felt that the state of their health was largely determined by the quality of the health care available to them. This attitude has fostered an unhealthy dependence upon the health care system and contributed to the skyrocketing costs. It should be obvious by now that while there is no simple solution to our health care problems, we would all be a lot better off if we accepted more personal responsibility for our health. While this shift would help ease the financial burden of health care, it might necessitate a more responsible coverage of medical news, in order to educate and enlighten the public on personal health issues.

Pharmacist Refusals:
A Threat to Women's Health

Marcia D. Greenberger and Rachel Vogelstein

Pharmacist refusals to fill prescriptions for birth control based on personal beliefs have been increasingly reported around the world. In the United States, reports of pharmacist refusals have surfaced in over a dozen states. These refusals have occurred at major drugstore chains like CVS and Walgreens and have affected everyone from rape survivors in search of emergency contraception to married mothers needing birth control pills. Pharmacists who refuse to dispense also often have refused to transfer a woman's prescription to another pharmacist or to refer her to another pharmacy. Other pharmacists have confiscated prescriptions, misled women about availability of drugs, lectured women about morality, or delayed access to drugs until they are no longer effective.

Pharmacist refusal incidents have also been reported in other countries. For example, a pharmacist at a popular London pharmacy chain recently refused to fill a woman's prescription for emergency contraception (EC), or the "morning-after pill," due to religious beliefs; two pharmacists refused to fill contraceptive prescriptions for women at a pharmacy in Salleboeuf, France; and in the small country town of Merriwa, Australia, the local pharmacist refuses to stock EC altogether.[1-3] Pharmacists for Life International, a group refusing to fill prescriptions for contraception, currently claims to have over 1600 members worldwide and represents members in 23 countries.[4]

Pharmacist refusals can have devastating consequences for women's health. Access to contraception is critical to preventing unwanted pregnancies and to enabling women to control the timing and spacing of their pregnancies. Without contraception, the average woman would bear between 12 and 15 children in her lifetime. For some women, pregnancy can entail great health risks and even life-endangerment. Also, women rely on prescription contraceptives for a range of medical reasons in addition to birth control, such as amenorrhea, dysmenorrhea, and endometriosis. Refusals to fill prescriptions for EC (a form of contraception approved by the U.S. Food and Drug Administration and relied on worldwide) are particularly burdensome, as EC is an extremely time-sensitive drug. EC is most effective if used within the first 12 to 24 hours after contraceptive failure, unprotected sex, or sexual assault. If not secured in a timely manner, this drug is useless. Rural and low-income women, as well as survivors of sexual assault, are at particular risk of harm.

In the United States, most states have an implied duty to dispense. Personal beliefs are omitted from the enumerated instances where pharmacists are authorized to refuse; such as where the pharmacist has concerns about therapeutic duplications, drug-disease contraindications, drug interactions, incorrect dosage, or drug abuse. In New Hampshire, the pharmacy regulations' Code of Ethics states that a pharmacist shall "[h]old the health and safety of patients to be of first consideration and render to each patient the full measure of his/her ability as an essential health practitioner."[5] Pharmacists who refuse to fill valid prescriptions based on personal beliefs do not hold patient health and safety as their first consideration.

Illinois explicitly charges pharmacies with a duty to ensure that women's prescriptions for birth control are filled without delay or interference.[6] Massachusetts and North Carolina have interpreted their laws to ensure that women's access to medication is not impeded by pharmacists' personal beliefs.[7,8] However, Arkansas, Georgia, Mississippi, and South Dakota explicitly grant pharmacists the right to refuse to dispense prescriptions for birth control based on personal beliefs.[9]

In addition, a small number of administrative and judicial bodies have considered challenges to pharmacist refusals. In the United States, the Wisconsin pharmacy board found that a pharmacist's failure to transfer a birth control prescription fell below the expected standard of care and constituted a danger to the health and welfare of the patient. The board formally reprimanded the pharmacist for his actions, charged him with the $20,000 cost of adjudication, and conditioned his license on provision of proper notification to his employer about anticipated refusals and his assurances about steps he will take to protect patient access to medication.[10]

Outside of the United States, the European Court of Human Rights rejected an appeal of a conviction of pharmacists under the French consumer code for a refusal to sell contraceptive pills. The Court held that the right to freedom of religion does not allow pharmacists to impose their beliefs on others, so long as the sale of contraceptives is legal.[2]

Some have questioned how such rules comport with the treatment of other medical professionals. In general, medical professionals have a duty to treat patients, with only limited exceptions. The majority of refusal laws apply to doctors and nurses and are limited to abortion services. Allowing pharmacists to refuse to dispense prescriptions for contraception would dramatically expand the universe of permissible refusals. Moreover, unlike doctors and nurses, pharmacists do not select or administer treatments or perform procedures. Therefore, pharmacists' involvement is not as direct, nor would patients' safety be potentially compromised in the same way as would be the case if a doctor or nurse were forced to perform a procedure that they personally oppose.

Since 1997, 28 states have introduced legislation that would permit pharmacists to refuse to dispense, and sometimes to refer or transfer, drugs on the basis of moral or religious grounds. Fifteen states have introduced such bills in the 2005 legislative session alone; while some are specific to contraception, others apply to all medication. These bills have implications for future refusals to fill prescriptions, such as in HIV regimens or treatments derived from embryonic stem cell research. On the other hand, bills have been introduced in four state legislatures and the U.S. Congress that would require pharmacists or pharmacies either to fill prescriptions for contraception or ensure that women have timely access to prescription medication in their pharmacies.

Some professional and medical associations have issued guidelines that protect women against pharmacist refusals. Value VIII of the *Code of Ethics* of the College of Pharmacists of British Columbia requires pharmacists to ensure "continuity of care in the event of . . . conflict with moral beliefs."[11] It permits pharmacists to refuse to dispense prescriptions based on moral beliefs, but only if there is another pharmacist "within a reasonable distance or available within a reasonable time willing to provide the service."

In the United States, several associations have issued similar, although not legally binding, policies. The American Public Health Association states that "[h]ealth systems are urged to establish protocols to ensure that a patient is not denied timely access to EC based on moral or religious objections of a health care provider."[12] The American Medical Women's Association has stated that "pharmacies should guarantee seamless delivery, without delay (within the standard practice for ordering), judgment, or other interference, of all contraceptive drugs and devices lawfully prescribed by a physician."[13]

The American Pharmacists Association (APhA) articulates a standard of professionalism in its *Code of Ethics* that is not legally binding. It mandates that pharmacists place "concern for the well-being of the patient at the center of professional practice"[14]. The code also emphasizes that pharmacists are "dedicated to protecting the dignity of the patient" and must "respect personal and cultural differences . . ."[14] This language precludes refusals, lectures, and other barriers erected by pharmacists who disagree with a woman's decision, made in consultation with her health-care provider, to use birth control. Some state pharmacy associations have similar codes.

However, the APhA has another policy that conflicts with these principles. It allows for refusals based on personal beliefs, as long as pharmacists refer prescriptions to another pharmacist or pharmacy.[15] The APhA has not formally explained how to square this policy with its ethical principles of patient-protective care, let alone with state laws and regulations.

Recommendations

Women must be provided timely access to prescription medication. One solution is to require pharmacists to dispense all drugs despite their personal beliefs, in line with their professional duties and ethical obligations. Another solution is to shift the duty to fill from pharmacists onto pharmacies. Under this approach, pharmacies would be charged with ensuring that prescriptions for all drugs are filled without delay or other interference. Such a requirement would allow pharmacies to make arrangements to accommodate the personal beliefs of individual pharmacists. However, active obstruction by pharmacists of women's access to prescription medication—such as withholding or delaying prescriptions or providing misinformation—should be deemed unethical or unprofessional conduct subject to legal sanction.

References and Notes

1. "I Won't Sell Pill, It's Against My Religion," *Sunday Mirror* (27 February 2005).
2. Pichon and Sajous v. France, App. No. 49853/99, Eur. Court H.R. (2001).
3. "U.S. Firm Ships Free Contraceptives to Condom-Deprived Australian Town," *Financial Times,* 31 March 2005 [source: Agence France-Presse].
4. See www.pfli.org/main.php?pfli=locations.
5. N.H. Code Admin. R. Ph. 501.01(b)(1) (2005).
6. Illinois Pharmacy Practice Act, § 1330.91 (j)(1) (2005).
7. Massachusetts Board of Pharmacy, letter on file with the National Women's Law Center, 6 May 2004.
8. Conscience concerns in pharmacist decisions, *North Carolina Board Pharm. Newsl.* **26** (3), 1 (2005), 1; available as item 2061 at www.ncbop.org/Newsletters/NC012005.pdf.
9. Ark. Code. Ann. § 20-16-304 (1973); Ga. Comp. R. & Regs. r. 480-5-.03(n) (2001); Miss. Code. Ann. § 41-107-1 (2004); S.D. Codified Laws § 36-11-70 (1998).
10. See www.naralwi.org/assets/files/noesendecision &finalorder.pdf
11. See www.bcpharmacists.org/standards/ethicslong/
12. American Public Health Association (APHA), Policy statement 2003-15 (APHA, Washington, DC, 2003).
13. American Medical Women's Association (AMWA), Statement of AMWA supporting pharmacies' obligation to dispense birth control (Alexandria, VA, 2005) (on file with the National Women's Law Center).
14. See www.aphanet.org/AM/Template.cfm ?Section=Pharmacy_ Practice&CONTENTID=2903&TEMPLATE=/CM/ HTMLDisplay.cfm.
15. S. C. Winckler, American Pharmacists Association (1 July 2004) (letter to the editor, unpublished); available at www.aphanet.org/AM/Template.cfm? Section=Public_Relations&Template=/CM/HTML Display. cfm&ContentID=2689.

The authors are with the National Women's Law Center, Washington, DC 20036, USA. For correspondence, e-mail: rlaser@nwlc.org.

From *Science Magazine,* June 10, 2005, pp. 1557–1558. Copyright © 2005 by American Association for the Advancement of Science. Reprinted by permission.

Curbing Medical Costs

Daniel Callahan

It is no secret that the United States has a scandalously large number of uninsured people, now up to 47 million and growing. That number is vivid and evocative, but it has overshadowed a far more serious issue: the steady escalation of health care costs, currently increasing at an annual rate of 7 percent. As a consequence, it is projected that the Medicare program will be bankrupt in nine years and overall health care costs will rise from the present $2.1 trillion to $4 trillion in 10 years.

Those rising costs are an important reason why the number of uninsured people keeps going up. Businesses find it harder and harder to pay for employee health benefits, and only 61 percent of employers even provide them (from a high of close to 70 percent a decade ago). The employers who do provide benefits are cutting them and forcing employees to pay more in the form of co-payments and deductibles. The 15 percent of Americans who are uninsured are surely faced with both health and financial threats. The cost problem, however, now threatens everyone else as well, including those assisted by Medicare and Medicaid.

Universal care is the only tried and effective way to control costs. The European health care systems do so effectively by means of a strong government hand.

Yet even if most people are aware of the dangers of cost escalation—and many know it from personal experience—it has not gripped the public imagination, the presidential candidates or the media with the force of the problem of the uninsured (even though recent public opinion polls indicate it is catching up). Candidates and others have proposed a number of detailed plans for universal care, but nothing comparable for cost control. There is a reason for that.

The problem of the uninsured is the popular problem and the problem of cost control the unpopular one. The former is popular because it is easy to empathize with millions of people who cannot get decent care. Cost control, by contrast, is unpopular, or, perhaps more precisely put, it is dodged and evaded as if it were a nasty political virus to be avoided. Consider what serious cost control will require: moving from a 7 percent annual cost growth down to 3 percent—a rate of inflation for health

care costs that is no greater than the annual rise from general inflation. This amounts to a cost reduction of $1.5 trillion over the next 10 years, settling in at $2.5 trillion in a decade. That would represent an enormous and unprecedented drop in annual costs for a health care system that has never, since World War II, seen anything more than a short and temporary decline from time to time. But this will mean that just about everyone will be forced to give up something, obliged to accept a different, more austere kind of health care.

There are at bottom only three ways to deal with the high cost of health care. One of them is to increase revenues for the system. With government programs such as Medicare, this means raising taxes sharply; with private insurance it means raising premiums. Another approach is to cut benefits drastically, giving people less care. Still another way is to force individuals to pay more out of pocket for their care. Not one of these strategies, if openly embraced, could possibly become popular. They would just be different ways of inflicting pain.

Controlling Medical Technology

The feature of cost escalation that ought to catch our eye most is the role of medical technology. Health care economists estimate that 40 percent to 50 percent of annual cost increases can be traced to new technologies or the intensified use of old ones. That means that control of technology is the most important factor in bringing costs down. Technology also happens to be the most beloved feature of American medicine. Patients expect it; doctors are given extensive training to use it; the medical industries make billions of dollars selling it; and the media love to write about it. The economic and social incentives to develop and make it widely available are powerful, and the disincentives so far are weak and almost useless.

Even among economists and others who concede that technology plays a central role in the cost problem, there is considerable ambivalence about how to deal with it. Technological innovation is as fundamental a feature of American medicine as it is of our industrial sector. After all, innovation has given us vaccines, antibiotics, advanced heart disease care, splendid surgical advances and increasingly effective cancer treatments. And many diseases and crippling medical conditions call for still more innovation. No wonder a distinguished economist from the Brookings Institution, Henry Aaron, who has prominently called attention to all the problems of technology, has written nonetheless that any effort to curb the introduction of new technologies "beyond what is required for safety and efficacy would be sheer madness."

If there is ambivalence in many quarters about managing technology costs, there is outright resistance to such attempts among many American physicians and medical industry associations. Those groups were heavily responsible in the 1980s and 1990s for killing two federal agencies designed to assess medical technology from a scientific and economic perspective. Medical groups opposed them on the grounds that studies of that kind could interfere with the doctor-patient relationship (only they can decide about treatment evidence), and that since life is priceless, any economic assessment would be immoral. Congress, which has never shown much enthusiasm for the control of technology costs, did the actual killing. Ever since the advent of Medicare in 1965, Congress has not allowed it to take costs into account in determining which technologies and treatments it will cover. The medical device industry has been blamed for that resistance. Meanwhile, the pharmaceutical industry has blocked price controls on drugs for many decades.

While it will be hard enough to get universal health care in this country, it will be even harder to control costs. The opposition to such control is politically more intransigent; and in the case of technology, the opposition is deeply rooted in American culture, whose obsession with health is not matched in any other society. Comparative public opinion surveys in Europe and the United States indicate a much greater belief in technology in this country. An astonishing 40 percent of Americans believe that medical technology can always save their lives; not nearly as many Europeans share that fantasy. The old line that Americans believe death is just one more disease to be cured is no longer a joke.

Cost-Cutting Ideas

Can anything be done about costs? A number of ideas have been floated about how to meet the challenge, most of them not rooted in any experience or evidence. The longtime favorite has been to eliminate waste and inefficiency, which is like trying to keep dust out of a house located on the edge of a desert. Medical information technology is a more recent candidate, along with increased efforts to advance disease prevention efforts, consumer-directed health care and disease management programs.

Those are all attractive ideas, but they share a common and crippling handicap. In our messy and fragmented mixture of public and private health care, there is no effective leverage, government or otherwise, to put in place good but often painful ideas. Government might manage to act on some of them, but only after a long and difficult fight. The private sector has never shown much capacity to do so; and given its market philosophy, it would surely resist government efforts to impose cost control mechanisms upon it.

Universal care is the only tried and effective way to control costs. The European health care systems do so effectively by means of a strong government hand. They use, among other things, price controls, negotiated physician fees, hospital budgets with limits on expenditures and stringent policies on the adoption and diffusion of new technologies. The net result is that they keep annual cost increases within the range of 3 percent to 4 percent, have better health outcomes than we do and achieve both at significantly less cost. With the exception of the United Kingdom and Italy—despite what many American conservatives say—there is little rationing and there are no waiting lists for care.

But that is Europe, and this is America. The methods we are inclined to use here to control costs are generally mild and do not promise anything near the reduction in costs needed. The methods the Europeans use, dependent upon government, work well but are culturally and politically unacceptable here. That is the fundamental dilemma in trying to think through the problem.

Consequences of Cost Control

We need a change in culture, not just in the management of health care. Since many of the effective means of controlling costs will be painful for us because of our fascination with technology, the resistance to change will be formidable. Effective control will force patients to give up treatments they may need, doctors to sacrifice to a considerable extent their ancient tradition of treating patients the way they see fit and industry to reduce its drive for profit. Hardly anyone will want to do such things. Liberals will hate it, because though they favor universal health care, they are also children of the Enlightenment, champions of endless scientific progress and technological innovation. Economic conservatives will despise it as government interference with market freedom and consumer choice. Social conservatives will see the necessary rationing as a form of social euthanasia, killing off the burdensome in the name of cold-hearted economics.

The pharmaceutical industry has successfully blocked price controls for many decades.

Many commentators argue that if health care is not reformed, our system will collapse. I doubt that will happen. Instead, there is likely to be gradual deterioration, tolerable enough for the affluent but bringing to everyone else a gradual loss of quality, with more people uninsured, more expensive insurance, more bankruptcies and economic pain from medical debts and more economic anxiety about getting sick.

The frustrating part of all this is that in principle, cost control is a problem that can be solved. There is indeed waste and inefficiency, enormous and absurd variation in costs of care from one geographical region to the next, a great deal of useless or only marginally useful treatment, great possibilities in disease prevention programs, far too few primary care physicians and geriatricians and far too many specialists. The fact that the European countries can control costs and limit technologies without harming health is a patent rebuke to our way of doing things.

Looking for Solutions

Can we get there from here? To do so, both a huge economic gap and an equally huge cultural gap must be closed. We have become accustomed to living (and dying) with an expensive and disorganized system that serves many ends other than health. It is a system designed for reckless affluence. It builds upon a model of health and medical progress that is open-ended and infinite in its aspirations. Suffering, aging and death are enemies to be conquered, at whatever the cost to other social needs.

With the help of intensive marketing by industry and daily media hype, we have become fearful hypochondriacs, sensitive to every ache and pain and always anxious about that undiagnosed cancer or heart disease just waiting to get us. Our standard for good health constantly rises. Whatever the state of our health, it is never good enough. However high our life expectancy, we remain forever hopeful for medical miracles and endlessly dissatisfied with our health.

The nation needs a good dialogue on health care reform, but one that moves beyond organizational and management schemes. They are important but no more so than some deeper matters.

Should death be seen as the greatest evil, which medicine should seek to combat, or would a good quality of life within a finite life span be a better goal?

Do the elderly need better access to intensive care units and more high-tech medicine to extend their lives, or better long-term and home care and improved economic and social support? Does it make any sense that the healthier we get in this country the more we spend on health care, not less? Should we be spending three times more of our gross domestic product on health care than on education (when 40 years ago it was about the same)?

Those are rhetorical questions. But they are the place to begin any serious discussion about the control of costs and technology. That discussion merits at least as much attention as does the plight of the uninsured; it will be harder to maintain and focus, but it is even more necessary.

DANIEL CALLAHAN, director of the international program at the Hastings Center in Garrison, N.Y., is the author of *Setting Limits: Medical Goals in an Aging Society* (1987) and co-author of *Medicine and the Market: Equality vs. Choice* (2006).

From *America*, March 10, 2008. Copyright © 2008 by America Magazine. All rights reserved. Reprinted by permission of America Press. For subscription information, visit www.americamagazine.org.

Thanks, But No Thanks

Why more doctors, medical schools and hospitals are just saying no to drug-company promotions.

Anne Underwood

Dr. Jonathan Mohrer, a New York internist, used to tolerate visits from drug-company representatives. The reps provided a break in the routine, brought free pens, lunches and drug samples, and, most important, answered questions about new medications. But as the number of visits swelled to as many as 10 a day, his patience wore thin. It finally snapped in the fall of 2004, when the heavily promoted painkiller Vioxx was withdrawn after clear evidence emerged that it increased the risk of heart attacks. "I'd been getting pitches for Vioxx almost every week, even while questions were being raised about it in medical journals," says Mohrer. He kicked the reps out and made it clear he wouldn't take their calls in the future. "It's been a real relief," he says. "I don't know how I juggled it all."

Mohrer is one of a number of doctors who are just saying no to drug-company promotions. Some belong to No Free Lunch, an organization that asks doctors to take a pledge not to receive drug-company representatives. Admittedly, their numbers are small. Founded in 1999, No Free Lunch has just 800 members out of 800,000 practicing physicians in this country. The American Medical Student Association (AMSA) has collected a similar number of pledges among the nation's 68,000 med students, but that's twice as many pledges as it had a year ago. And increasing numbers of hospitals, health-care systems, medical schools and even states are starting to institute restrictive policies. Minnesota has already set limits on gifts, and three other states are weighing similar bills. "There's growing evidence that these relationships color doctors' prescribing practices, even if doctors think they don't," says Dr. Karen Antman, dean of Boston University's medical school, which last month instituted a ban on all gifts and lunches from drug reps and allows reps to visit only if invited.

It's no secret that Big Pharma spends megabucks marketing to physicians. In 2004, the total ran to $23 billion, including $15.9 billion in free drug samples, according to the Pharmaceutical Research and Manufacturers of America (PhRMA). Drug reps provide "solid, scientific, FDA-approved information on the safety and efficacy of our drugs," says Dr. Cathryn Clary, vice president of Pfizer. "So many medicines are getting label updates all the time, it's hard to keep current."

But critics say sales reps do a lot more than educate. They come armed with information from databases telling them individual physicians' prescribing practices. They know before a visit whether a doctor prescribes a competitor's drug—and whether he switches after a sales call. They also bring gifts. True, PhRMA instituted voluntary guidelines in 2002 banning big-ticket items, like harbor cruises and golf outings. But social scientists say that trivial gifts like pens create a sense of obligation, too—all the more so when the friendly person who drops them off, along with free food for the staff, is a regular visitor. It doesn't hurt that the drug logos on pens and notepads keep a drug in the doctor's mind. Even free samples, which patients love (and sometimes depend on), aren't as philanthropic as they seem, given that they're often for the company's newest, most expensive medicines—particularly drugs like birth-control pills or heart medications that a patient could potentially take for years. Once a patient starts taking a drug that works, he wants to stay on it—an obvious boon to manufacturers.

What's the problem with that? Possibly none. The result may be as inconsequential as a physician's prescribing one drug instead of a me-too pill from a competitor. But the bulk of the reps' efforts target pricey new medications—which ultimately drives up costs for consumers. And, critics say, newer isn't necessarily better. In many cases, older, cheaper drugs are just as effective. Occasionally, they're even safer. Serious side effects may be discovered only after pills have come to market, as the withdrawal of the painkiller Vioxx and the recent controversy over the diabetes drug Avandia show.

Serious side effects may be discovered only after promoted drugs get to market.

Fortunately, for doctors who kick the habit, there are independent sources of up-to-date information, such as The Medical Letter on Drugs and Therapeutics—a sort of Consumer Reports for drugs that takes no advertising and costs only $100 a year. Still, reps are nothing if not persistent. Dr. Robert Goodman, the founder of No Free Lunch, recently found several of them parked in front of his rep-free New York clinic. From the open tailgate of their SUV, they were promoting their products and handing out bagels and cream cheese to doctors "like a coffee truck at a construction site," he says. He didn't ask why they were there. He didn't need to.

From *Newsweek,* October 29, 2007. Copyright © 2007 by Newsweek, Inc. All rights reserved. Used by permission and protected by the Copyright Laws of the United States. The printing, copying, redistribution, or retransmission of the Material without express written permission via PARS International Corp. is prohibited.

The Silent Epidemic—
The Health Effects of Illiteracy

ERIN N. MARCUS, MD, MPH

He came in for a "tune-up." He was 64 years old, with a "history of noncompliance," according to the resident, and he hadn't taken his diabetes or cardiac medications for weeks. We weren't quite sure why. He was alert, he appeared to be intelligent and interested in getting well, and he was able to get his prescriptions filled at a reduced cost. Before he went home, we explained why he needed to take his medicines and reviewed the frequency and doses with him several times. He told us he would follow up with his doctor (though he couldn't remember the doctor's name or telephone number) and left the hospital with a handwritten discharge summary.

Five months later, he appeared at the community clinic. He said he was taking his medications, but he wasn't sure of their names or how often he took them. A medical student and I reviewed the regimen again. The student typed up simple instructions in big letters for him to follow, as well as a list of dates and times at which he should record his blood sugar levels. We asked him to come back in two weeks.

When he returned, the student saw him first—and made a diagnosis that no one else had considered: illiteracy. The clue lay in the jumbled mess of his glucose log. Many of the sugar values were written next to future dates. We quietly asked him to read his list of medications aloud. Haltingly, he told us he couldn't do it. Born in the rural South, he had left school in the second grade. He lived alone. He had been able to support himself as a gas-station attendant and handyman, but he had never learned to read.

We were stunned. We had tried to avoid jargon and to use simple language in explaining our instructions, and he had seemed to understand everything we had told him. He had seen scores of doctors, nurses, and social workers over the years without anyone's guessing he had a reading problem.

Although we had been blind to his illiteracy, our patient's problem is not uncommon. The National Assessment of Adult Literacy (NAAL), a large survey conducted by the National Center for Education Statistics, recently estimated that 14 percent of adults in the United States have a "below basic" level of "prose literacy"—defined as the ability to use "printed and written information to function in society, to achieve one's

goals, and to develop one's knowledge and potential."[1] The NAAL describes "below basic" skills as "no more than the most simple and concrete literacy skills," specifying that adults with this level of prose literacy range from being nonliterate in English to being able to locate easily identifiable information in short, commonplace prose text—able to find out, for example, "what a patient is allowed to drink before a medical test." They generally cannot, say, find "in a pamphlet for prospective jurors an explanation of how people were selected for the jury pool." Like my patient, 55 percent of those in the lowest prose-literacy group had not finished high school.

On the basis of the NAAL results, 12 percent of U.S. adults are estimated to have below basic "document literacy," the ability to read and understand documents such as transportation schedules and drug or food labels—they may be able to sign a form, but they cannot use "a television guide to find out what programs are on at a specific time." In addition, 22 percent of adults are estimated to have below basic "quantitative literacy," the ability to perform fundamental quantitative tasks—they may be able to sum the numbers on a bank deposit slip, but they cannot compare the ticket prices for two events. Older adults fared poorest on the NAAL: 23 percent of those more than 64 years of age had below basic prose literacy, 27 percent below basic document literacy, and 34 percent below basic quantitative skills.

There is also a growing body of research on health literacy, the ability to comprehend and use medical information.

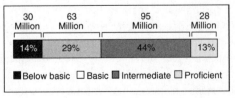

Prose Literacy Levels among U.S. Adults in 2003. Percentages are based on a sample of 18,102 household respondents and 1156 prison inmates. Data are from the National Assessment of Adult Literacy.

Survey results indicate that more than a third of English-speaking patients and more than half of primarily Spanish-speaking patients at U.S. public hospitals have low health literacy. One analysis found that Medicare enrollees with low health literacy were more likely than enrollees with adequate health literacy to use the emergency room and to be admitted as inpatients.[2]

Patients with reading problems may avoid outpatient doctors' offices and clinics because they are intimidated by paperwork, according to Joanne Schwartzberg, director of aging and community health at the American Medical Association and editor of a textbook on health literacy. "Emergency rooms are user-friendly if you don't read," she pointed out, "because somebody else asks the questions and somebody else fills out the form."

The exact relation between literacy and health is still unclear, but people with low literacy are more likely to report having poor health, and are more likely to have diabetes and heart failure, than those with adequate literacy.[3,4] Some studies have found correlations between literacy and measures of disease such as glycated hemoglobin levels in people with diabetes.[3] Of course, factors other than literacy (such as educational level, income, primary language, sex, and age) affect the management of many conditions, and whereas "some studies have attempted to control for income and social circumstances . . . many didn't," according to Darren DeWalt, an internist at the University of North Carolina who has reviewed the evidence for the Agency for Healthcare Research and Quality.

Many researchers describe low literacy as a silent epidemic: despite its high prevalence, many physicians and other health care workers remain unaware that their patients may have reading problems. "I think most doctors are blind to the problem," said Barry D. Weiss, a professor of family and community medicine at the University of Arizona. "It's hard for them to believe."

Patients with poor literacy skills often are ashamed of their problem and are adept at hiding it. In one study, more than two thirds of patients with low literacy in one public hospital said they had never told their spouses about it. Nearly a fifth said they had never told anyone. Forty percent of the patients with low literacy said they felt shame about it.[5] "A clinical psychologist once told me that the shame experienced by people with literacy problems is comparable to the shame experienced by incest victims," said Ruth Parker, a professor of medicine at Emory University, who coauthored the study. "In our society, it is very embarrassing not to know. Nobody wants to look dumb, especially not in front of their doctor."

Weiss advocates routine screening for literacy as a new "vital sign." He has created a brief, bilingual literacy-screening test that entails asking patients six questions about a nutrition label. He recommends that physicians screen some of their patients to assess literacy levels and then tailor the way they talk with patients accordingly. "The average doctor who's thinking he or she is talking in simple, plain language probably isn't," he said.

"It may be more practical to screen a sample of patients to see what's needed."

But routine screening is controversial. Some worry that it takes too long, embarrasses patients, and could stigmatize those with low literacy. Moreover, in an era of "pay for performance," physicians might avoid low-literacy patients, viewing them as time-consuming and difficult to treat. Many literacy experts say that physicians often perceive inquiring about reading ability as opening Pandora's box, releasing a sprawling, unwieldy problem that they haven't been trained to handle and that is beyond the scope of a 15-minute office visit. "Physicians are not prepared to know what [their] immediate response should be," said Dean Schillinger, an internist at San Francisco General Hospital who has conducted several studies of physicians and health literacy. He added that the health care system does not help physicians who treat low-literacy patients.

Some experts advocate an approach to communication similar to universal precautions for preventing HIV infection. Health care workers, they say, should assume that all patients have a limited understanding of medical words and concepts, whether or not they have passable general-reading skills. Schwartzberg advocates that physicians organize their discussions with patients around three key points per visit and use a teach-back approach, asking patients to explain what they have been told.

Parker, a general internist, routinely carries an empty pill bottle in her pocket when she works in the clinic. "I tell patients, 'This is not your medication, but if it were, tell me how you would take it,' " she said. "It's never been validated [as a screening test], but I pick up a lot of people who can't do it, and it's an immediate way for me to know, does this patient need help?"

Other interventions such as educational videotapes, simplified brochures, and color-coded medication schedules have had mixed results in improving the health of patients with low literacy, according to Michael Pignone, an internist and associate professor at the University of North Carolina. Pignone and other researchers have shown that disease-management programs specifically designed for low-literacy patients with diabetes and congestive heart failure—approaches involving simply written educational materials or reminders, individualized educational sessions, and teach-back methods—can be effective in reducing symptoms and improving disease markers such as glycohemoglobin levels. A variety of professional groups have launched initiatives to improve patients' health literacy—as well as physicians' skills in communicating with low-literacy patients.

With the help of a social worker, our patient enrolled in an adult reading program, which he attends regularly. Three years later, it's not clear that he always takes his medications as prescribed. But he feels that the literacy program has been useful in helping him to decipher his pill labels and to function in the world. And these days, I think twice whenever I explain anything to a patient—or jot down instructions on a pad of paper.

Notes

1. Kutner M, Greenberg E, Baer J. A first look at the literacy of America's adults in the 21st century. Washington, D.C.: National Center for Education Statistics, Department of Education, December 2005. (Accessed July 6, 2006, at http://nces.ed.gov/naal/.)

2. Howard DH, Gazmararian J, Parker RM. The impact of low health literacy on the medical costs of Medicare managed care enrollees. Am J Med 2005;118:371–7. [Erratum, Am J Med 2005;118:933.]

3. Dewalt DA, Berkman ND, Sheridan S, Lohr KN, Pignone MP. Literacy and health outcomes: a systematic review of the literature. J Gen Intern Med 2004;19:1228–39.

4. Wolf MS, Gazmararian JA, Baker DW. Health literacy and functional health status among older adults. Arch Intern Med 2005;165:1946–52.

5. Parikh NS, Parker RM, Nurss JR, Baker DW, Williams MV. Shame and health literacy: the unspoken connection. Patient Educ Couns 1996;27:33–9.

DR. MARCUS is an assistant professor of clinical medicine in the Division of General Internal Medicine at the University of Miami Miller School of Medicine, Miami.

From *The New England Journal of Medicine*, July 27, 2006, pp. 339–341. Copyright © 2006 by Massachusetts Medical Society. All rights reserved. Reprinted by permission.

Incapacitated, Alone and Treated to Death

JOSEPH SACCO, MD

M r. Green lay in the bed next to the window, 15 floors above the Cross-Bronx Expressway. Fifty-nine years old and suffering from AIDS-related dementia, he was bedbound, permanently tethered to a ventilator and, though conscious, unaware of his medical condition. In medico-legal parlance, he was incapacitated: unable to understand the consequences of his decisions and unable to direct the doctors caring for him.

The view from his bedside was impressive—a thousand acres of worn, low-slung apartment buildings set off by the massed arc of Manhattan, rising from the distance like the Emerald City.

That no friend or family member would ever share this view was another of his mounting misfortunes. Referred to the hospital from a nursing home for fever and weight loss—he was so thin that the skin of his chest would not even hold EKG leads—he had no identified relatives or friends. His personal history had vanished into the maze of health care facilities that had been his home for more than a year. Other than name, Social Security number and date of birth, his life story had disappeared.

Mr. Green was one of thousands of New Yorkers—physically devastated, mentally depleted, without hope of recovery and without surrogates—for whom the prolongation of life at all costs was the only legally sanctioned course of treatment. Even if friends or relatives were found, New York prohibits the withholding or withdrawing of life-sustaining treatment without a signed health care proxy or "clear and convincing" evidence of a patient's wishes. A "do not resuscitate" order can be put in place by doctors, but only in the absence of identified surrogates and only if resuscitation is considered futile.

Other states, to varying extents, allow family members, friends or guardians to make the decision about life support, even without knowledge of a patient's prior wishes. A few states grant it to the doctor in the absence of such surrogates. A treatment that preserves a heartbeat but offers no hope of recovery—long-term ventilator support in a vegetative state, say—may be withdrawn. New York permits no such possibility. Physicians

not wanting to find themselves at the center of precedent-setting test cases on patients' rights will treat, treat and treat, no matter the cost to the patient or their own souls.

Mention the idea of withholding or withdrawing medical care from patients who cannot express their wishes, and people get uncomfortable. Advocacy groups use the term "medical killing," and despite the hyperbole, their concerns are merited. Doctors have no right to judge the value of a life. Many patients want their lives prolonged, regardless of prognosis, quality or need for invasive treatment.

Yet a 2007 study found that doctors in intensive-care units across the country commonly withheld or withdrew life support in critically or terminally ill patients who lacked surrogates, without knowledge of their wishes. Most such decisions were made by a single physician, without regard to hospital policy, professional society recommendations or state law. In other words, doctors are withholding treatment from this vulnerable population, a practice that is neither regulated nor publicly recognized.

Many things influenced the patient's care. Just not his own wishes.

Mr. Green's monetary value cannot be underestimated as an influence on his care. He was a valuable commodity. A ventilator-dependent patient, especially one undergoing the surgical incision necessary for long-term vent support, is among the highest-paying under Medicare's prospective hospital reimbursement system; his need for skilled care outside the hospital made him a lucrative nursing home patient.

Prognosis is not a factor in this equation. Forever on life support without hope of recovery, Mr. Green would develop pneumonias, urinary infections and other complications, each requiring transfer from the nursing home to the hospital, stabilization and transfer back again. The providers would be reimbursed for each of these procedures.

Extraordinary advances have been made in the treatment of H.I.V. Still, Mr. Green's dementia worsened, as did his terrible wasting and bedsores. In July, despite a full volley of high-tech interventions, he died, without ever having done anything volitional, never mind eating, talking or making eye contact. His well-intentioned hospital and doctors, fully aware of his dismal prognosis, continued the excruciating process of inserting pencil-thick IV catheters and cleaning fist-size bed sores.

No one asked if Mr. Green wanted these interventions, assuming instead that to do otherwise was both unethical and illegal, and he was treated to death. Modern American medicine owed him a better way.

JOSEPH SACCO is director of the palliative medicine consultation service at Bronx Lebanon Hospital Center.

From *The New York Times*, October 7, 2009. Copyright © 2009 by The New York Times Company. Reprinted by permission via PARS International.

UNIT 9

Consumer Health

Unit Selections

Key Points to Consider

- What do you know about medical tourism?

- Why is it risky to try and kill all germs?

- What are the risks associated with getting a tattoo?

- What should consumers look for when choosing health insurance?

Student Website
www.mhcls.com

Internet References

FDA Consumer Magazine
   http://www.fda.gov/fdac
Global Vaccine Awareness League
   http://www.gval.com

For many people, the term "consumer health" conjures up images of selecting health care services and paying medical bills. While these two aspects of health care are indeed consumer health issues, the term consumer health encompasses all consumer products and services that influence the health and welfare of people. A definition this broad suggests that almost everything we see or do may be construed to be a consumer health issue, whether it's related to products or discussions such as those related to the concept of getting enough sleep. In many ways consumer health is an outward expression of our health-related behaviors and decision-making processes, and as such, is based on our desire to make healthy choices, be assertive, and be in possession of accurate information on which to base our decisions.

Consumer health issues addressed in this section include the increasing number of Americans who travel overseas to combine surgery or medical treatments with sightseeing. These travelers find that the costs of many treatments are much lower than in the United States. And, they can also seek those treatments that are not yet available back home. During the past few years, nearly a half million Americans went overseas each year for medical and dental treatment, a number that's expected to rise.

An unrelated topic that is of concern is the use of antimicrobial soaps and gels to kill germs. Jerry Adler and Jeneen Interlandi discuss the latest research into the relationship between humans and the microbes that cover their bodies. Many of these germs are not harmful and some are actually beneficial. Unfortunately, harmful germs are being strengthened by exposure to sanitizers and antibiotics used by a society obsessed with health and hygiene.

Other issues in this section include an overview on the need for adequate sleep. Since the invention of electric lights,

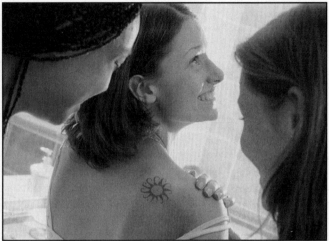

© image100/Corbis

Americans have increasingly gotten by with less sleep. Unfortunately, sleep deprivation is linked to mortality and overall health status. Two other topics address the safety of getting tattooed and the adequacy of many health insurance plans.

The health-conscious consumer seeks to be as informed as possible when making dietary and medical decisions—but the best intentions come to no avail when consumers base their decisions on inaccurate information, old beliefs, or media hype that lacks a scientific base. Knowledge (based on accurate information) and critical thinking are the key elements required to become proactive in managing your daily health concerns.

Dentists Frown at Overuse of Whiteners

Natasha Singer

Kevin Ross, a psychologist in Queens, is a serial tooth whitener. He started out seven years ago with custom-fitted bleaching trays, the kind dentists sell. When his teeth became sensitive, he switched to over-the-counter whitening strips, which use less bleach. These were gentler, but not as effective. So earlier this year Mr. Ross upgraded to professional-strength whitening strips dispensed by his dentist.

"I insist on having my teeth as white as possible," he said. "I guess it's like skinny people who always think they could be a little skinnier. I'd like to get another whitening treatment tomorrow."

But when Mr. Ross recently asked for a new set of whitening strips, his dentist said no. "I had to cut him off temporarily," said Dr. Marc M. Liechtung, who practices in New York City, "because his teeth are as white as they are going to get. It's our job not to indulge them when they want touch-ups they don't need."

Mr. Ross is not even the most avid whitener among Dr. Liechtung's patients. Some, Dr. Liechtung said, come back "like drug addicts pleading, 'Doc, sell me more just this once.'" "Meanwhile, on their own, they use every type of drugstore whitening product: not only the strips but also whitening toothpaste, floss, rinse and chewing gum.

More and more, dentists like Dr. Liechtung are putting their foot down for fear that these patients may be overexposing themselves to bleach. "In the long run," Dr. Liechtung said, "chronic whiteners could end up causing themselves tooth damage."

Dentists generally consider whitening to be a safe treatment when patients, following a proper dental exam, choose a bleaching product from a reputable brand, adhere to package instructions and don't overdo it. But tooth bleaching was never intended to become a daily grooming habit like shampooing or shaving. And some dentists suspect that uninterrupted whitening, using a hodgepodge of high-strength products, not only will make teeth more sensitive, but may also cause permanent damage to tooth enamel and gum tissue.

Until more studies have been done to assess the potential side effects of constant bleaching, these dentists say, consumers should take care to avoid going overboard.

"We see younger and younger patients wanting whiter and whiter teeth," said Dr. Bruce A. Matis, the director of the Clinical Research Section at Indiana School of Dentistry in Indianapolis. "We'll know in 10 years if they've damaged their teeth."

A fondness for pearly white teeth is ancient. In the Bible, Jacob hopes that his son Judah will have "teeth white with milk." But never in history have paper-white teeth been as popular or easy to obtain as they are now. The market for dentist-dispensed tooth whitening products and in-office treatments is expected to reach more than $2 billion this year, up from $435 million in 2000, according to a report from Mintel International Group, a market research firm. Mintel expects sales of over-the-counter whitening kits to reach $351 million in 2005, up from $38 million five years ago.

All this bleaching has made teeth so white that manufacturers of dental materials used for bonding and filling have had to create ever-lighter shades to match them. The very whitest are an unnatural color that did not exist before bleaching, a shade dentists have nicknamed "Regis white."

Given that even short-term whitening can cause temporary tooth sensitivity and gum irritation, some dentists speculate that continuous bleaching could erode tooth enamel or cause gum inflammation. Some people's teeth have even taken on a translucent blue or gray color around the edges, dentists say.

Many clinical studies have indicated it is safe for teeth to be bleached—either professionally or with name-brand do-it-yourself kits—once or twice a year. Procter & Gamble, maker of Crest Whitestrips, has also done research on the safety of uninterrupted bleaching using the company's products; one of its clinical trials, conducted with researchers at Tufts University in Boston, found it was safe to use Whitestrips twice a day for six months.

Today's 'Regis white' may be tomorrow's gray, or worse.

Still, some dentist say that when people routinely use high-strength bleaches, or use whitening products in every step of their oral-care routine, it may add up to a level of exposure to bleaching agents that goes beyond what has been studied.

"We don't know how the body handles regular use of high concentrations of peroxide," said Dr. Van B. Haywood, a professor at the School of Dentistry at the Medical College of Georgia in Augusta, who in 1989 was an author of the first paper published on the effectiveness and safety of overnight bleaching trays.

The peroxides used in tooth bleach, hydrogen peroxide and carbamide peroxide (which contains hydrogen peroxide) produce free radicals that can damage cells of the gums or pulp inside teeth, said Dr. Yiming Li, the director of the Center for Dental Research at Loma Linda University School of Dentistry in California. "The lower your overall exposure," Dr. Li said, "the lower your risk."

Because of the unknown risks of high peroxide exposure, some dentists advise pregnant women as well as cancer patients and smokers (who are at risk of developing cancer) to avoid tooth whitening altogether.

Some dentists say certain over-the-counter bleaching products are riskier than professional whitening treatments because the bleach more easily strays from the teeth to the rest of the mouth. Ill-fitting one-size-fits-all trays easily leak bleaching material onto the gums and down the throat, Dr. Matis said.

Dentists say they prevent such leaks. "We protect the gums by painting on a semiplastic barrier, so no bleaching material touches the soft tissue," said Dr. Laurence R. Rifkin, a dentist in Beverly Hills, Calif. "We also make custom-fitted trays for home use that keep the whitening gel in close contact with your teeth."

In Europe only whitening products that are no more than one-tenth of a percent peroxide may be sold over the counter. Earlier this year, after examining the potential risks, the European Union's Scientific Committee on Consumer Products concluded that higher-strength bleaching is safe only when it is supervised by a dentist.

American products are much more powerful and getting stronger all the time, raising the risk of overexposure to bleach, dentists say. Fifteen years ago the first trays dispensed by dentists used gels that were 10 percent carbamide peroxide, equivalent to about 3 1/3 percent hydrogen peroxide. Today, Discus Dental Nite White ACP Deluxe Kit, dispensed by dentists, contains 22 percent carbamide peroxide gel (about 7 percent hydrogen peroxide).

The Minute White Laser Speed Tooth Whitening System, sold on the QVC shopping channel, includes a 22 percent carbamide peroxide whitener. And the strongest bleaching strips sold by dentists now contain 14 percent hydrogen peroxide gels.

"Once you get above 15 percent carbamide, you are pushing the envelope," Dr. Haywood said.

Manufacturers counter that it is the amount of gel used, rather than the strength of its bleaching agent, that determines whether a product is safe. The gel in Crest Whitestrips Premium, for example, is 10 percent hydrogen peroxide, but the overall amount is small, the company said.

"The gel on each strip is as thin as two or three pieces of paper," said Dr. Robert W. Gerlach, a principal scientist at Procter & Gamble. "A tray-based system uses 4 to 10 times as much peroxide. And a whitening mouthwash could contain up to 20 times as much peroxide." Consumers often do not know how much bleach over-the-counter whiteners contain, however, because manufacturers are not required to quantify it on the label. Some dentists say that practice endangers consumers.

"The consumer cannot make an informed decision without concentrations listed on the labels," Dr. Matis said.

Dentists do not agree on how often their patients should use today's powerful whiteners. After his patients have completed their initial 10- to 14-day tray bleaching treatment, Dr. Rifkin permits them to wear the trays again once or twice a year for one- or two-day touch-ups. Dr. Matis advises patients to wait one to three years. And Dr. Haywood says that once a decade may be enough for some people.

Try telling that to Dale Michele Asti, a boutique owner in Beverly Hills who uses her 22 percent carbamide peroxide bleaching tray several times a week.

"I admit I'm obsessed," said Ms. Asti, a patient of Dr. Rifkin. "Whitening has become part of my routine when I'm getting ready for a date. I'll do it to make my smile sparkle while I'm shaving my legs or putting on makeup."

When told of Ms. Asti's habit, Dr. Rifkin said: "She shouldn't be doing that."

"It's not going to make her teeth any whiter," he added, "and it's potentially irritating. I may have to limit her number of whitening kits."

From *The New York Times*, November 17, 2005. Copyright © 2005 by The New York Times Company. Reprinted by permission via PARS International.

Medicial Tourism:
What You Should Know

From international outsourcing to in-home visits, doctors and patients are reinventing the way medicine is viewed and practiced at home and around the world.

LORENE BURKHART AND LORNA GENTRY

I n 2006, West Virginia lawmaker Ray Canterbury made headlines across the country when he introduced House Bill 4359, which would allow enrollees in the state government's health plan to travel to foreign countries for surgery and other medical services. In fact, not only would the bill allow for such a choice, it encourages it; those choosing to go to an approved foreign clinic for a procedure covered by the plan would have all of their medical and travel expenses (including those of one companion) paid, plus be given 20 percent of the savings they racked up by having the procedure done overseas, rather than here at home.

Canterbury's bill drew attention to a growing international boom in medical tourism—an industry with special appeal for many of America's 61 million uninsured or underinsured citizens. At prices as much as 80 to 90 percent lower than those here, hospitals in countries such as Costa Rica, Thailand, India, and the Philippines offer a wide range of healthcare procedures in accommodations equal to or even better than their American counterparts. Some estimate that 500,000 Americans went overseas for medical treatment in 2006 alone, and that medical tourism could become a $40 billion industry by 2010.

Overseas Surgery?
What You Should Know

According to Canterbury and other proponents of medical service outsourcing, the idea is all about competition. Proponents believe the rate of healthcare inflation in this country, at almost four times the rate of overall inflation, has placed an unsustainable burden on the American economy.

"The best way to solve this problem is to rely on market forces," Canterbury writes. "My bills are designed to force domestic healthcare companies to compete for our business."

It's hard to argue with the economics of medical outsourcing. According to MedicalTourism.com, the cost of typical heart bypass surgery in the United States is $130,000. The same operation is estimated to cost approximately $10,000 in India, $11,000 in Thailand, and $18,500 in Singapore. A $43,000 hip replacement in an American hospital could be performed for $9,000 in India, or for $12,000 in either Thailand or Singapore. Even adding the costs of travel and lodging, consumers stand to save real money by traveling overseas for these and many other types of routine surgery, including angioplasties, knee replacements, and hysterectomies.

Of course, many people have serious concerns about the idea of shopping overseas for invasive medical procedures. What about the quality of the service? Follow up care? And what happens if something goes terribly wrong?. Those backing the business—including employers and lawmakers desperately seeking ways to cut the cost of employer-sponsored medical care—are quick to answer these concerns.

Most of the foreign medical facilities courting Western tourists are state-of-the-art facilities that offer luxurious accommodations and individual around-the-clock nursing attention. Thailand's Bumrungrad Hospital, for example, offers five-star hotel quality rooms, a lobby that includes Starbucks and other restaurants, valet parking, an international staff and interpreters, a travel agent, visa desk, and a meet-and-greet service at Bangkok's Suvarnabhumi Airport. In a 2007 report broadcast on NPR, an American woman told how when her doctor in Alaska announced that she needed double knee replacements at a cost of $100,000, she replied that she couldn't afford the treatment. Her doctor recommended that she wait four years, when she would be eligible for Medicare. Instead, the woman opted for treatment at Bumrungrad, where the two knee replacements cost $20,000 (including the services of two physicians, an anesthesiologist, and physical therapy), and she was able to recover in the hospital's luxurious surroundings with her husband at her side. Her husband, who underwent surgery in the United States the previous year, couldn't believe the amount of attention his wife received from her doctors and nurses, whom he said were in almost constant attendance.

Why is all of this lavish treatment and high-quality care so much cheaper abroad than here? We only need to look at all of the other services the United States has outsourced in the past decade to find the first part of the answer to that question: In places like Thailand and India—two popular destinations for cardiac, orthopedic, and cosmetic surgery—salaries are much lower than in the United States. Further, most services are provided under one roof, and patients select and pay for their medical services up front—no insurance billing. Medical malpractice liability insurance and claims caps in some foreign countries also help keep costs down.

But how safe are foreign medical facilities? Bumrungrad Hospital is accredited by the Joint Commission International (the same organization that accredits U.S. hospitals) and has over 200 U.S. board-certified physicians. And that hospital isn't unique in the world of international medicine. Increasing numbers of medical tourism facilities are staffed by American- and European-trained physicians and backed by well-funded research facilities. Dubai, already a luxury travel destination, is preparing to enter the business of international medical practice and research in a very serious way. Its 4.1 million square-foot Dubai Healthcare City is slated to open in 2010 and will offer academic medical research facilities, disease treatment, and wellness services backed by the oversight of a number of international partners, including a new department of the Harvard School of Medicine.

Good News for Patients Might Be Bad News for U.S. Hospitals

Most baby boomers love to travel, and many are only too happy to combine foreign travel experiences with low-cost and high-value medical procedures. And many insurance companies are eyeing medical outsourcing, too, as a way to cut costs for both enrollees and their employers. Blue Cross/Blue Shield of South Carolina, for example, has begun working with Bumrungrad to provide overseas alternatives for healthcare to its members.

Of course, one or two horrific medical mishaps alone could seriously damage the medical tourism industry. Most foreign countries don't support malpractice litigation to the extent that we do in the United States, and fears of the "what ifs" are keeping many private individuals and organizations from plunging in until they have a few more years to observe the medical outsourcing industry in action. For now, however, foreign medical facilities are eager to maintain standards high enough to avoid any claims of malpractice. And many Americans with our fondness for bargains and luxury are more than willing to give those facilities an opportunity to prove their worth.

Medical tourism is good news for patients, but it could pose consequences for America's already-ailing hospital system. If patients travel to foreign lands to avoid pricey surgeries at home, what kind of financial "hit" will American hospitals face? At 2007's International Medical Tourism Conference in Las Vegas, hospital physicians and administrators from around the globe gathered to discuss the issues surrounding medical tourism and its impact on the healthcare industry. In an interview about the conference, Sparrow Mahoney, chief executive officer of MedicalTourism.com and conference co-chair, admitted that American medical facilities are now in direct competition with their foreign competitors. "Hospitals will feel a pinch," she said.

Yes, We Make House Calls

All of us have experienced the frustrating and sometimes frightening wait for medical care that we desperately need. We have a raging fever and are told that the doctor can see us in three days. If we choose instead to go to the emergency room of a nearby hospital, we may wait for hours in a roomful of equally ill and distressed people with their impatient spouses, parents, or screaming children, and the constant chiming of cell phones. If our doctor agrees to "work us in," we're faced with an only slightly less daunting process, requiring what might be an hour or so wait. When we finally see a doctor, we're rushed through a few minutes of evaluation, given a prescription, and sent on our way—typically worn out and much worse for the wear of the experience.

But many Americans are opting out of this tribal experience and choosing instead to pay an annual fee (typically, $3,000 to $30,000 above insurance costs) to retain the personalized, private care of a family physician. The "boutique" healthcare movement began in the early 1990s in Seattle, Washington, and has since spread to urban areas around the nation. Instead of waiting days, weeks, or even months for an appointment that fits the doctor's schedule, members of these plans schedule medical visits at their convenience.

Need a house call? Not a problem with most boutique or "concierge" plans. Members have their doctor's cell phone number and can simply call to arrange for the doctor to come to their home. If a plan member needs to see a specialist or go to the emergency room, he or she is accompanied by a plan physician—and no rushing through appointments.

Although many primary care physicians have caseloads of as many as 3,000 to 5,000 patients, doctors in boutique plans might have no more than a few hundred patients under their care; Seattle retainer medicine pioneer MD^2 (pronounced "MD Squared") limits its doctor loads to no greater than 50 patients.

Some retainer plans require that members also carry insurance, while others refuse to process insurance payments at all. In a 2005 report on boutique medicine by CBS5 News in California, one doctor complained that he had lost patience with insurance companies that require reams of tedious paperwork and billing regulations, then reimburse at 20 percent of his billing rate. "I went to medical school to be a doctor and take care of patients," says Dr. Jordan Shlain of the San Francisco group On Call. "I didn't take one class on billings, on insurance company shenanigans and the HMO grip."

Although some concierge medical services charge fees aimed squarely at the middle class, most admit that their fees put them out of the range of many people. FirstLine Personal Health Care, in Indianapolis, charges members an annual retainer of a few thousand dollars in return for 24-hour access to one of the plan's doctors, unlimited office visits, and a small keychain hard drive loaded with their medical records. Even though their fees are modest in comparison with some concierge medical services, FirstLine doctors Kevin McCallum and Timothy Story know that many patients they saw prior to forming the service won't be able to afford membership.

Like other doctors around the country, however, McCallum and Story believe that retainer medicine offers the only option for family medicine doctors trying to escape the grinding demands of escalating practice costs and patient caseloads. With many family physicians around the country retiring early and medical students avoiding the low pay and high demands of a typical family practice, retainer-fee medical groups might be the most viable way to keep the "good old family doctor" in business.

We have yet to see what will happen when the average American is financially excluded from most family medicine clinics and groups—a fate that may occur in the not-so-distant future. Dr. Kevin Grumbach of the University of California at San Francisco was in family practice for more than 20 years and now worries that the rush to boutique medical services is threatening our nation's system of medical care.

"I have grave concerns," he told the CBS5 news reporter, "that . . . we are as a profession abandoning the need of the vast majority of Americans . . . . It's the middle class people that are increasingly left behind in an increasingly inequitable system."

From *The Saturday Evening Post*, January/February 2008. Copyright © 2008 by Meitus Gelbert Rose LLP. Reprinted by permission.

Caution: Killing Germs May Be Hazardous to Your Health

Our war on microbes has toughened them. Now, new science tells us we should embrace bacteria.

JERRY ADLER AND JENEEN INTERLANDI

Behold yourself, for a moment, as an organism. A trillion cells stuck together, arrayed into tissues and organs and harnessed by your DNA to the elemental goals of survival and propagation. But is that all? An electron microscope would reveal that you are teeming with other life-forms. Any part of your body that comes into contact with the outside world—your skin, mouth, nose and (especially) digestive tract—is home to bacteria, fungi and protozoa that outnumber the cells you call your own by 10, or perhaps a hundred, to one.

Their ancestors began colonizing you the moment you came into the world, inches from the least sanitary part of your mother's body, and their descendants will have their final feast on your corpse, and join you in death. There are thousands of different species, found in combinations "as unique as our DNA or our fingerprints," says Stanford biologist David Relman, who is investigating the complex web of interactions microbes maintain with our digestive, immune and nervous systems. Where do you leave off, and they begin? Microbes, Relman holds, are "a part of who we are."

Relman is a leader in rethinking our relationship to bacteria, which for most of the last century was dominated by the paradigm of Total Warfare. "It's awful the way we treat our microbes," he says, not intending a joke; "people still think the only good microbe is a dead one." We try to kill them off with antibiotics and hand sanitizers. But bacteria never surrender; if there were one salmonella left in the world, doubling every 30 minutes, it would take less than a week to give everyone alive diarrhea. In the early years of antibiotics, doctors dreamed of eliminating infectious disease. Instead, a new paper in The Journal of the American Medical Association reports on the prevalence of Methicillin-resistant Staphylococcus aureus (MRSA), which was responsible for almost 19,000 deaths in the United States in 2005—about twice as many as previously thought, and more than AIDS. Elizabeth Bancroft, a leading epidemiologist, called this finding "astounding."

As antibiotics lose their effectiveness, researchers are returning to an idea that dates back to Pasteur, that the body's natural microbial flora aren't just an incidental fact of our biology, but crucial components of our health, intimate companions on an evolutionary journey that began millions of years ago. The science writer Jessica Snyder Sachs summarizes this view in four words in the title of her ground-breaking new book: "Good Germs, Bad Germs." Our microbes do us the favor of synthesizing vitamins right in our guts; they regulate our immune systems and even our serotonin levels: germs, it seems, can make us happy. They influence how we digest our food, how much we eat and even what we crave. The genetic factors in weight control might reside partly in their genes, not ours. Regrettably, it turns out that bacteria exhibit a strong preference for making us fat.

Our well-meaning war on microbes has, by the relentless process of selection, toughened them instead. When penicillin began to lose its effectiveness against staph, doctors turned to methicillin, but then MRSA appeared—first as an opportunistic infection among people already hospitalized, now increasingly a wide-ranging threat that can strike almost anyone. The strain most commonly contracted outside hospitals, dubbed USA300, comes armed with the alarming ability to attack immune-system cells. Football players seem to be especially vulnerable: they get scraped and bruised and share equipment while engaging in prolonged exercise, which some researchers believe temporarily lowers immunity. In the last five years outbreaks have plagued the Cleveland Browns, the University of Texas and the University of Southern California, where trainers now disinfect equipment almost hourly. The JAMA article was a boon to makers of antimicrobial products, of which about 200 have been introduced in the United States so far this year. Press releases began deluging newsrooms, touting the benefits of antibacterial miracle compounds ranging from silver to honey. Charles Gerba, a professor of environmental microbiology at the University of Arizona, issued an ominous warning that teenagers were catching MRSA by sharing cell phones. Gerba is a consultant to the makers of Purell hand sanitizer, Clorox bleach and the Oreck antibacterial vacuum cleaner, which uses ultraviolet light to kill germs on your rug.

To be sure, MRSA is a scary infection, fast-moving and tricky to diagnose. Hunter Spence, a 12-year-old cheerleader from Victoria, Texas, woke up one Sunday in May with pain in her left leg. "I think I pulled a calf muscle," she told her mother, Peyton. By the next day, the pain was much worse and she was running a low-grade fever, but there was no other sign of infection. A doctor thought she might have the flu. By Wednesday her fever was 103 and the leg pain was unbearable. But doctors at two different community hospitals couldn't figure out what was wrong until Friday, when a blood culture came up positive for MRSA. By the time she arrived at Driscoll Children's Hospital in Corpus Christi—by helicopter—her temperature was 107 and her pulse 220. Doctors put her chance of survival at 20 percent.

Hunter needed eight operations over the next week to drain her infections, and an intravenous drip of two powerful new antibiotics, Zyvox and Cubicin. She did survive, and is home now, but her lung capacity is at 35 percent of normal. "We are seeing more infections, and more severe infections" with the USA300 strain, says Dr. Jaime Fergie, who treated her at Driscoll. In many cases, there's no clue as to how the infection was contracted, but a study Fergie did in 2005 of 350 children who were seen at Driscoll for unrelated conditions found that 21 percent of them were carrying MRSA, mostly in their noses. Then all it may take is a cut . . . and an unwashed hand.

And there are plenty of unwashed hands out there; Gerba claims that only one in five of us does the job properly, getting in all the spaces between the fingers and under the nails and rubbing for at least 20 seconds. Americans have been obsessed with eradicating germs ever since their role in disease was discovered in the 19th century, but they've been partial to technological fixes like antibiotics or sanitizers rather than the dirty work of cleanliness. Nancy Tomes, author of "The Gospel of Germs," believes the obsession waxes and wanes in response to social anxiety—about diseases such as anthrax, SARS or avian flu, naturally, but also about issues like terrorism or immigration that bear a metaphoric relationship to infection. "I can't protect myself from bin Laden, but I can rid myself of germs," she says. "Guarding against microbes is something Americans turn to when they're stressed." The plastic squeeze bottle of alcohol gel, which was introduced by Purell in 1997, is a powerful talisman of security. Sharon Morrison, a Dallas real-estate broker with three young daughters, estimates she has as many as 10 going at any time, in her house, her car, her purse, her office and her kids' backpacks. She swabs her grocery cart with sanitizing wipes and, when her children were younger, she would bring her own baby-seat cover from home and her own place mats to restaurants. Sales of Purell last year were $90 million, so she's clearly not alone. There's no question it kills germs, although it's not a substitute for washing; the Centers for Disease Control website notes that alcohol can't reach germs through a layer of dirt. Alcohol gels, which kill germs by drying them out, don't cause the kind of resistance that gives rise to superbugs like

Bacteria's Base

By the time you turn 2, mircobes have colonized every inch of your body. Some regions are more densely populated than others.

Sharing Intelligence

How resistant bacteria spreads:

1. **Armed:** Some bacteria—but not all—carry extra genes that make them resistant to certain antibiotics.
2. **Dangerous Liaisons:** They can pass on these resistant genes by connecting to their nonresistant neighbors through a protein tube.
3. **Building Ranks:** As antibiotics kill off the vulnerable bacteria, the resistant ones thrive, and continue to pass their genes along.

The Hiding Places

The Mouth is made up of dozens of distinct microbial neighborhoods. Each tooth has its own species and strains.

The Appendix is now thought to be stockpiling gut microbes to replenish your intestine in the event of an illness.

The Gut houses more microbes than all other body parts combined. These bugs aid digestion and produce nutrients.

The Groin supplies most people with their first microbial residents, acquired as you pass through the birth canal.

The Skin is covered in different species of friendly staphylococcus that may help keep infectious strains from getting in.

Hospitalized by Staph

Methicillin-resistant Staphylococcus aureus hospital stays, 1993–2005

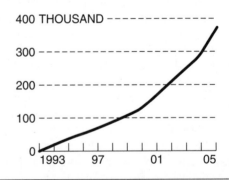

MRSA. But they're part of the culture of cleanliness that's led to a different set of problems.

In terms of infectious disease, the environment of the American suburb is unquestionably a far healthier place than most of the rest of the world. But we've made a Faustian bargain with our antibiotics, because most researchers now believe that our supersanitized world exacts a unique price in allergies, asthma and autoimmune diseases, most of which were unknown to our ancestors. Sachs warns that many people drew precisely the wrong conclusion from this, that contracting a lot of diseases in childhood is somehow beneficial. What we need is more exposure to the good microbes, and the job of medicine in the years to come will be sorting out the good microbes from the bad.

That's the goal of the Human Microbiome Project, a five-year multinational study that its advocates say could tell us almost as much about life as the recently completed work of sequencing the human genome. One puzzling result of the Human Genome Project was the paltry number of genes it found—about 20,000, which is only as many as it takes to make a fruit fly. Now some researchers think some of the "missing" genes may be found in the teeming populations of microbes we host.

And the microbe project—which as a first step requires sampling every crevice and orifice of 100 people of varying ages from a variety of climates and cultures—is "infinitely more complex and problematic than the genome," laments (or boasts) one of its lead researchers, Martin Blaser of NYU Medical School. Each part of the body is a separate ecosystem, and even two teeth in the same mouth can be colonized by different bacteria. In general, researchers know what they'll find— *Escherechia* (including the ubiquitous microbial Everyman, *E. coli*) in the bowel, lactobacilli in the vagina and staphylococcus on the skin. But the mix of particular species and strains will probably turn out to be unique to each individual, a product of chance, gender (men and women have different microbes on their skin but are similar in their intestines) and socioeconomic status and culture. (Race seems not to matter much.) Once the microbes establish themselves they stay for life and fight off newcomers; a broad-spectrum antibiotic may kill most of them but the same kinds usually come back after a few weeks. The most intriguing question is how microbes interact with each other and with our own cells. "There is a three-way conversation going on throughout our bodies," says Jane Peterson of the National Human Genome Research Institute. "We want to listen in because we think it will fill in a lot of blanks about human health—and human disease."

The vast majority of human microbes live in the digestive tract; they get there by way of the mouth in the first few months of life, before stomach acid builds to levels that are intended to kill most invaders. The roiling, fetid and apparently useless contents of the large intestine were a moral affront to doctors in the early years of modern medicine, who sought to cleanse them from the body with high-powered enemas. But to microbiologists, the intestinal bacteria are a marvel, a virtual organ of the body which just happens to have its own DNA. Researchers at Duke University claim it explains the persistence of the human appendix. It serves, they say, as a reservoir of beneficial microbes which can recolonize the gut after it's emptied by diseases such as cholera or dysentery.

Microbes play an important role in digestion, especially of polysaccharides, starch molecules found in foods such as potatoes or rice that may be hundreds or thousands of atoms long. The stomach and intestines secrete 99 different enzymes

for breaking these down into usable 6-carbon sugars, but the humble gut-dwelling *Bacterioides theta* produces almost 250, substantially increasing the energy we can extract from a given meal.

Of course, "energy" is another way of saying "calories." Jeffrey Gordon of the University of Washington raised a colony of mice in sterile conditions, with no gut microbes at all, and although they ate 30 percent more food than normal mice they had less than half the body fat. When they were later inoculated with normal bacteria, they quickly gained back up to normal weight. "We are finding that the nutritional value of food is pretty individualized," Gordon says. "And a big part of what determines it is our microbial composition."

We can't raise humans in sterile labs, of course, but there's evidence that variations between people in their intestinal microbes correspond to differences in body composition. And other factors appear to be at work besides the ability to extract calories from starch. Bacteria seem able to adjust levels of the hormones ghrelin and leptin, which regulate appetite and metabolism. Certain microbes even seem to be associated with a desire for chocolate, according to research by the Nestlé Research Center. And a tiny study suggests that severe emotional stress in some people triggers an explosion in the population of B. theta, the starch-digesting bacteria associated with weight gain. That corresponds to folk wisdom about "stress eating," but it is also a profoundly disturbing and counterintuitive observation that something as intimate as our choice between a carrot and a candy bar is somehow mediated by creatures that are not us.

But these are the closest of aliens, so familiar that the immune system, which ordinarily attacks any outside organism, tolerates them by the trillions—a seeming paradox with profound implications for health. The microbes we have all our lives are the ones that colonize us in the first weeks and months after birth, while our immune system is still undeveloped; in effect, they become part of the landscape. "Dendritic" (treelike) immune cells send branches into the respiratory and digestive tracts, where they sample all the microbes we inhale or swallow. When they see the same ones over and over, they secrete an anti-inflammatory substance called interleukin-10, which signals the microbe-killing T-cells: stand down.

And that's an essential step in the development of a healthy immune system. The immune reaction relies on a network of positive and negative feedback loops, poised on a knife edge between the dangers of ignoring a deadly invader and overreacting to a harmless stimulus. But to develop properly it must be exposed to a wide range of harmless microbes early in life. This was the normal condition of most human infants until a few generations ago. Cover the dirt on the floor of the hut, banish the farm animals to a distant feedlot, treat an ear infection with penicillin, and the inflammation-calming interleukin-10 reaction may fail to develop properly. "Modern sanitation is a good thing, and pavement is a good thing," says Sachs, "but they keep kids at a distance from microbes." The effect is to tip the immune system in the direction of overreaction, either to outside stimuli or even to the body's own cells. If the former, the result is allergies or asthma. Sachs writes that "children who receive antibiotics in the first year of life have more than double the rate of allergies and asthma in later childhood." But if the immune system turns on the body itself, you see irritable bowel syndrome, lupus or multiple sclerosis, among the many autoimmune diseases that were virtually unknown to our ancestors but are increasingly common in the developed world.

That is the modern understanding of the "Hygiene Hypothesis," first formulated by David Strachan in 1989. In Strachan's original version, which has unfortunately lodged in the minds of many parents, actual childhood illness was believed to exert a protective effect. There was a brief vogue for intentionally exposing youngsters to disease. But researchers now believe the key is exposure to a wide range of harmless germs, such as might be found in a playground or a park.

Microbes synthesize vitamins, and regulate immune systems and even serotonin levels. Germs, it seems, can make you happy.

The task is complicated, in part because some bacteria seem to be both good and bad. The best-known is *Helicobacter pylori*, a microbe that has evolved to live in the acid environment of the stomach. It survives by burrowing into the stomach's mucous lining and secreting enzymes that reduce acidity. Nobel laureates Barry Marshall and Robin Warren showed it could cause gastric ulcers and stomach cancer. But then further studies discovered that infection with H. pylori was protective against esophageal reflux and cancer of the esophagus, and may also reduce the incidence of asthma. H. pylori, which is spread in drinking water and direct contact among family members, was virtually universal a few generations ago but is now on the verge of extinction in the developed world. The result is fewer ulcers and stomach cancer, but more cancer of the esophagus—which is increasing faster than any other form of cancer in America—more asthma, and . . . what else? We don't know. "H. pylori has colonized our guts since before humans migrated out of Africa," says Blaser. "You can't get rid of it and not expect consequences."

Blaser questions whether eliminating H. pylori is a good idea. Someday, conceivably, we might intentionally inoculate children with a bioengineered version of H. pylori that keeps its benefits without running the risk of stomach cancer. There is already a burgeoning market for "probiotics," bacteria with supposed health benefits, either in pill form or as food. Consumers last year slurped down more than $100 million worth of Dannon's Activia, a yogurt containing what the website impressively calls "billions" of beneficial microbes in every container. The microbes are a strain of *Bifidobacterium animalis*, which helps improve what advertisers delicately call "regularity," a fact Dannon has underscored by rechristening the species with its trademarked name "*Bifidus regularis*." Other products contain *Lactobacillus casei*, which is supposed to stimulate production of infection-fighting lymphocytes. Many others on the market are untested and of dubious value. Labels that claim antibiotic resistant ought to be considered a warning, not a boast. Bacteria swap genetic material among themselves, and the last thing you want to do is introduce a resistant strain, even of a beneficial microbe, into your body.

And there's one more thing that microbes can do, perhaps the most remarkable of all. *Mycobacterium vaccae*, a soil microbe found in East Africa that has powerful effects on the immune system, was tested at the University of Bristol as a cancer therapy. The results were equivocal, but researchers made the startling observation that patients receiving it felt better regardless of whether their cancer was actually improving. Neuroscientist Chris Lowry injected mice with it, and found, to his amazement, that it activated the serotonin receptors in the prefrontal cortex—in other words, it worked like an antidepressant, only without the side effects of insomnia and anxiety. Researchers believe *M. vaccae* works through the interleukin-10 pathway, although the precise mechanism is uncertain. But there is at least the tantalizing, if disconcerting, suggestion that microbes may be able to manipulate our happiness. Could the hygiene hypothesis help explain the rise in, of all things, depression? We're a long way from being able to say that, much less use that insight to treat people. But at least we are asking the right questions: not how to kill bacteria, but how to live with them.

With **Matthew Philips**, **Raina Kelley** and **Karen Springen**.

From *Newsweek*, October 29, 2007. Copyright © 2007 by Newsweek, Inc. All rights reserved. Used by permission and protected by the Copyright Laws of the United States. The printing, copying, redistribution, or retransmission of the Material without express written permission via PARS International Corp. is prohibited.

Tattoos: Leaving Their Mark

Getting one is pretty safe these days, but what if you have second thoughts and want a tattoo removed? Even today's pinpoint lasers may not get rid of it entirely.

People have been getting tattoos for millennia, but only recently has tattooing entered the American mainstream. In a 2004 telephone survey of Americans ages 18 to 50, a quarter of those interviewed said they had a tattoo. Now it's probably more.

With acceptance has come safety, although there's still a chance of infection, so it's important that equipment be sterilized and that tattooists wash their hands and wear gloves. In 2004 and 2005, 44 people were infected with methicillin-resistant *Staphylococcus aureus* (MRSA) by unlicensed tattooists, some of whom fashioned guitar string into needles and used ink from printer cartridges for dye.

The flip side to the popularity of tattoos is increased demand for removal. Laser treatments work, but they're expensive, time-consuming, and may not erase the tattoo completely.

Bad Reactions

Tattoos are more or less permanent because the ink is injected into the dermis, the relatively stable level of skin beneath the epidermis, the outermost layer that's continually flaking off. They've been described as tiny, ink-filled puncture wounds; indeed, tattoos used to be created manually by jabbing a needle into the skin, and they are still done that way illicitly in prisons and elsewhere. But legal tattooists now depend on machines to rapidly inject the ink to just the right depth, about half a millimeter below the surface of the skin. Even with these machines, getting a tattoo may hurt.

Because there's usually some bleeding, the possibility of getting a blood-borne disease exists for both the tattoo artists and their customers. In the 1950s, New York City banned tattooing after a dramatic increase in tattoo-related hepatitis cases. An Australian study published last year found a link between hepatitis C infections and getting a tattoo in prison, but American health officials have said that there are no data so far in this country linking tattoos to transmission of hepatitis C.

A bigger problem than infections may be the allergic reactions and skin growths.

Some people get henna tattoos, especially while on vacation, because they fade in a couple of weeks. By itself, henna isn't a problem, but a chemical called paraphenylenediamine is sometimes added to intensify the color. Several case reports describe people having an allergic reaction to henna tattoos because of this darkening agent. Henna-based hair dyes have caused red and itchy scalps for the same reason.

The permanent inks can also be trouble. The mercury in red pigments made with mercuric sulfide (cinnabar) has caused allergic reactions.

Some people have developed strange skin growths—none full-fledged cancers—from permanent tattoos. Earlier this year, University of Maryland researchers described the case of a 38-year-old man who had a keratoacanthoma, a benign squamous cell growth, sprout from his month-old tattoo. Last year, doctors in Kansas City reported a case involving a 59-year-old woman who developed a different type of growth, called a pseudoepitheliomatous hyperplasia, in a two-year-old tattoo.

Lasering It Away

The permanence of tattoos is part of the attraction, but more than a few people have had regrets. Sometimes it's not a frivolous situation: cancer patients may get small tattoos to mark the spot where radiation is to be delivered. After their treatments are over, they want the marks removed.

In the past, dermatologists physically removed skin tissue to get rid of a tattoo, cutting or abrading it away. Now they depend on lasers to target and break apart the pigment particles so they get carried away by the lymphatic system. The lasers work in bursts that are nanoseconds long, so damage to nearby tissue is limited. Different wavelengths are used, depending on the color of the ink. Some colors—black, blue—are much easier to remove than others—yellow, orange. Local anesthesia is often needed, and there may be some bleeding.

Laser treatment is a big advance, but it's far from perfect. Many tattoos can't be completely removed: a realistic goal is 75% "clearing." Sometimes the tattoo may turn darker, rather than disappear, because the ink contains titanium dioxide or ferric oxide. The pigments used in tattoos to outline the eyes and lips (sometimes called permanent makeup) can be especially hard to remove. Up to 20 treatments may be needed. In people with dark skin, there's a danger of the skin turning white, so only lasers with a certain wavelength should be used. Allergic reactions may occur as the pigment particles get liberated from the dermis. Meanwhile, demand is growing for bigger, more complex and vibrantly colored tattoos that will be even harder to remove.

For these and other reasons, there's interest in tattoo inks that will stay sharp but can be removed more easily. The inks developed by Freedom-2, a New Jersey company, are a possibility. They come encapsulated in tiny polymer spheres and leave the skin quickly after a laser beam bursts open the sphere. Results from animal experiments are impressive. Whether they will work as well in humans and be accepted by tattoo artists and their customers has yet to be determined.

Excerpted from *Harvard Health Letter,* March 2008. Copyright © 2008 by the President and Fellow of Harvard College. Reprinted with permission via Copyright Clearance Center. www.health.harvard.edu/health

Hazardous Health Plans

Coverage gaps can leave you in big trouble.

Many people who believe they have adequate health insurance actually have coverage so riddled with loopholes, limits, exclusions, and gotchas that it won't come close to covering their expenses if they fall seriously ill, a *Consumer Reports* investigation has found.

At issue are so-called individual plans that consumers get on their own when, say, they've been laid off from a job but are too young for Medicare or too "affluent" for Medicaid. An estimated 14,000 Americans a day lose their job-based coverage, and many might be considering individual insurance for the first time in their lives.

But increasingly, individual insurance is a nightmare for consumers: more costly than the equivalent job-based coverage, and for those in less-than-perfect health, unaffordable at best and unavailable at worst. Moreover, the lack of effective consumer protections in most states allows insurers to sell plans with "affordable" premiums whose skimpy coverage can leave people who get very sick with the added burden of ruinous medical debt.

Just ask Janice and Gary Clausen of Audubon, Iowa. They told us they purchased a United Healthcare limited benefit plan sold through AARP that cost about $500 a month after Janice lost her accountant job and her work-based coverage when the auto dealership that employed her closed in 2004.

"I didn't think it sounded bad," Janice said. "I knew it would only cover $50,000 a year, but I didn't realize how much everything would cost." The plan proved hopelessly inadequate after Gary received a diagnosis of colon cancer. His 14-month treatment, including surgery and chemo-therapy, cost well over $200,000. Janice, 64, and Gary, 65, expect to be paying off medical debt for the rest of their lives.

For our investigation, we hired a national expert to help us evaluate a range of real policies from many states and interviewed Americans who bought those policies. We talked to insurance experts and regulators to learn more. Here is what we found:

- Heath insurance policies with gaping holes are offered by insurers ranging from small companies to brand-name carriers such as Aetna and United Healthcare. And in most states, regulators are not tasked with evaluating overall coverage.
- Disclosure requirements about coverage gaps are weak or nonexistent. So it's difficult for consumers to figure out in advance what a policy does or doesn't cover, compare plans, or estimate their out-of-pocket liability for a medical catastrophe. It doesn't help that many people who have never been seriously ill might have no idea how expensive medical care can be.
- People of modest means in many states might have no good options for individual coverage. Plans with affordable premiums can leave them with crushing medical debt if they fall seriously ill, and plans with adequate coverage may have huge premiums.
- There are some clues to a bad policy that consumers can spot. We tell you what they are, and how to avoid them if possible.
- Even as policymakers debate a major overhaul of the health-care system, government officials can take steps now to improve the current market.

Good Plans vs. Bad Plans

We think a good health-care plan should pay for necessary care without leaving you with lots of debt or high out-of-pocket costs. That includes hospital, ambulance, emergency-room, and physician fees; prescription drugs; outpatient treatments; diagnostic and imaging tests; chemotherapy, radiation, rehabilitation and physical therapy; mental-health treatment; and durable medical equipment, such as wheelchairs. Remember, health insurance is supposed to protect you in case of a catastrophically expensive illness, not simply cover your routine costs as a generally healthy person. And many individual plans do nowhere near the job.

For decades, individual insurance has been what economists call a "residual" market—something to buy only when you have run out of other options. The problem, according to insurance experts we consulted, is that the high cost of treatment in the U.S., which has the world's most expensive health-care system, puts truly affordable, comprehensive coverage out of the reach of people who don't have either deep pockets or a generous employer. Insurers tend to provide this choice: comprehensive coverage with a high monthly premium or skimpy coverage at a low monthly premium within the reach of middle- and low-income consumers.

More consumers are having to choose the latter as they become unemployed or their workplace drops coverage. (COBRA, the federal program that allows former employees to continue with the insurance from their old job by paying the full monthly premium, often costs $1,000 or more each month for family coverage. The federal government is temporarily subsidizing 65 percent of those premiums for some, but only for a maximum of nine months.) *Consumer Reports* and others label as "junk insurance" those so-called affordable individual plans with huge coverage gaps. Many such plans are sold throughout the nation, including policies from well-known companies.

Decent insurance covers more than just routine care.

Aetna's Affordable Health Choices plans, for example, offer limited benefits to part-time and hourly workers. We found one such policy that covered only $1,000 of hospital costs and $2,000 of out-patient expenses annually.

The Clausens' AARP plan, underwritten by insurance giant United Health Group, the parent company of United Healthcare, was advertised as "the essential benefits you deserve. Now in one affordable plan." AARP spokesman Adam Sohn said, "AARP has been fighting for affordable, quality health care for nearly a half-century, and while a fixed-benefit indemnity plan is not perfect, it offers our members an option to help cover some portion of their medical expenses without paying a high premium."

Nevertheless, AARP suspended sales of such policies last year after Sen. Charles Grassley, R-Iowa, questioned the marketing practices. Some 53,400 AARP members still have policies similar to the Clausens' that were sold under the names Medical Advantage Plan, Essential Health Insurance Plan, and Essential Plus Health Insurance Plan. In addition, at least 1 million members are enrolled in the AARP Hospital Indemnity Insurance Plan, Sohn said, an even more bare-bones policy. Members who have questions should first call 800-523-5800; for more help, call 888-687-2277. (Consumers Union, the nonprofit publisher of *Consumer Reports,* is working with AARP on a variety of health-care reforms.)

United American Insurance Co. promotes its supplemental health insurance as "an affordable solution to America's health-care crisis!" When Jeffrey E. Miller, 56, of Sarasota, Fla., received a diagnosis of prostate cancer a few months after buying one of the company's limited-benefit plans, he learned that it would not cover tens of thousands of dollars' worth of drug and radiation treatments he needed. As this article went to press, five months after his diagnosis, Miller had just begun treatment after qualifying for Florida Medicaid. A representative of United American declined to comment on its products.

Even governments are getting into the act. In 2008, Florida created the Cover Florida Health Care Access Program, which Gov. Charlie Crist said would make "affordable health coverage available to 3.8 million uninsured Floridians." But many of the basic "preventive" policies do not cover inpatient hospital treatments, emergency-room care, or physical therapy, and they severely limit coverage of everything else.

7 Signs a Health Plan Might Be Junk

Do Everything in Your Power to Avoid Plans with the Following Features:

Limited benefits. Never buy a product that is labeled "limited benefit" or "not major medical" insurance. In most states those phrases might be your only clue to an inadequate policy.

Low overall coverage limits. Health care is more costly than you might imagine if you've never experienced a serious illness. The cost of cancer or a heart attack can easily hit six figures. Policies with coverage limits of $25,000 or even $100,000 are not adequate.

"Affordable" premiums. There's no free lunch when it comes to insurance. To lower premiums, insurers trim benefits and do what they can to avoid insuring less healthy people. So if your insurance was a bargain, chances are good it doesn't cover very much. To check how much a comprehensive plan would cost you, go to *ehealthinsurance.com,* enter your location, gender, and age as prompted, and look for the most costly of the plans that pop up. It is probably the most comprehensive.

No coverage for important things. If you don't see a medical service specifically mentioned in the policy, assume it's not covered. We reviewed policies that didn't cover prescription drugs or outpatient chemotherapy but didn't say so anywhere in the policy document—not even in the section labeled "What is not covered."

Ceilings on categories of care. A $900-a-day maximum benefit for hospital expenses will hardly make a dent in a $45,000 bill for heart bypass surgery. If you have to accept limits on some services, be sure your plan covers hospital and outpatient medical treatment, doctor visits, drugs, and diagnostic and imaging tests without a dollar limit. Limits on mental-health costs, rehabilitation, and durable medical equipment should be the most generous you can afford.

Limitless out-of-pocket costs. Avoid policies that fail to specify a maximum amount that you'll have to pay before the insurer will begin covering 100 percent of expenses. And be alert for loopholes. Some policies, for instance, don't count co-payments for doctor visits or prescription drugs toward the maximum. That can be a catastrophe for seriously ill people who rack up dozens of doctor's appointments and prescriptions a year.

Random gotchas. The AARP policy that the Clausens bought began covering hospital care on the second day. That seems benign enough, except that the first day is almost always the most expensive, because it usually includes charges for surgery and emergency-room diagnostic tests and treatments.

The Wild West of Insurance

Compounding the problem of limited policies is the fact that policyholders are often unaware of those limits—until it's too late.

"I think people don't understand insurance, period," said Stephen Finan, associate director of policy at the American Cancer Society Cancer Action Network. "They know they need it. They look at the price, and that's it. They don't understand the language, and insurance companies go to great lengths to make it incomprehensible. Even lawyers don't always understand what it means."

Case in point: Jim Stacey of Fayetteville, N.C. In 2000, Stacey and his wife, Imelda, were pleased to buy a plan at what they considered an "incredible" price from the Mid-West National Life Insurance Co. of Tennessee. The policy's list of benefits included a lifetime maximum payout of up to $1 million per person. But after Stacey learned he had prostate cancer in 2005, the policy paid only $1,480 of the $17,453 it cost for the implanted radioactive pellets he chose to treat the disease.

"To this day, I don't know what went wrong," Stacey said about the bill.

We sent the policy, along with the accompanying Explanation of Benefit forms detailing what it did and didn't pay, to Karen Pollitz, research professor at the Georgetown University Health Policy Institute. We asked Pollitz, an expert on individual health insurance, to see whether she could figure out why the policy covered so little.

"The short answer is, 'Beats the heck out of me,'" she e-mailed back to us. The Explanation of Benefit forms were missing information that she would expect to see, such as specific billing codes that explain what treatments were given. And there didn't seem to be any connection between the benefits listed in the policy and the actual amounts paid.

Contacted for comment, a spokeswoman for HealthMarkets, the parent company of Mid-West National, referred us to the company website. It stated that the company "pays claims according to the insurance contract issued to each customer" and that its policies "satisfy a need in the marketplace for a product that balances the cost with the available benefit options." The spokeswoman declined to answer specific questions about Stacey's case, citing patient privacy laws.

One reason confusion abounds, Pollitz said, is that health insurance is regulated by the states, not by the federal government, and most states (Massachusetts and New York are prominent exceptions) do not have a standard definition of what constitutes health insurance.

"Rice is rice and gasoline is gasoline. When you buy it, you know what it is," Pollitz said. "Health insurance —who knows what it is? It is some product that's sold by an insurance company. It could be a little bit or a lot of protection. You don't know what is and isn't covered. Nothing can be taken for granted."

How to Protect Yourself

Seek out comprehensive coverage. A good plan will cover your legitimate health care without burdening you with oversized debt.

Want Better Coverage? Try Running for Congress

President Barack Obama says Americans should have access to the kind of health benefits Congress gets. We detail them below. Members of Congress and other U.S. government employees can receive care through the Federal Employees Health Benefits Program. Employees choose from hundreds of plans, but the most popular is a national Blue Cross and Blue Shield Preferred Provider Organization plan. Employee contributions for that plan are $152 per person, or $357 per family, per month.

Plan Features

- No annual or lifetime limits for major services
- Deductible of $300 per person and $600 per family
- Out-of-pocket limit of $5,000 per year with preferred providers, which includes most deductibles, co-insurance, and co-payments

Covered Services

- Inpatient and outpatient hospital care
- Inpatient and outpatient doctor visits
- Prescription drugs
- Diagnostic tests
- Preventive care, including routine immunizations
- Chemotherapy and radiation therapy
- Maternity care
- Family planning
- Durable medical equipment, orthopedic devices, and artificial limbs
- Organ and tissue transplants
- Inpatient and outpatient surgery
- Physical, occupational, and speech therapy
- Outpatient and inpatient mental-health care

"The idea of 'Cadillac' coverage vs. basic coverage isn't an appropriate way to think about health insurance," said Mila Kofman, Maine's superintendent of insurance. "It has to give you the care you need, when you need it, and some financial security so you don't end up out on the street."

What you want is a plan that has no caps on specific coverages. But if you have to choose, pick a plan offering unlimited coverage for hospital and outpatient treatment, doctor visits, drugs, and diagnostic and imaging tests. When it comes to lifetime coverage maximums, unlimited is best and $2 million should be the minimum. Ideally, there should be a single deductible for everything or, at most, one deductible for drugs and one for everything else. And the policy should pay for 100 percent of all expenses once your out-of-pocket payments hit a certain amount, such as $5,000 or $10,000.

If you are healthy now, do not buy a plan based on the assumption that you will stay that way. Don't think you can safely

The Real Cost of Illness Can Be Staggering . . .

Few Americans realize how much care costs. Coverage gaps can leave you in debt.

Condition	Treatment	Total Cost
Late-stage colon cancer	124 weeks of treatment, including two surgeries, three types of chemotherapy, imaging, prescription drugs, hospice care.	$285,946
Heart attack	56 weeks of treatment, including ambulance, ER workup, angioplasty with stent, bypass surgery, cardiac rehabilitation, counseling for depression, prescription drugs.	$110,405
Breast cancer	87 weeks of treatment, including lumpectomy, drugs, lab and imaging tests, chemotherapy and radiation therapy, mental-health counseling, and prosthesis.	$104,535
Type 2 diabetes	One year of maintenance care, including insulin and other prescription drugs, glucose test strips, syringes and other supplies, quarterly physician visits and lab, annual eye exam.	$5,949

. . . and Out-of-Pocket Expenses Can Vary Widely

With its lower premium and deductible, the California plan at right would seem the better deal. But because California, unlike Massachusetts, allows the sale of plans with large coverage gaps, a patient there will pay far more than a Massachusetts patient for the same breast cancer treatments, as the breakdown below shows.

Massachusetts Plan	California Plan
Monthly premium for any 55-year-old: $399	**Monthly premium for a healthy 55-year-old:** $246
Annual deductible: $2,200	**Annual deductible:** $1,000
Co-pays: $25 office visit, $250 outpatient surgery after deductible, $10 for generic drugs, $25 for nonpreferred generic and brand name, $45 for nonpreferred brand name	**Co-pays:** $25 preventive care office visits
	Co-insurance: 20% for most covered services
Co-insurance: 20% for some services	**Out-of-pocket maximum:** $2,500, includes hospital and surgical co-insurance only.
Out-of-pocket maximum: $5,000, includes deductible, co-insurance, and all co-payments	**Exclusions and limits:** Prescription drugs, most mental-health care, and wigs for chemotherapy patients not covered. Outpatient care not covered until out-of-pocket maximum satisfied from hospital/surgical co-insurance.
Exclusions and limits: Cap of 24 mental-health visits, $3,000 cap on equipment	
Lifetime benefits: Unlimited	**Lifetime benefits:** $5 million

Service and Total Cost	Patient Pays	Patient Pays
Hospital	$0	$705
Surgery	$981	$1,136
Office visits and procedures	$1,833	$2,010
Prescription drugs	$1,108	$5,985
Laboratory and imaging tests	$808	$3,772
Chemotherapy and radiation therapy	$1,987	$21,113
Mental-health care	$950	$2,700
Prosthesis	$0	$350
Total $104,535	$7,668	$37,767

Source: Karen Pollitz, Georgetown University Health Policy Institute, using real claims data and policies. Columns of figures do not add up exactly because all numbers are rounded.

go without drug coverage, for example, because you don't take any prescriptions regularly today. "You can't know in advance if you're going to be among the .01 percent of people who needs the $20,000-a-month biologic drug," said Gary Claxton, a vice president of the nonprofit Kaiser Family Foundation, a health-policy research organization. "What's important is if you get really sick, are you going to lose everything?"

Consider trade-offs carefully. If you have to make a trade-off to lower your premium, Claxton and Pollitz suggest opting for a higher deductible and a higher out-of-pocket limit rather than fixed dollar limits on services. Better to use up part of your retirement savings paying $10,000 up front than to lose your whole nest egg paying a $90,000 medical bill after your policy's limits are exhausted.

What Lawmakers Need to Do Next

Consumers Union, the nonprofit publisher of *Consumer Reports,* has long supported national health-care reform that makes affordable health coverage available to all Americans. The coverage should include a basic set of required, comprehensive health-care benefits, like those in the federal plan that members of Congress enjoy. Insurers should compete for customers based on price and the quality of their services, not by limiting their risk through confusing options, incomplete information, or greatly restricted benefits.

As reform is developed and debated, Consumers Union supports these changes in the way health insurance is presented and sold:

Clear terms. All key terms in policies, such as "out-of-pocket" and "annual deductible," should be defined by law and insurers should be required to use them that way in their policies.

Standard benefits. Ideally, all plans should have a uniform set of benefits covering all medically necessary care, but consumers should be able to opt for varying levels of cost-sharing. Failing that, states should establish a menu of standardized plans, as Medicare does for Medigap plans. Consumers would then have a basis for comparing costs of plans.

Transparency. Policies that insurers currently sell should be posted in full online or available by mail upon request for anyone who wants to examine them. They should be the full, legally binding policy documents, not just a summary or marketing brochure. In many states now, consumers can't see the policy document until after they have joined the plan. At that point, they're legally entitled to a "free look" period in which to examine the policy and ask for a refund if they don't like what they see. But if they turn the policy back in, they face the prospect of being uninsured until they can find another plan.

Disclosure of costs. Every plan must provide a standard "Plan Coverage" summary that clearly displays what is—and more important, is not—covered. The summary should include independently verified estimates of total out-of-pocket costs for a standard range of serious problems, such as breast cancer treatment or heart bypass surgery.

Moreover, reliable information should be available to consumers about the costs in their area of treating various medical conditions, so that they have a better understanding of the bills they could face without adequate health coverage.

With such a high deductible, in years when you are relatively healthy you might never collect anything from your health insurance. To economize on routine care, take advantage of free community health screenings, low-cost or free community health clinics, immediate-care clinics offered in some drugstores, and low-priced generic prescriptions sold at Target, Walmart, and elsewhere.

Look for a plan that doesn't cap your coverage.

If your financial situation is such that you can afford neither the higher premiums of a more comprehensive policy nor high deductibles, you really have no good choices, Pollitz said, adding, "It's why we need to fix our health-care system."

Check out the policy and company. You can, at least, take some steps to choose the best plan you can afford. First, see "7 signs a health plan might be junk" to learn to spot the most dangerous pitfalls and the preferred alternatives.

Use the Web to research insurers you're considering. The National Association of Insurance Commissioners posts complaint information online at *www.naic.org.*

Entering the name of the company and policy in a search engine can't hurt either. Consumers who did that recently would have discovered that Mid-West National was a subsidiary of HealthMarkets, whose disclosure and claims handling drew many customers' ire. Last year, Health-Markets was fined $20 million after a multi state investigation of its sales practices and claims handling.

Don't rely on the salesperson's word. Jeffrey E. Miller, the Florida man whose policy failed to cover much of his cancer treatment, recalls being bombarded with e-mail and calls when he began shopping for insurance. "The salesman for the policy I bought told me it was great, and I was going to be covered, and it paid up to $100,000 for a hospital stay," he said. "But the insurance has turned out to pay very little."

Pollitz advises anyone with questions about their policy to ask the agent and get answers in writing. "Then if it turns out not to be true," she said, "you can complain."

Copyright © 2009 by Consumers Union of U.S., Inc. Yonkers, NY 10703-1057, a nonprofit organization. Reprinted with permission from the May 2009 issue of CONSUMER REPORTS® for educational purposes only. No commercial use or reproduction permitted. www.ConsumerReports.org.

UNIT 10

Contemporary Health Hazards

Unit Selections

Key Points to Consider

- What diseases are most likely to have an environmental link?

- Why are more and more women being diagnosed with COPD?

- What are the risks associated with contracting MRSA?

- How does noise affect health?

- Is swine flu a serious concern or are we overreacting?

Student Website
www.mhcls.com

Internet References

Centers for Disease Control: Flu
   http://www.cdc.gov/flu
Food and Drug Administration Mad Cow Disease Page
   http://www.fda.gov/oc/opacom/hottopics/bse.html
Environmental Protection Agency
   http://www.epa.gov

This unit examines a variety of health hazards that Americans face on a daily basis and includes topics ranging from environmental health issues to newly emerging, or rather, reemerging infectious illnesses. During the 1970s and 1980s, Americans became deeply concerned about environmental changes that affected the air, water, and food we take in. While some improvements have been observed in these areas, much remains to be done, as new areas of concern continue to emerge. Global warming is responsible for climatic changes, including an increase in the number of weather disasters such as hurricanes. Global warming and its relationship to disease is discussed in "Climate Change and Your Health."

Another area of concern has to do with the relationship between loud noise and health. Author Elizabeth Svoboda discusses how noise plays a role in triggering violent tendencies, aggression, heart problems, hearing impairments, and decreased productivity. Yet another environmentally linked condition is the potential health dangers of bisphenol A, a common chemical found in plastic bottles and containers.

We face newly recognized diseases such as Methicillin-Resistant *Staphlococcus aureus,* Avian Flu, Severe Acute Respiratory Syndrome (SARS), AIDS, West Nile Virus, and Mad Cow. Some of these diseases may have their causes rooted in environmental factors. Environmental Author Zach Patton discusses the changes in the way AIDS is treated and perceived. In "Methicillin-Resistant *Staphlococcus aureus,*" author Priya Sampathkumar addresses the growing health problem related to this drug-resistant bacterial infection. It is a particular concern among the institutionalized elderly and in any place where many people are in close contact with each other. Similarly, swine flu has recently emerged, or reemerged,

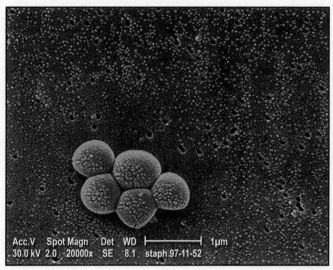

© CDC/Janice Carr

and is causing concerns over whether or not it will be the next pandemic.

While this unit focuses on exogenous factors that influence our state of health, it is important to remember that health is a dynamic state representing the degree of harmony or balance that exists between endogenous and exogenous factors. This concept of balance applies to the environment as well. Due to the intimate relationship that exists between people, animals, and their environment, it is impossible to promote the concept of wellness without also safeguarding the quality of our environment, both the physical and the social.

When Government Makes Us Sick

GLENN DAVIDSON

Like many Americans, I pick up an energy bar from time to time without giving a moment's thought to my safety before eating it. Earlier this year, that choice hit me with a case of **salmonella** poisoning. Across the country, the outbreak caused by tainted **peanuts** plunged hundreds of young and elderly people into medical trauma and tragically led to nine deaths.

I confidently consume processed food products—as do millions of other Americans—because I assume that regulators, especially the Food and Drug Administration, are on the case ensuring our safety.

Yet FDA failed miserably to protect the public in the case of **salmonella**-laced peanut products, and it wasn't the first or only instance. The public has a right to know what FDA knew about the Georgia peanut plant that was responsible, how far back the agency knew it, and why officials didn't take immediate action to shut down the entire chain of contaminated products that went to market from the plant at the first warning sign.

FDA is making the case that the manufacturer is to blame, and there's no doubt that the company is primarily at fault. But can we accept FDA's conclusion that food safety in the United States is a matter of industry self-policing? If private industry had a strong track record of compliance and FDA had a record of challenging internal tests or punishing companies that abuse the system, maybe then such a system could be defended.

But FDA's recent record on food and consumer product safety is dismal:

A peer-reviewed report (http://www.ehjournal.net/content/8/1/2) in the journal *Environmental Health* found that high fructose corn syrup is commonly tainted with trace levels of mercury. The lead author of the study, Renee Dufault, was an FDA researcher who was aware of the results in 2005, then went public after retiring from the agency in 2008.

Researchers at the University of Rochester in New York say in a study (http://www.ehponline.org/members/2009/0800376/0800376.pdf) released in January that bisphenol A, which is used to make plastic and suspected of causing cancer, stays in the body much longer than previously thought. In 2008, FDA declared the chemical safe for all use in an assessment that contained language from reports written on behalf of chemical-makers or others with a financial stake in BPA.

According to a Jan. 23 article (http://www.govexec.com/dailyfed/0109/012309cdam2.htm) by Government Executive.com's sister publication *CongressDaily,* "Earlier this month, a group of FDA scientists wrote to President Obama's transition team a letter similar to one they sent Rep. John Dingell, D-Mich., in October claiming FDA brass interferes with the medical-device review process to push through approvals based on faulty and unethical evidence."

It's no wonder the Government Accountability Office recently put FDA on its high-risk list, noting the agency's regulatory scope has expanded while resources to conduct that mission have not kept pace. There's no question FDA's mission should be reviewed and, when appropriate, get more funding to fulfill it.

But there are other important questions that go beyond agency funding levels. Why weren't food safety experts empowered to act on reports of problems at the Georgia peanut factories in real time? Why were the reports of respected scientists ignored in the instance of high fructose corn syrup? Why were industry groups allowed to write public safety reports on BPA? And why were political appointees interfering with a scientific review process about medical devices?

All these examples support a chilling similarity of failure—every one of them resulting from the federal government's broken human capital management system, which isn't merely wasting taxpayer dollars, but also is putting the health and safety of Americans at risk every day.

If only these problems were confined to FDA, we could sweep out its system and replace it with that of a better performing agency. Unfortunately, there are no examples of better performing government agencies, only more examples of failure—from the Federal Emergency Management Agency's tragic incompetence in New Orleans to NASA's ignored red flags before the space shuttle Columbia disaster to collapsed bridges, poorly explained prescription drug programs and financial systems run amok. The list goes on in today's newspapers.

The Bush administration's command-and-control approach to governance is largely responsible for the sad state of federal management. The White House persistently pushed its agenda down to departments and agencies rather than involving people in the decision-making process or creating market forces that help drive decisions. All management improvement initiatives were led centrally, resulting in a backlash among the rank and file.

This is the federal government President Obama has inherited. New marching orders and higher morale are good things, and a larger federal workforce probably is a necessity. But if the president doesn't act quickly to overhaul the way people are managed in all agencies, change the culture and change it fast, everything he tries to do—from health care reform to energy independence projects—could be imperiled.

Only the Office of Personnel Management has the governmentwide scope to deal with these issues in a comprehensive and continuous manner. OPM must become, at all levels and in all ways, part of the larger human resources community. While public sector HR management poses distinct challenges, it overlaps far more with the broader world of HR management than many in the public sector acknowledge or practice. OPM should stop being insular and isolated and come to understand what's going on in the public and private sectors.

By focusing on getting the most out of its workforce, the federal government would make major, long-overdue investments in effective government. Good, cost-effective government starts with staying out of the news and making what Americans expect to be routine, routine again.

All Americans ask is that the next time we pick up a piece of peanut butter candy or drink from a plastic container, please, no surprises.

GLENN DAVIDSON is managing director of EquaTerra's public sector practice, serving federal, state and local government clients. In the public sector he was chief of staff for former Virginia Gov. L. Douglas Wilder and legislative director for former Ohio Congressman Ron Mottl.

From *Government Executive*, March 6, 2009. Copyright © 2009 by National Journal. Reprinted by permission.

From Smoking Boom, A Major Killer of Women

DENISE GRADY

For Jean Rommes, the crisis came five years ago, on a Monday morning when she had planned to go to work but wound up in the hospital, barely able to breathe. She was 59, the president of a small company in Iowa. Although she had quit smoking a decade earlier, 30 years of cigarettes had taken their toll.

After several days in the hospital, she was sent home tethered to an oxygen tank, with a raft of medicines and a warning: "If I didn't do something, life was going to continue to be a pretty scary experience."

Ms. Rommes has chronic obstructive pulmonary disease, or C.O.P.D., a progressive illness that permanently damages the lungs and is usually caused by smoking. Once thought of as an old man's disease, this disorder has become a major killer in women as well, the consequence of a smoking boom in the 1950s, '60s and '70s. The death rate in women nearly tripled from 1980 to 2000, and since 2000, more women than men have died or been hospitalized every year because of the disease.

"Women started smoking in what I call the Virginia Slims era, when they started sponsoring sporting events," said Dr. Barry J. Make, a lung specialist at National Jewish Medical and Research Center in Denver. "It's now just catching up to them."

Chronic obstructive pulmonary disease actually comprises two illnesses: one, emphysema, destroys air sacs deep in the lungs; the other, chronic bronchitis, causes inflammation, congestion and scarring in the airways. The disease kills 120,000 Americans a year, is the fourth leading cause of death and is expected to be third by 2020. About 12 million Americans are known to have it, including many who have long since quit smoking, and studies suggest that 12 million more cases have not been diagnosed. Half the patients are under 65. The disease has left some 900,000 working-age people too sick to work and costs $42 billion a year in medical bills and lost productivity.

"It's the largest uncontrolled epidemic of disease in the United States today," said Dr. James Crapo, a professor at the National Jewish Medical and Research Center.

Experts consider the statistics a national disgrace. They say chronic lung disease is misdiagnosed, neglected, improperly treated and stigmatized as self-induced, with patients made to feel they barely deserve help, because they smoked. The disease is mired in a bog of misconception and prejudice, doctors say. It is commonly mistaken for asthma, especially in women, and treated with the wrong drugs.

Although incurable, it is treatable, but many patients, and some doctors, mistakenly think little can be done for it. As a result, patients miss out on therapies that could help them feel better and possibly live longer. The therapies vary, but may include drugs, exercise programs, oxygen and lung surgery.

Incorrectly treated, many fall needlessly into a cycle of worsening illness and disability, and wind up in the emergency room over and over again with pneumonia and other exacerbations— breathing crises like the one that put Ms. Rommes in the hospital—that might have been averted.

"Patients often come to me with years of being under treated," said Dr. Byron Thomashow, the director of the Center for Chest Disease at New York-Presbyterian/Columbia hospital.

Still others are overtreated for years with steroids like prednisone, which is meant for short-term use and if used too much can thin the bones, weaken muscles and raise the risk of cataracts.

Adequate treatment means drugs, usually inhaled, that open the airways and quell inflammation—preventive medicines that must be used daily, not just in emergencies. It is essential to quit smoking.

Patients also need antibiotics to fight lung infections, vaccines to prevent flu and pneumonia and lessons on special breathing techniques that can help them make the most of their diminished lungs. Some need oxygen, which can help them be more active and prolong life in severe cases. Many need dietary advice: obesity can worsen symptoms, but some with advanced disease lose so much weight that their muscles begin to waste. Some people with emphysema benefit from surgery to remove diseased parts of their lungs.

Above all, patients need exercise, because shortness of breath drives many to become inactive, and they become increasingly weak, homebound, disabled and depressed. Many could benefit from therapy programs called pulmonary rehabilitation, which combine exercise with education about the disease, drugs and nutrition, but the programs are not available in all parts of the country, and insurance coverage for them varies.

"I have a complicated, severe group of patients, but I will swear to you that very few wind up in hospitals," Dr. Thomashow said. "I treat aggressively. I use the medicines, I exercise all of them. You can make a difference here. This is an example of how we're undertreating this entire disease."

Little-Known Epidemic

Researchers say there is so little public awareness of how common and serious C.O.P.D. is that the O might as well stand for "obscure" or "overlooked."

The disease may not be well known, but people who have it are a familiar sight. They are the ones who cannot climb half a flight of stairs without getting winded, who have a perpetual smoker's cough or wheeze, who need oxygen to walk down the block or push a cart through the supermarket. Some grow too weak and short of breath to leave the house. The flu or even a cold can put them in the hospital. In advanced stages, the lung disease can lead to heart failure.

"This is a disease where people eventually fade away because they can no longer cope with life," said Grace Anne Dorney Koppel, who has chronic lung disease. (Ms. Dorney Koppel, a lawyer, is married to Ted Koppel.) "My God, if you don't have breath, you don't have anything."

Most cases, about 85 percent, are caused by smoking, and symptoms usually start after age 40, in people who have smoked a pack a day for 10 years or more. In the United States, 45 million people smoke, 21 percent of adults. Only about 20 percent of smokers develop chronic lung disease.

The illness is not the same as asthma, but some patients have asthma along with their other lung problems. Most have a combination of emphysema and chronic bronchitis. In about one-sixth of cases, emphysema is the main problem. Women are far more likely than men to develop chronic bronchitis, and are less prone to emphysema. Some studies have suggested that women's lungs are more sensitive than men's to the toxins in smoke.

Worldwide, these lung diseases kill 2.5 million people a year. An article in September in The Lancet, a medical journal, said that "if every smoker in the world were to stop smoking today, the rates of C.O.P.D. would probably continue to increase for the next 20 years." The reason is that although quitting slows the disease, it can develop later.

Cigarettes are the major cause worldwide, but other sources are important in developing countries, especially smoke from indoor fires that burn wood, coal, straw or dung for heating and cooking. Women and children are most likely to be exposed. Outdoor air pollution plays less of a part: it can aggravate existing disease, but is believed to cause only 1 percent of cases in rich countries and 2 percent in poorer ones. Occupational exposures in cotton mills and mines may contribute.

Researchers have differed about whether passive smoking plays a role, but a Lancet article in September predicted that in China, among the 240 million people who are now over 50, 1.9 million who never smoked will die from chronic lung disease— just from exposure to other people's smoke.

Many patients with lung disease have other illnesses as well, like heart disease, acid reflux, hypertension, high cholesterol, sinus problems or diabetes. Compared with other smokers, those with C.O.P.D. are more likely to develop lung cancer as well. Researchers suspect that all the ailments stem partly from the same underlying condition, widespread inflammation, a reaction by the immune system that can affect blood vessels, organs and tissues all over the body.

Lung disease can creep up insidiously, because human beings have lung power to spare. Millions of airways, with enough surface area to cover a tennis court, provide so much reserve that most people would not notice it if they lost the use of a third or even half of a lung. But all that extra capacity can hide an impending disaster.

"If it comes on gradually, the body can adjust," said Dr. Neil Schachter, a lung specialist and professor at Mount Sinai Medical Center in New York. "Some of these patients are at oxygen levels where you and I would be gasping for breath."

People adjust psychologically as well, cutting back their activities, deciding perhaps that they just do not enjoy sports anymore, that they are getting older, gaining weight or a bit out of shape. But at some point the body can no longer compensate, and denial does not work anymore.

"It's like trying to breathe through a straw," Dr. Schachter said. "It's very uncomfortable."

By then, half a lung might be ruined. On a CT scan, he said, the lungs may look "moth-eaten," full of holes where tissue has been destroyed.

Often, the diagnosis is not made until the disease is advanced. Even though breathing tests are easy to perform and recommended for high-risk patients like former and current smokers, many doctors do not bother. People who do get a diagnosis frequently are not taught how to use the inhalers that are the mainstay of treatment. Access to pulmonary rehabilitation is limited because Medicare has left coverage decisions to the states. Some programs have shut down, and there are bills in the House and Senate that would require pulmonary rehabilitation to be covered by Medicare. Medicare may also reduce coverage for home oxygen.

Meanwhile, billions are spent on treating exacerbations, episodes of severe breathing trouble that are often caused by colds, flu or other respiratory infections.

A recent study of 1,600 consecutive hospitalizations for chronic lung disease in five New York hospitals found that once patients were in the hospital, their treatment was generally correct, Dr. Thomashow said. But "most upsetting," he said, was that the majority had been incorrectly treated before going to the hospital.

For many, trying to control the disease, rather than be controlled by it, is a daily struggle. Diane Williams Hymons, 57, a social service consultant and therapist in Silver Spring, Md., has had lifelong problems with bronchitis, allergies and asthma. In the last five or 10 years, her breathing difficulties have worsened, but she was told only three years ago that she had C.O.P.D. It motivated her to give up cigarettes, after smoking for more than 30 years.

"I have good days, and days that aren't as great," she said. "I sometimes have trouble walking up steps. I have to stop and catch my breath."

She is "usually fine" when sitting, she said.

Her mother, also a former smoker with chronic lung disease, has been in a pulmonary rehabilitation program. Ms. Williams Hymons's doctor has not recommended such a program for her, but she has no idea why. They have discussed surgery to remove part of her lungs, which helps some people with emphysema, but she said no decision had been made yet because it is not clear whether her main problem is emphysema or asthma. She is not sure what her prognosis is.

A Risky Approach

Ms. Williams Hymons has been taking prednisone pills for years, something both she and her doctor know is risky. But when she tries to cut back, the disease flares up. She has many side effects from the drug.

"My bone density is not looking real good," she said. "I have cramps in my hands and feet, weight gain and bloating, the moon face, excess facial hair, fat deposits between my shoulder blades. Yes, I have those."

She has broken two ribs just from coughing, probably because the prednisone has thinned her bones, she said. She went to a hospital for the rib pain last year and was given so much asthma medication to stop the coughing that it caused abnormal heart rhythms. She wound up in the cardiac unit for five days, and now says "never again" to being hospitalized.

Her doctor orders regular bone density tests.

"I know he's concerned, like I'm concerned," Ms. Williams Hymons said, "but we can't seem to kind of get things under control."

A recent study of 25 primary care practices around the United States treating chronic lung disease found that most did not perform spirometry, a simple breathing test used to diagnose or monitor the disease, even when they had the equipment to do so. The test takes only a few minutes, but doctors said there was not enough time during the usual 15-minute visit. Similarly, the practices did not offer much help with smoking cessation.

The author of the study (published in August in The American Journal of Medicine), Pamela L. Moore, said many of the doctors felt unable to help smokers quit, and believed that as long as patients kept smoking, treatments for lung disease would be for nought. But Dr. Moore said research had found that people are more likely to quit or start cutting back if doctors recommend it.

Labeling the disease self-induced is "an unbelievably painful concept," Dr. Thomashow said. "Patients blame themselves, their family blames them, we even have evidence that health providers blame them."

Shame and Blame

Indeed, a patient at a clinic in Manhattan, with nasal oxygen tubing attached to equipment in a backpack, said, "This is one of the evils you must suffer for the things we did in our life."

Smoking also contributes to heart disease, Dr. Thomashow said, and yet people "don't waste time blaming the patient."

"This disease quite frankly has an image problem," said Dr. James Kiley, the director of lung research at the National Heart,

Lung and Blood Institute, which started a campaign last January to educate people about the disease.

In one way or another every patient seems to have encountered what John Walsh, president of the C.O.P.D. Foundation, calls the "shame and blame" attached to this disease.

It is a familiar theme to Ms. Dorney Koppel, who agreed to become a spokeswoman for the institute's education campaign. She was surprised to be asked to help, she said, because the campaign needed a celebrity, and she is merely married to one. She asked the person who invited her, whether there were no famous people with C.O.P.D.

"I was told, 'None who will admit it,'" she said.

Ms. Dorney Koppel, who is candid about being a former smoker, calls the illness the Rodney Dangerfield of diseases.

"You don't get no respect," she said. "I have to pay publicly for my sins. I have paid."

Like many patients, Ms. Rommes has both emphysema and chronic bronchitis, along with asthma. She had symptoms for years before receiving the correct diagnosis.

She began smoking in college during the 1960s, when she was 18. People whom she admired smoked, and it seemed cool. She smoked for 30 years.

When she quit in 1992, it was not because she thought she was ill, but because she realized that she was organizing her day around chances to smoke. But she almost certainly was ill. She was only 50, but climbing a flight of stairs left her winded. From what she found in medical dictionaries, she began to suspect she had lung disease.

By 2000 she was so short of breath that she consulted her doctor about it.

He gave her a spirometry test. In one second, healthy adults should be able to blow out 80 percent of the total they can exhale; her score was 34 percent, which, she knows now, indicated moderate to severe lung disease.

"I honestly don't know whether he knew," she said of her doctor. "I suspect he did, but he didn't call it emphysema."

"He put me on a couple of inhalers and he called it asthma," Ms. Rommes said. "I sort of ignored the whole thing, because the inhalers did make me feel better. I started to gain some weight, and things got progressively worse."

She cannot help wondering now if she could have avoided becoming so desperately ill, if she had only known sooner what a dangerous illness she had.

The turning point came in February 2003 when she tried to take a shower and found that she could not breathe. The steam all but suffocated her. She managed to drive from her home in Osceola, Iowa, to her doctor's office, struggle across the parking lot like someone climbing a mountain and collapse, gasping, onto a couch inside the clinic. Her blood oxygen was perilously low, two-thirds of normal, even when she was given oxygen. The hospital was next door, and her doctor had her admitted immediately.

Fear and Anger

She had Type 2 diabetes as well as lung disease, and her doctor told her that losing weight would help both illnesses. But she said, "He made it pretty clear that he didn't think I would or could."

After Early Success, Operations to Remove Damaged Tissues Have Fallen Sharply

Intently watching the rise and fall of Madeline Gallagher's abdomen as she lay on the operating table, Dr. Mark Ginsburg said, "Her diaphragm is finally moving. That's a really good sign."

He had just removed 30 percent of each of her lungs. Now, he said, she was breathing normally, for the first time in many years.

"It's counterintuitive," he said. "Patients have poor lung function, and you help them by taking out part of their lungs."

Mrs. Gallagher, 65, has emphysema, first diagnosed in 1993. She had smoked for 35 years, starting when she was 15, and quit in 1992. Initially not severe, the disease worsened over the years until cleaning the house, shopping, just walking down the street became a struggle. More and more, she needed oxygen. Pneumonia put her in the hospital twice. Already thin, she lost 15 pounds, a danger sign in emphysema.

On Oct. 17, at New York-Presbyterian/Columbia hospital, she had lung-volume reduction surgery. It is not a cure, but has been found to help certain people with emphysema—possibly 10 percent—those with such poor lung function that they can barely exercise, and with disease mostly localized to parts of the lungs that can be removed. With the surgery many feel better, and some also live longer.

Lungs damaged by emphysema lose their elasticity and trap stale air. As a result, they can enlarge, or hyperinflate, to 150 percent of their normal size, or more, preventing the diaphragm from moving normally. Instinctively, patients begin working other muscles to compensate, and sometimes become barrel-chested or raise their shoulders so much that they look like they are wearing shoulder pads. On X-rays, abnormally wide spaces between the ribs are a telltale sign of the disease. Doctors and nurses can spot patients in waiting rooms, sitting straight up on the edges of their seats, leaning on their hands with elbows stiff and shoulders up as if they are about to push off. But no matter how hard they try, they cannot take in enough air.

In theory, by cutting away the most diseased tissue, the operation should stop some of the air trapping, and by restoring the lungs to their proper size, it should let the diaphragm work so that the chest can move more normally.

The surgery has had a rocky history. Reports of fantastic recoveries made it popular in the 1990s, but health officials wanted a rigorous study. A government-sponsored experiment began in 1996, and ultimately found the operation beneficial only for some types of emphysema, and useless or even harmful in others. In 2003, Medicare decided to cover it only for people like those who had done well in the study, and only at experienced hospitals.

The number of operations has fallen sharply, from thousands a year to under 200 in 2006. Some researchers praise the outcome as a triumph of data over wishful thinking, but others say that the pendulum has swung too far, and that many patients who could be helped are missing out.

Meanwhile, researchers are experimenting with valves and other devices that are implanted in the lungs through scopes passed down the throat, without cutting through the chest. The devices are meant to vent trapped air into the airways, where it can be exhaled, and to deflate diseased parts of the lungs—without having to cut out any tissue. In some cases, the implants might replace surgery, but they might also help patients who are not candidates for the surgery.

After Mrs. Gallagher's second bout with pneumonia, doctors recommended lung-volume reduction, and she agreed to it in the hope that it would give her back some of her life—let her be more active, take trips with her husband, keep up with her grandchildren.

Dr. Ginsburg operated through tiny slits, rather than opening the entire chest. He inserted a camera, and guided by a monitor, cut away a cellphone-size slab of each lung. The operation took about 90 minutes.

"We did exactly what we wanted to do," Dr. Ginsburg said. "The question is, will it work?" Ideally, the operation can set the clock back three to five years, he said, but added, "At the end of the day she's only as good as what she has left."

Mrs. Gallagher had a rough recovery. She spent 10 days in the hospital, twice as long as expected. She had trouble breathing and could not keep food down, which worried her family because she was already frail.

A few days after leaving the hospital, she was supposed to resume exercising in a pulmonary rehabilitation program that had begun before the surgery. Her daughter wondered how she would manage, when she was too weak even to dress herself.

But she bounced back quickly. Two weeks later, she said, "I'm doing terrific," adding that she had just walked 25 minutes on a treadmill without needing oxygen, something she could not do before. Her appetite was back, and she had polished off a dinner of veal parmesan and baked ziti.

"My breathing isn't as shallow as it used to be," Mrs. Gallagher said. "I can take a deeper breath. I'm very, very happy."

Motivated by fear and anger, she began riding an exercise bike, walking on a treadmill, lifting weights at a gym and eating only 1,200 to 1,500 calories a day, mostly lean meat with plenty of vegetables and fruit.

"I kind of came to the conclusion that if I didn't, I probably wasn't going to be around," Ms. Rommes said. "I wasn't ready to check out. And my husband was beginning to show the signs of Alzheimer's disease. I knew that if I couldn't continue to manage our affairs, it wasn't going to work out."

By December 2003, her efforts were starting to pay off. She went from needing oxygen around the clock to using it only for sleeping, and by January 2005 she no longer needed it at all. She was able to lower the doses of her inhalers and diabetes medicines. By February 2005, she had lost 100 pounds.

The daily exercise also helped her deal with the stress of her husband's illness. He died in June.

"I had no clue that exercise would do as much for ability to breathe as it did," she said, adding that it helped more than the drugs, which she described as "really pretty minimal."

She is hooked on exercise now, getting up every morning at 5 A.M. to walk for 45 minutes on the treadmill. She goes at it hard enough to break a sweat, wearing a blood oxygen monitor to make sure her level does not dip too low (if it does, she slows down or uses special breathing techniques to bring it up). She walks outdoors, as well, and three times a week, she works out with weights at a gym.

"Exercise is absolutely essential, and it's essential to start it as soon as you know you have C.O.P.D.," she said.

Exercise does not heal or strengthen the lungs themselves, but it improves overall fitness, which people with lung disease need desperately because their shortness of breath leads to inactivity, muscle wasting and loss of stamina.

"Both my pulmonologist and my regular doctor have made it really, really clear to me that I have not increased my lung capacity at all," Ms. Rommes said. "But I've improved the mechanics. I've done everything I know how to do to make the lung capacity as efficient as possible. That's the key for me; I know there are lots of people with this disease who don't exercise, who I guess just give up."

She realizes that she has two serious chronic diseases that could shorten her life. But it does not worry her much, she said, because she figures she is doing everything she can to take care of herself, and would rather spend her time enjoying life—work, reading, opera, traveling, children and grandchildren.

"I will tell pretty much anybody that I have emphysema," Ms. Rommes said. "They say, 'Did you smoke?' I say, 'Yes I did, for 30 years, and I quit in 1992.' Maybe it's why I've attacked this the way I did. O.K., I did it to myself, and so I better do everything I can to get out of it. We all do things in our lives that are stupid, and then you do what you can to fix it."

From *The New York Times*, November 29, 2007. Copyright © 2007 by The New York Times Company. Reprinted by permission via PARS International.

Sound the Alarm? A Swine Flu Bind

Lawrence K. Altman, MD

For all that scientists have learned about influenza since the catastrophic pandemic of 1917–19, one thing has not changed: the predictably unpredictable nature of the viruses that cause it.

The sudden detection of the new swine influenza virus, A(H1N1), occurred just as scientists were focusing wary eyes on behavioral changes observed in another virus, the A(H5N1) bird flu strain, in Egypt. Virologists have tracked the avian virus since its discovery in Hong Kong in 1997.

A new virus could lead to a pandemic. Then again . . .

The World Health Organization said over the weekend that the new swine flu virus had the potential to cause another pandemic, but that it had no way of knowing whether it actually would.

The W.H.O. and public-health agencies like the Centers for Disease Control and Prevention find themselves in a delicate balance, obliged to provide information about potentially lethal diseases without causing panic.

Although health officials have held exercises to prepare for pandemics and outbreaks caused by bioterrorism, they have yet to master the necessary communications skills. They are in a "damned if they do, damned if they don't" situation.

A decision about travel restrictions or advisories, for example, could affect trade and finances at a time of economic chaos. If the public health emergency declared by the W.H.O. and the Obama administration turns out to be a false alarm, officials will be ridiculed for unnecessarily worrying millions of people—perhaps even for creating fear to justify their budgets.

If a pandemic materializes, some of the same critics are very likely to blame officials for failing to prevent it.

History teaches that the influenza virus mutates to cause worldwide spread about twice a century, on average. But scientists have yet to figure out what causes the mutations, when they will occur and what makes certain viruses more lethal than others.

Epidemiologists know that the number of cases reported in the days just after detection of a new strain can be deceiving, just as early returns can be in political elections.

To evaluate outbreaks, they need, among other things, accurate information about the numbers of cases; where they are occurring; the age distribution of those infected; and what contact they might have had with one another. At this stage of the swine flu investigation, such data are sorely lacking.

Most mystifying are why reported deaths have occurred only in Mexico so far and why confirmed cases reported elsewhere are mild. The disparity cannot be explained by any apparent biological factors. Could it instead reflect reporting bias?

For example, Mexican authorities may be more likely to look for swine flu in hospitals than authorities in other countries—who may be focusing on less vulnerable populations, like travelers. By contrast, those other countries might not have had time to concentrate on deaths in hospitals.

Occasionally, alerts of a new virus, or a mutation of an old one, come from a laboratory. More often, fatalities are the first clue.

But high initial death rates often fall as officials find that the causative microbe also causes mild, even symptomless cases. Officials may learn that the outbreak has gone on silently for weeks, even months.

H1N1 appears to be passed easily from person to person, and reports from the United States suggest that some cases may be mild and therefore may go undetected, allowing the disease to spread further.

In contrast, avian flu has killed 257 of the 421 people who have contracted it. But it has shown little ability to pass from person to person, mainly infecting poultry, and some experts suggest that there may be something about the H5N1 virus that makes it inherently less transmissible among people.

SARS, or severe acute respiratory syndrome, is easily spread and virulent. In a 2003 outbreak in Hong Kong, it killed 299 of the 1,755 people it infected.

Health authorities there are aggressively applying the lessons they learned from SARS. While Mexico struggles to confirm cases of swine flu and sends samples to the United States, Hong Kong is already performing swift genetic tests on patient samples and will have laboratories doing so at six local hospitals by Thursday.

In an influenza outbreak, standard surveillance, or disease monitoring, is crucial. That effort can determine how many of the confirmed cases are mild or fatal, painting a more accurate picture of the virulence.

As part of the exercise, epidemiologists, virologists and other health workers also interview patients and doctors, and they test many samples. The goal is to answer a list of questions, including these:

- Whether deaths occur in the early or late stages of the infection.
- Whether those who died also had certain underlying ailments, and which ones.
- Whether infected patients respond to standard anti-influenza drugs.
- Whether they develop secondary bacterial infections, and if so, what kinds.
- Whether the incubation period—the time it takes to develop symptoms after exposure to a mutated virus—differs from that for known influenza viruses, usually one to three days.

- Whether the new virus mainly strikes healthy individuals or has a predilection for people with certain diseases.
- What percentage of those infected might have been protected by prior influenza shots.

For the new swine influenza virus, it is too soon to know the answers. And as scientists are all too keenly aware, they have been wrong before.

In 1976, after a small outbreak of swine influenza at Fort Dix in New Jersey, public-health officials persuaded President Gerald R. Ford and Congress to mount a nationwide immunization campaign that came in for widespread criticism. Yet 60 years earlier, an influenza virus that apparently started as a mild outbreak in the spring came back in a giant storm months later.

Which model will the swine influenza virus follow? Scientists can only prepare for the worst and hope for the best.

Keith Bradsher contributed reporting from Hong Kong.

From *The New York Times,* April 28, 2009. Copyright © 2009 by The New York Times Company. Reprinted by permission via PARS International.

Chemical in Plastic Bottles Fuels Science, Concern—and Litigation

VALERIE JABLOW

A common chemical denominator in the stuff of modern life—helmets, CDs, baby bottles, sunglasses, cell phones, can coatings, and dental sealants—is the focus of increasing scientific and legislative scrutiny, as well as lawsuits. More than 20 cases have been filed, mostly since April, against manufacturers and sellers of baby and water bottles containing bisphenol A (BPA).

BPA, studied in the 1930s as an estrogen mimic, came into commercial use in the 1950s after scientists discovered that it could make clear, hard, yet not easily breakable plastic compounds called polycarbonates. These plastics, along with epoxy resin can linings containing BPA, have become ubiquitous in food uses, where they are prized for their durability. Today, more than 6 billion pounds of BPA is produced each year; the United States alone accounts for more than a third of worldwide production.

But BPA's association with food has attracted controversy. Although the FDA had maintained that the chemical did not leach out of containers made with it, in 1999 scientists began using more sensitive testing techniques, allowing them to measure very low levels of BPA.

Studies since then have measured the chemical in a variety of human tissues, including placenta, cord blood, fetal blood, and urine. The Centers for Disease Control and Prevention (CDC) found that nearly 93 percent of people tested had measurable levels of BPA in their urine, with children having the highest levels.

The Centers for Disease Control and Prevention found that nearly 93 percent of people tested had measurable levels of BPA in their urine, with children having the highest levels.

Scientists believe that most human exposure comes from diet, through the leaching of BPA from can linings and polycarbonate water bottles and baby bottles. Researchers have shown that leaching occurs at a higher rate when the bottles are heated, such as for warming milk or formula or for hot-water washing or sterilizing of baby bottles.

All of which may be cause for concern—depending on who you talk to.

In testimony before the House Subcommittee on Commerce, Trade, and Consumer Protection on June 10, Marian Stanley, senior director of the American Chemistry Council, a trade group for the plastics industry, concluded a presentation of BPA studies by noting that "no restriction on [BPA's] uses in current applications is warranted at this time." Stanley said studies showing low-dose effects of BPA in animals were "unvalidated."

But in April, a draft report on BPA by the National Toxicology Program (NTP) noted that such low doses produce in fetal and young animals changes in "behavior and the brain, prostate gland, mammary gland, and the age at which females attain puberty." Because those low doses are similar to human exposure levels, the report raised "some concern for neural and behavioral effects in fetuses, infants, and children at current human exposures" and "some concern" about how BPA exposure in young children might affect their prostate and mammary glands and the onset of puberty in females.

The NTP—a joint program of agencies within the FDA, CDC, and National Institutes of Health—concluded that "the possibility that bisphenol A may alter human development cannot be dismissed."

The NTP draft came in the wake of more than 150 low-dose BPA studies in animals showing harmful effects ranging from cancer to genital malformations to early puberty. Other studies found high levels of the chemical in human amniotic fluid and showed that fetuses cannot metabolize BPA.

After the NTP issued the draft report, Sen. Charles Schumer (D-N.Y.) proposed legislation banning BPA in children's products, and Reps. John Dingell (D-Mich.) and Bart Stupak (D-Mich.) asked four infant formula makers to stop using the chemical in their packaging. In June, Rep. Edward Markey (D-Mass.) proposed legislation to prohibit the use of BPA in all food and beverage containers.

Several polycarbonate bottle manufacturers, including Playtex and Nalgene, have said they will use alternatives to BPA, and Wal-Mart and Toys "R" Us are in the process of pulling BPA-containing items for babies from store shelves. The California senate in May passed a bill to ban BPA from food or beverage containers for children younger than three.

The FDA, which regulates containers that come into contact with food, is not yet raising alarm bells. Norris Alderson, an associate commissioner for science at the agency, testified at the June congressional hearing that the FDA is reviewing the use of BPA in food containers, but that currently it is satisfied that "exposure levels to BPA from these materials . . . are below those that may cause health effects."

The FDA has been criticized for relying on two studies, both funded by the chemical industry, to arrive at this conclusion. Dingell and Stupak are investigating that connection.

Class Actions

Lawsuits against the makers of polycarbonate baby bottles and covered "sippy" cups for toddlers (including Gerber, Avent, and Playtex) have been filed in several states, including Arkansas, California, Connecticut, Illinois, Kansas, Missouri, and Washington. Most have been filed in federal court and claim that the sale of products containing BPA violates various state consumer protection acts. None of the claims allege personal injury.

Other claims include breach of express and implied warranties, defective design, failure to warn, false and misleading advertising, fraudulent concealment, intentional and negligent misrepresentation, unfair and deceptive business practices, and unjust enrichment. The cases seek reimbursement to consumers who bought the products, in addition to punitive and actual damages.

Although most of the BPA lawsuits emerged earlier this year, the first—a California class action against makers and retailers of plastic baby bottles and cups—was filed in 2007. (*Ganjei v. Ralphs*, No. 367732 (Cal., Los Angeles Co. Super. filed Mar. 12, 2007).) The lead plaintiffs are five children with varying disorders—including congenital genital injury, attention deficit hyperactivity disorder, premature puberty, and Down syndrome—who used polycarbonate baby bottles and cups. Although the complaint does not say that BPA caused the children's disabilities, it alleges that most of their conditions are associated with exposure to BPA.

Stephen Murakami, a Jericho, New York, lawyer who is handling the class action, said proving specific causation is not yet possible. But, he noted, "the primary suspect group are infants and children, who are most susceptible to the dose of estrogen-like chemical [BPA] during critical times during their development. It changes them permanently. They're not equipped to handle that level of estrogen that affects their brain and sexual development."

The first class action concerning the use of BPA in water bottles was filed in April, also in California. The lead plaintiff, a mother of two daughters who also used the bottles, claims that the company violated the California Business and Professions Code by "omitting, suppressing, and withholding material information regarding the bottles' BPA-related risks," according to the complaint. (*Felix-Lozano v. Nalge Nunc Intl. Corp.*, No. 08-cv-854 (E.D. Cal. filed Apr. 22, 2008).)

The defendant, Nalge Nunc International, notes on its website that it believes that its water bottles containing BPA "are safe for their intended use." Meanwhile, the company is phasing out the use of the chemical in its bottles because of consumer requests for alternative materials, it says.

In May, a group of plaintiff attorneys asked the district court in the Northern District of Illinois to consolidate 13 similar class actions filed in seven federal districts. One of the lawyers, Scott Poynter of Little Rock, Arkansas, noted that the classes would be hard to certify if they included personal injury claims.

Cause and Effect

Causation—and BPA's effects in humans—is a point of frequent debate. In 1987, the EPA said a BPA exposure level of 50 micrograms per kilogram per day (micrograms/kg/day) was safe in humans, based on animal experiments then available showing that 1,000 times that amount in rodents caused weight loss.

Today, the BPA level known to cause birth defects in pregnant mice is 2.4 micrograms/kg/day. But the level in humans that is harmful remains uncertain and contentious, in large part because few human studies have been conducted.

And some studies have reached different conclusions about human and animal harm from BPA. Why the disparity? A 2005 review of many studies found that one factor may be the researchers' funding source. In 94 of 104 published studies on BPA funded by the government, researchers found that doses of less than 50 milligrams/kg/day had significant effects. But none of 11 industry-funded studies found significant effects at those doses.

Almost everyone involved in the issue agrees that further study of BPA in humans is needed. Meanwhile, the chemical's ubiquity will likely continue to cause powerful clashes. For instance, attempts to pass or enact legislation banning BPA in Maryland, Minnesota, and San Francisco have failed. The plastics industry even sued San Francisco when it attempted to enact its ban.

Some BPA critics say the industry's reach affects official government statements on the chemical as well. In 2007, the Center for the Evaluation of Risks to Human Reproduction, part of NTP, assembled a nonexpert panel to look at 500 BPA studies. But the company hired to compile the data was also doing work for Dow Chemical, a BPA maker.

Although the company was fired from the project, the panel concluded that most people were safe because exposure levels were below those set by the government. (It did note some concern for BPA in young children and fetuses.)

Then, in June, the NTP draft report on BPA underwent peer review by the program's Board of Scientific Counselors, made up of 19 researchers from academia, pharmaceutical companies, and biological research firms. One board member works for Dow Chemical, and all are appointed by the secretary of the Department of Health and Human Services.

The board voted to lower the concern expressed in the NTP draft—from "some concern" to "minimal concern"—for BPA's effects on young children's mammary glands and puberty onset in females. The NTP's final report is due at the end of the summer.

From *Trial Magazine,* August 2008. Copyright © 2008 by Trial Magazine. Reprinted by permission.

HIV Apathy

New drugs have changed HIV from a terminal to a chronic illness. To counter complacency, health officials are pushing to make testing more widespread.

ZACH PATTON

On a rainy day last June, local officials in Washington, D.C., gathered under tents erected on a public plaza to be tested for HIV. The District of Columbia's health department was kicking off a sweeping new effort to encourage city residents to take action against the disease. With banners, music and mobile-testing units, officials hoped the launch event and the campaign would help raise local awareness about HIV—and help the city address its most pressing health concern.

Washington has the nation's highest rate of new AIDS cases, and the city's goal—HIV testing for every resident between the ages of 14 and 84, totaling over 400,000 people—was unprecedented in its scope. City officials said the campaign, which also included distributing an initial 80,000 HIV tests to doctors' offices, hospitals and health clinics, would enable them to get a better idea of how many residents are infected with HIV. And making such screenings routine, they hoped, would help erase the stigma against getting tested for the disease.

Six months later, though, the effort was faltering. Fewer than 20,000 people had been tested. Many of the HIV test kits expired before they were distributed, forcing the city to throw them away. Others were donated to the Maryland health department to use before they went bad. And the city still lacked a comprehensive plan for ensuring effective treatment for those residents who test positive for the disease.

It's not all bad news. The District nearly tripled the number of sites offering free HIV screenings, and the Department of Corrections began screening all inmates for HIV. And the city improved its disease-surveillance technique, recording information on behaviors and lifestyles, in addition to counting the number of new HIV cases.

But D.C.'s struggle to meet its goals underscores a challenge common to local health officials across the country. More than a million U.S. residents are infected with HIV, and one-quarter of them don't know it, experts estimate. Diagnosis rates of HIV have stabilized in recent years, but large

cities continue to grapple with much higher rates. They're dealing with higher incidents of the risky behaviors—drug use and unprotected sex, particularly gay sex—that tend to spread the disease. But they're also trying to battle something less tangible: complacency. Antiretroviral drugs have largely changed HIV from a terminal illness into a chronic one. And the fears associated with AIDS have faded over the past 20 years. As health officials work to combat HIV, they're finding that their hardest fight is the one against apathy.

Testing Laws

The first test for the human immunodeficiency virus was licensed by the FDA in March 1985. It was quickly put into use by blood banks, health departments and clinics across the country. But HIV testing at that time faced some major obstacles, which would continue to thwart HIV policies for much of the following two decades. For one, it usually took two weeks to obtain lab results, requiring multiple visits for patients waiting to see if they had HIV. Many patients—in some places, as many as half—never returned for the second visit. Another barrier was that, at the time, a diagnosis of the disease was a death sentence. With no reliable drugs to slow the progression of HIV into AIDS, and with an attendant stigma that could decimate a person's life, many people just didn't want to know if they were HIV-positive. "The impact of disclosure of someone's HIV-positive status could cost them their job, their apartment and their social circle," says Dr. Adam Karpati, assistant commissioner for HIV/AIDS Prevention & Control for the New York City health department. "In a basic calculus, the value to the patient was questionable. Knowing their status could only maybe help them, but it could definitely hurt them."

Because of that stigma and the seriousness of a positive diagnosis, many cities and states developed rigorous measures to ensure that testing was voluntary and confidential, and that it included a full discussion of the risks associated with the disease. That meant requiring written consent in order to perform tests, and mandatory pre- and post-test counseling. "A lot of the laws were, appropriately, concerned with confidentiality and protecting people's rights," Karpati says.

Two major developments have since changed the method—and the purpose—of HIV testing. First, the development of antiretroviral drugs in the mid-1990s has lessened the impact of HIV as a fatal disease. And in the past two or three years, advancements in testing technology have effectively eliminated the wait time for receiving results. Rapid tests using a finger-prick or an oral swab can be completed in 20 minutes, meaning nearly everyone can receive results within a single visit.

Those changes, along with aggressive counseling and education about risk-prevention measures, helped stabilize the rate of HIV diagnosis. After peaking in 1992, rates of AIDS cases leveled off by 1998. Today, about 40,000 AIDS cases are diagnosed every year. Data on non-AIDS HIV infection rates are much harder to come by, but they seem to have stabilized as well.

The problem, however, remains especially acute in urban areas. While health experts take pains to stress that HIV/AIDS is no longer just a "big city" problem, the fact is that 85 percent of the nation's HIV infections have been in metropolitan areas with more than half a million people. "Urban areas have always been the most heavily impacted by the HIV epidemic, and they continue to be," says Jennifer Ruth of the Centers for Disease Control and Prevention. Intravenous drug use, risky sexual behavior and homosexual sex all contribute to higher HIV rates, and they are all more prevalent in urban areas. But cities face other complicating factors as well, including high poverty rates and residents with a lack of access to medical care, which exacerbate the challenges of HIV care.

Prevention Fatigue

Nowhere is that more evident than in Washington, D.C., where an estimated one in every 20 residents is HIV-positive. That's 10 times the national average. But that figure is only a rough guess. The truth is that health officials don't even know what the city's HIV rate is. Last year's campaign was supposed to change that. By setting a goal to test nearly all city residents, District health officials hoped to make HIV screening a routine part of medical care. In the process, the health department hoped it could finally get a handle on just how bad the crisis was. "We've had problems in the past, I'll be the first to say," says D.C. health department director Dr. Gregg A. Pane. "But we have galvanized interest and action, and we've highlighted the problem in a way it hasn't been before."

The effort stumbled, though. The Appleseed Center for Law and Justice, a local public advocacy group, has issued periodic report cards grading the District's progress

on HIV. The most recent assessment, published six months into last year's testing push, found mismanagement and a lack of coordination with the medical community. The District was testing substantially more people than it had been, but the number was still falling far short of officials' goal. "D.C. took a great step forward, but it takes more than just a report announcing it," says Walter Smith, executive director for the Appleseed Center. "You have to make sure there's a plan."

What D.C. did achieve, however, was a fundamental shift in the way health officials perceive the HIV epidemic. "This is a disease that affects everyone," says Pane. "It's our No. 1 public health threat, and treating it like a public health threat is the exact right thing to do."

That paradigm change has been happening in health departments across the country. Last year, the CDC made waves when it announced new recommendations for treating HIV as an issue of public health. That means testing as many people as possible, making HIV testing a routine part of medical care, and removing the barriers to getting tested. Washington was the first city to adopt the CDC's recommendations for comprehensive testing, but other cities have also moved to make testing more routine. San Francisco health officials dropped their written-consent and mandatory-counseling requirements for those about to be tested. New York City has been moving in a similar direction, although removing the written-consent rule there will require changing state law. Many health officials think that since testing has become so easy and social attitudes about the disease have shifted, the strict testing regulations adopted in the 1980s are now cumbersome. The protections have become barriers.

Officials also are moving away from "risk-assessment testing," in which doctors first try to identify whether a patient falls into a predetermined high-risk category. "What has evolved is that, with an epidemic, risk-based testing is not sufficient," says New York City's Karpati. "Now there's a general move toward comprehensive testing." Privacy advocates and many AIDS activists oppose the shift away from individual protections. Yes, the stigma isn't what it used to be, they say, but it still exists. HIV isn't like tuberculosis or the measles, so they believe health officials shouldn't treat it like it is.

But even if officials could strike the perfect balance between public health and private protection, there's another factor that everyone agrees is thwarting cities' efforts to combat HIV. Call it burnout or complacency or "prevention fatigue." In an age when testing consists of an oral swab and a 20-minute wait, and an HIV-positive diagnosis means taking a few pills a day, health officials are battling a growing sense of apathy toward the disease. "The very successes we've made in the past 20 years have hurt us, in a sense," Karpati says. "We don't have hospital wards full of HIV patients. We don't have people dying as much. There's a whole new generation of folks growing up who don't remember the fear of the crisis in the 1980s."

That casual attitude toward the disease can lead to riskier behavior and, in turn, more infections. With HIV and AIDS disproportionately affecting low-income residents, any increase in infections places an additional burden on governments. And while prescription drugs have made the disease more manageable, the fact is that 40 percent of the new HIV diagnoses in the nation are still made within a year of the infection's progressing to AIDS—which is usually too late for medicine to do much good. As cities try to fight HIV complacency through refined testing policies and a focus on comprehensive testing, residents will have increasingly widespread access to tests for the disease. But for health officials, the greatest challenge will be getting the right people to care.

ZACH PATTON can be reached at zpatton@governing.com

From *Governing*, February 2007, pp. 48–50. Copyright © 2007 by Governing. Reprinted by permission.

Methicillin-Resistant *Staphylococcus aureus*

The Latest Health Scare

PRIYA SAMPATHKUMAR

For decades, methicillin-resistant *Staphylococcus aureus* (MRSA) has been the most commonly identified multidrug-resistant pathogen in many parts of the world, including the United States. Recently, it has become the focus of intense media attention. Some of this attention stems from a recent article in the *Journal of the American Medical Association* that provided estimates of MRSA infections annually in the United States.[1] (The occurrence of the word "staph" increased by 10-fold in the 2 weeks after this report.[2]) In addition, both health care safety initiatives (eg, Joint Commission National Patient Safety Goals, Institute for Healthcare Improvement) and consumer groups (eg, American Association of Retired Persons, StopHospitalInfection.org) have begun calling for hospitals to do more to reduce MRSA infections. Legislation related to hospital infections, including measures targeting MRSA control and public reporting of MRSA infections, is being introduced in many states and at the federal level.[3–5] Finally, increasing reports of MRSA occurring in community settings, eg, day care centers, schools, and sports teams, along with several reports of deaths in previously healthy children and young adults, have also prompted fears that we are now facing a new "superbug."

Historical Background

Staphylococcus aureus is one of the most successful and adaptable human pathogens. Its remarkable ability to acquire antibiotic resistance has contributed to its emergence as an important pathogen in a variety of settings. In the preantibiotic era, *S aureus* infections were associated with very high mortality. When penicillin was first introduced in the early 1940s, much of its success was in the treatment of *S aureus* bloodstream infections. However, as early as 1942 the first strains of penicillin-resistant *S aureus* were detected in hospitals (Table 1). These subsequently spread into the community; by 1960, most *S aureus* strains both in hospitals and in the community were resistant to penicillin. Shortly after the introduction in 1959 of methicillin, a semisynthetic penicillin, resistance to it emerged; the first hospital outbreak of MRSA was reported in 1963.[6] Initially spreading widely in Europe, India, and Australia, MRSA strains were detected in the United States in the late 1960s.[7] By the 1980s, MRSA had become firmly established in US hospitals, and rates of MRSA infection have since continued to increase. In large US hospitals, MRSA rates (the proportion of all *S aureus* isolates that are MRSA) increased from 4% in the 1980s to 50% in the late 1990s. According to National Nosocomial Infections Surveillance data, the increase in MRSA rates in intensive care units was even greater, reaching 60% in 2003.[8]

Nosocomial MRSA is remarkable for its clonal pattern of spread. Currently, 5 major MRSA clones account for approximately 70% of MRSA isolates in hospitals in the United States, South America, and Europe. The major cause of this clonal spread is infection control lapses by health care professionals. The traditional risk factors for MRSA acquisition include previous hospitalization, antibiotic use, residence in long-term care facilities, and long-term hemodialysis. Increasing use of vancomycin to treat MRSA led to the emergence of *S aureus* with intermediate resistance to vancomycin (VISA) and then vancomycin-resistant *S aureus* (VRSA) in the 1990s.[9,10] Fortunately, VISA and VRSA infections have been sporadic, and intense infection control measures have ensured that they did not circulate widely in health care settings.

In the early 1980s, several instances of community-onset MRSA were reported in the upper Midwest. Because many of these early cases involved intravenous drug users or people with serious underlying disease, it was thought that the infections were acquired during contact with health care personnel. However, in the 1990s serious MRSA infections were reported in patients with no prior contact with the health care system, heralding the onset of community-acquired MRSA (CA-MRSA) outbreaks. The seriousness of CA-MRSA was highlighted by a report in 1999 of 4 deaths in children infected with CA-MRSA in Minnesota and South Dakota.[11] Since then, many reports have described CA-MRSA infections, particularly in children, and CA-MRSA is a growing problem worldwide. Clusters of CA-MRSA have been reported in correctional facilities,[12] professional sports teams,[13] high school athletes,[14] day care centers,[15] healthy newborns,[16] military personnel,[17, 18] and tattoo recipients.[19] The term "health care-acquired MRSA" (HA-MRSA) has been used to differentiate the earlier hospital strains of MRSA from these newer CA-MRSA strains.

Table 1 Timeline of *Staphylococcus aureus* Infection and Resistance

Year	Event
1940	Penicillin introduced
1942	Penicillin-resistant *Staphylococcus aureus* appears
1959	Methicillin introduced; most *S aureus* strains in both hospital and community settings are penicillin resistant
1961	Methicillin-resistant *S aureus* appears
1963	First hospital outbreak of methicillin-resistant *S aureus* (MRSA)
1968	First MRSA strain in US hospitals
1970s	Clonal spread of MRSA globally, very high MRSA rates in Europe
1982	4% MRSA rate in the United States
1980s, early 1990s	Dramatic decreases in MRSA rates due to search-and-destroy programs in Northern Europe
	By 1999, <1% MRSA rate in the Netherlands; that rate has been sustained to date despite increasing MRSA rates in other parts of the world
1996	Vancomycin-resistant *S aureus* (VRSA) reported in Japan
1997	Approximately 25% MRSA rate in US hospitals; vancomycin use increases; vancomycin-intermediate *S aureus* (VISA) appears; serious community-acquired MRSA (CA-MRSA) infections reported; pediatric deaths reported
2002	First clinical infection with VRSA in the United States
2003	MRSA rates continue to increase; approximately 60% MRSA rate in intensive care units; outbreaks of CA-MRSA (predominantly USA 300 clone) reported in numerous community settings and also implicated in hospital outbreaks
2006	>50% of staphylococcal skin infections seen in emergency departments caused by CA-MRSA
	HA-MRSA rate continues to increase
	Distinction between HA-MRSA and CA-MRSA on epidemiological basis becomes increasingly difficult
2007	"The Year of MRSA?"
	Report of active, population-based surveillance for invasive MRSA done in 2004–2005 estimates 95,000 invasive MRSA infections and 19,000 deaths from MRSA per year
	Continued reports in the medical literature and the lay press about severe CA-MRSA infections
	Several states pass or are considering legislation regarding control of MRSA and public reporting of MRSA rates
	Strategies to control MRSA, including public reporting of MRSA infections, are hotly debated; "staph" and MRSA become household words

Differences between HA-MRSA and CA-MRSA

A review article by Kowalski et al[20] contrasted the features of CA-MRSA and HA-MRSA. To summarize, HA-MRSA and CA-MRSA strains carry different types of the gene complex known as staphylococcal chromosome cassette mec (SCC mec), which contains the mecA gene that confers methicillin resistance. Health care-acquired MRSA strains carry SCC mec types I, II, and III and tend to be multidrug resistant. They typically cause bloodstream and postoperative wound infections along with nosocomial pneumonia in hospitalized patients.

In contrast, CA-MRSA strains carry SCC mec type IV and V and usually cause skin and soft tissue infections in community-dwelling children and adults. The most common clinical presentations are furuncles, superficial abscesses, and boils that are often mistakenly attributed to spider bites. Like HA-MRSA, CA-MRSA also spreads clonally, and the USA 300 clone is the predominant strain circulating in the United States.[21] Although resistant to methicillin and other β-lactam antibiotics (eg, penicillin, cephalosporins, carbapenems), CA-MRSA often remains sensitive to many other classes of antibiotics, including trimethoprim-sulfamethoxazole and tetracyclines. Resistance to macrolides, clindamycin, and fluoroquinolones varies by region. In addition to skin infections, cases of severe necrotizing pneumonia (including postinfluenza pneumonia) and necrotizing fasciitis caused by CA-MRSA have been described.[22,23] Many cases of necrotizing pneumonia and some soft tissue infections have been characterized by rapid progression to septic shock and death. Most CA-MRSA strains carry the Panton-Valentine leukocidin gene. This gene could play a role in the pathogenesis of more severe infection, especially pneumonia.[24] Community-acquired MRSA strains are also associated with production of other toxins, such as staphylococcal enterotoxin A, B, C, and H, which are capable of causing illness resembling toxic shock syndrome in animal models[25,26] and could play a role in severe human infections.

The epidemiological differences between these strains are becoming increasingly blurred. Community-acquired MRSA strains are making their way into health care settings, and several outbreaks of nosocomial infections with these strains have been reported.[27–30] They are also becoming increasingly drug resistant[31] and are spreading rapidly within defined populations and in select geographical regions, particularly in large urban centers. In some metro-politan areas, CA-MRSA accounts for as high as 80% of all *S aureus* infections seen in emergency departments.[21]

Prevalence of *S aureus* and MRSA

Staphylococcus aureus is a common colonizer of the skin and the nose. A 2001–2002 population-based study in the United States showed that the prevalence of nasal colonization with *S aureus* and with MRSA was 31.6% and 0.84%, respectively,[32] meaning that there are approximately 2.3 million MRSA-colonized people in the United States. Women, people older than 65 years, those with diabetes mellitus, or those who have been in long-term care in the preceding year are more likely to be colonized with MRSA. Two nasal *S aureus* carriage patterns can be distinguished: persistent and intermittent. The density of *S aureus* in the nose is highest in persistent carriers, as is its colonization of other body sites, including the hands, axillae, and perineal regions.

Although the relationship between colonization and infection is not completely understood, both are associated with intrinsic host factors, as well as the strain of *S aureus*. Nasal colonization with *S aureus* is a risk factor for subsequent infection. Both higher rates of *S aureus* nasal carriage and subsequent higher rates of infection have been associated with many underlying diseases or conditions, including insulin-dependent diabetes mellitus, long-term dialysis, intravenous drug abuse, repeated injections for allergies, liver cirrhosis, liver transplant, human immuno-deficiency virus infection, and hospitalization. Also correlated with higher *S aureus* infection rates are activities leading to skin lesions such as contact sports. The common factor between these conditions seems to be the repeated violation of the skin or mucosa as anatomical barriers.

Impact of MRSA

Patients colonized with MRSA are more likely to develop infections than patients colonized with methicillin-sensitive *S aureus* (MSSA).[33] Methicillin-resistant *S aureus* infections lengthen hospital stays (by an average of 10 days) and are associated with a 2.5-fold higher mortality rate and increased health care costs.[34,35] A diagnosis of *S aureus* infection accounts for an estimated 292,000 hospitalizations per year in the United States.[36] In 2005, approximately 94,000 persons were diagnosed as having invasive (ie, serious) MRSA infections, an estimated 19,000 of whom died. Of these MRSA infections, 86% were health care acquired and 14% were community acquired.[1] The annual cost of treating MRSA in hospitalized patients in the United States has been estimated to be between $3.2 and $4.2 billion.[37]

Transmission and Control of MRSA

In health care settings, MRSA is transmitted from patient to patient primarily via health care professionals' hands. It can survive on surfaces for days to weeks; hence, contaminated patient care equipment can play a role in transmission.[38] The factors that promote transmission of MRSA in community settings have been called the *5 Cs* and are summarized in Table 2. Although the strategies to control HA-MRSA and true CA-MRSA share many features, they differ in some respects. Rates of infection with both these organisms can be reduced by good antibiotic stewardship, which will prevent the selection of MRSA from among a population of *S aureus*. Good hand hygiene practices will limit person-to-person transmission and decrease the pool of persons who are colonized. In health care settings, active surveillance cultures to identify patients with MRSA, contact precautions (use of gown and gloves while caring for these patients), and good environmental cleaning have been proposed as additional strategies to limit MRSA transmission[39, 40] In selected patients, decolonization could help reduce infection. However, widespread use of decolonization is not recommended because it is expensive, its benefit is usually short lived (most patients become recolonized during the next few months), and it carries the risk of promoting resistance to agents, such as mupirocin, that are used in decolonizing regimens.

In July 2004, Mayo Clinic Rochester expanded its MRSA control program. In addition to isolating patients known to be carriers of MRSA and electronically flagging their records so that isolation procedures could be reinstituted on readmission, staff members began to screen high-risk patients for MRSA and preemptively isolated them until negative culture results were obtained. In the 36 months after institution of this program, rates of MRSA rates decreased by 25% (ie, from 42% to 29% of *S aureus* isolates) (unpublished data). Several Scandinavian countries have reduced MRSA infection rates to less than 2% through intensive infection control programs and have successfully maintained these low rates over the past several years.[41, 42]

Physicians can help control the spread of CA-MRSA in communities by encouraging hand hygiene, maintaining a high degree of suspicion for MRSA as an etiologic agent when treating skin and soft tissue infections, knowing local rates of CA-MRSA (public health departments might be able to provide these data), emphasizing the importance of hygiene to patients with MRSA, and discouraging the sharing of personal items such as towels and razors. Draining lesions should be kept covered, and return to team sports should be limited until the lesion has healed or can be adequately covered. Flu shots (especially in children) could be helpful in reducing the risk of postinfluenza bacterial pneumonia with MRSA.

Table 2 Factors Associated with Community-Acquired Methicillin-Resistant *Staphylococcus aureus* Transmission (The 5 Cs)

- Crowded living conditions
- Frequent skin-to-skin Contact
- Compromised skin
- Sharing Contaminated personal items such as towels and razors
- Lack of Cleanliness

Treatment Options

Selection of initial antibiotic regimens should be guided by the local prevalence of MRSA, the presence of health care-associated risk factors, and the severity and type of clinical presentation. For severe infections, intravenous vancomycin should be included in initial empiric therapy. Microbiological data and antibiotic susceptibility testing should be used to guide subsequent therapy. First approved in 1958, vancomycin became standard therapy for MRSA in the 1960s. Its advantages include its good safety profile, the long experience with its use, and its relatively infrequent dosing regimen. Disadvantages include the need for intravenous administration and monitoring of levels in critically ill patients and in those with changing renal function. In addition, the molecule is large, limiting its penetration into tissues. Recently, there have been reports of vancomycin failure due to either relative vancomycin resistance or MRSA infections in sites that have poor vancomycin penetration.[43, 44]

Overall, vancomycin remains standard treatment for MRSA; however, some alternatives have recently received Food and Drug Administration approval and could be good options in selected patients, including linezolid (a synthetic oxazolidinone), tigecycline (a derivative of minocycline), and daptomycin (a cyclic lipopeptide). Daptomycin should be avoided in the treatment of MRSA-associated pneumonia because it is inactivated by pulmonary surfactant. Additional agents that appear promising include dalbavancin, a semisynthetic lipoglycopeptide that can be dosed once a week, and ceftobiprole, an investigational cephalosporin.

For soft tissue CA-MRSA infections, surgical drainage is crucial, with antibiotics serving as adjunctive therapy. Severe infections should be managed with intravenous antibiotics as aforementioned. Oral antibiotics can be used for less severe infections in the outpatient setting. For initial empiric therapy, oral trimethoprim-sulfamethoxazole is a good choice. Other alternatives include minocycline, clindamycin, or a macrolide antibiotic, depending on local susceptibility patterns.

In summary, MRSA is a growing public health problem. Initially, it was feared that HA-MRSA, long a cause of health care-associated infections, would escape into community settings. Instead, in the past few years, CA-MRSA strains that are genetically different from HA-MRSA have appeared, are now circulating widely in many communities, and are causing a wide variety of infections, ranging from minor skin infections to rapidly progressive, life-threatening ones. Ironically, these more virulent CA-MRSA strains have been imported from the community into health care settings and have been responsible for outbreaks of infections in hospitals. Infection control measures have been successful in limiting the spread of MRSA in many parts of the world, and most hospitals in the United States are increasing MRSA control activities to improve patient safety and quality of care.

Currently, the health care industry is under increasing scrutiny by both the public and governmental agencies. Medicare and other groups have threatened not to reimburse for hospital-acquired infections. Legislation is being considered or has already been passed in some states mandating the reporting of health care-acquired infection rates and separate reporting of MRSA rates. The spread of MRSA and other drug-resistant organisms can be limited by infection control measures. It is time that we, as health care professionals, incorporate proven infection control measures such as hand hygiene and the use of appropriate personal protective equipment (gowns and gloves) into our daily patient care routines. The next influenza pandemic might or might not happen in our lifetime. The MRSA pandemic is here.

Notes

1. Klevens RM, Morrison MA, Nadle J, et al, Active Bacterial Core surveillance (ABCs) MRSA Investigators. Invasive methicillin-resistant *Staphylococcus aureus* infections in the United States. *JAMA*. 2007;298(15): 1763–1771.

2. Pitts L Jr. Media fall victim to the journalism of fear. LJWorld.com. November 5, 2007. Available at: http://www2.ljworld.com/news/2007/nov/05/media_fall_victim_journalism_fear/. Accessed November 7, 2007.

3. Staph outbreak prompts legislation. *Chicago Tribune*. October 29, 2007. Available at: www.chicagotribune.com/news/local/chi-durbinoct29,0,6847984.story?coll=chi_tab01_layout. Accessed November 7, 2007.

4. Hester T. NJ law requires hospitals to report infections. *The Philadelphia Inquirer*. November 1, 2007. Available at: www.philly.com/inquirer/health_science/daily/20071101_N_J__law_requires_hospitals_to_report_infections.html. Accessed November 7, 2007.

5. Gormley M. States consider new laws to fight spread of staph infections. *Press and Sun Bulletin*, Greater Binghampton, NY. October 27, 2007. Available at: http://forums.pressconnects.com/viewtopic.php?t=11922. Accessed November 7, 2007.

6. Stewart GT, Holt RJ. Evolution of natural resistance to the newer penicillins. *Br Med J*. 1963; 1(5326):308–311.

7. Barrett FF, McGehee RFJr, Finland M. Methicillin-resistant *Staphylococcus aureus* at Boston City Hospital: bacteriologic and epidemiologic observations. *N Engl J Med*. 1968;279(9):441–448.

8. National Nosocomial Infections Surveillance (NNIS) System Report, data summary from January 1992 through June 2004, issued October 2004. *Am J Infect Control*. 2004;32(8):470–485.

9. Centers for Disease Control and Prevention (CDC). Update: *Staphylococcus aureus* with reduced susceptibility to vancomycin—United States, 1997 [published correction appears in *MMWR Morb Mortal Wkly Rep*. 1997;46(35):851]. *MMWR Morb Mortal Wkly Rep*. 1997;46(35):813–815.

10. Centers for Disease Control and Prevention (CDC). *Staphylococcus aureus* resistant to vancomycin—United States, 2002. *MMWR Morb Mortal Wkly Rep.* 2002;51(26):565–567.

11. Centers for Disease Control and Prevention (CDC). Four pediatric deaths from community-acquired methicillin-resistant *Staphylococcus aureus*—Minnesota and North Dakota, 1997–1999. *JAMA.* 1999;282(12):1123–1125.

12. Centers for Disease Control and Prevention (CDC). Methicillin-resistant *Staphylococcus aureus* infections in correctional facilities—Georgia, California, and Texas, 2001–2003. *MMWR Morb Mortal Wkly Rep.* 2003;52(41):992–996.

13. Kazakova SV, Hageman JC, Matava M, et al. A clone of methicillin-resistant *Staphylococcus aureus* among professional football players. *N Engl J Med.* 2005;352(5):468–475.

14. Lindenmayer JM, Schoenfeld S, O'Grady R, Carney JK. Methicillin-resistant *Staphylococcus aureus* in a high school wrestling team and the surrounding community. *Arch Intern Med.* 1998;158(8):895–899.

15. Jensen JU, Jensen ET, Larsen AR, et al. Control of a methicillin-resistant *Staphylococcus aureus* (MRSA) outbreak in a day-care institution. *J Hosp Infect.* 2006 May;63(1):84–92. Epub 2006 Mar 15.

16. Centers for Disease Control and Prevention (CDC). Community-associated methicillin-resistant *Staphylococcus aureus* infection among healthy newborns—Chicago and Los Angeles County, 2004. *MMWR Morb Mortal Wkly Rep.* 2006;55(12):329–332.

17. Beilman GJ, Sandifer G, Skarda D, et al. Emerging infections with community-associated methicillin-resistant *Staphylococcus aureus* in outpatients at an Army Community Hospital. *Surg Infect (Larchmt).* 2005 Spring;6(1):87–92.

18. Pagac BB, Reiland RW, Bolesh DT, Swanson DL. Skin lesions in barracks: consider community-acquired methicillin-resistant *Staphylococcus aureus* infection instead of spider bites. *Mil Med.* 2006;171(9):830–832.

19. Centers for Disease Control and Prevention (CDC). Methicillin-resistant *Staphylococcus aureus* skin infections among tattoo recipients—Ohio, Kentucky, and Vermont, 2004–2005. *MMWR Morb Mortal Wkly Rep.* 2006;55(24):677–679.

20. Kowalski TJ, Berbari EF, Osmon Dr. Epidemiology, treatment, and prevention of community-acquired methicillin-resistant *Staphylococcus aureus* infections. *Mayo Clin Proc.* 2005;80(9):1201–1208.

21. King MD, Humphrey BJ, Wang YF, Kourbatova EV, Ray SM, Blumberg HM. Emergence of community-acquired methicillin-resistant *Staphylococcus aureus* USA 300 clone as the predominant cause of skin and soft-tissue infections. *Ann Intern Med.* 2006;144(5):309–317.

22. Centers for Disease Control and Prevention (CDC). Severe methicillin-resistant *Staphylococcus aureus* community-acquired pneumonia associated with influenza—Louisiana and Georgia, December 2006—January 2007. *MMWR Morb Mortal Wkly Rep.* 2007;56(14):325–329.

23. Miller LG, Perdreau-Remington F, Rieg G, et al. Necrotizing fasciitis caused by community-associated methicillin-resistant *Staphylococcus aureus* in Los Angeles. *N Engl J Med.* 2005;352(14):1445–1453.

24. Labandeira-Rey M, Couzon F, Boisset S, et al. *Staphylococcus aureus* Panton-Valentine leukocidin causes necrotizing pneumonia. *Science.* 2007 Feb 23;315(5815):1130–1133. Epub 2007 Jan 18.

25. McCollister BD, Kreiswirth BN, Novick RP, Schlievert PM. Production of toxic shock syndrome-like illness in rabbits by *Staphylococcus aureus* D4508: association with enterotoxin A. *Infect Immun.* 1990;58(7):2067–2070.

26. Omoe K, Ishikawa M, Shimoda Y, Hu DL, Ueda S, Shinagawa K. Detection of *seg, seh,* and *sei* genes in *Staphylococcus aureus* isolates and determination of the enterotoxin productivities of *S. aureus* isolates harboring *seg, seh,* or *sei* genes. *J Clin Microbiol.* 2002;40(3):857–862.

27. David MD, Kearns AM, Gossain S, Ganner M, Holmes A. Community-associated methicillin-resistant *Staphylococcus aureus*: nosocomial transmission in a neonatal unit. *J Hosp Infect.* 2006 Nov;64(3):244–250. Epub 2006 Aug 22.

28. Davis SL, Rybak MJ, Amjad M, Kaatz GW, McKinnon PS. Characteristics of patients with healthcare-associated infection due to SCCmec type IV methicillin-resistant *Staphylococcus aureus*. *Infect Control Hosp Epidemiol.* 2006 Oct;27(10):1025–1031. Epub 2006 Sep 19.

29. Schramm GE, Johnson JA, Doherty JA, Micek ST, Kollef MH. Increasing incidence of sterile-site infections due to non-multidrug-resistant, oxacillin-resistant *Staphylococcus aureus* among hospitalized patients. *Infect Control Hosp Epidemiol.* 2007 Jan;28(1):95–97. Epub 2006 Dec 20.

30. Seybold U, Kourbatova EV, Johnson JG, et al. Emergence of community-associated methicillin-resistant *Staphylococcus aureus* USA300 genotype as a major cause of health care-associated blood stream infections. *Clin Infect Dis.* 2006 Mar 1;42(5):647–656. Epub 2006 Jan 25.

31. Han LL, McDougal LK, Gorwitz RJ, et al. High frequencies of clindamycin and tetracycline resistance in methicillin-resistant *Staphylococcus aureus* pulsed-field type USA300 isolates collected at a Boston ambulatory health center. *J Clin Microbiol.* 2007 Apr;45(4):1350–1352. Epub 2007 Feb 7.

32. Graham PL III, Lin SX, Larson EL. A US population-based survey of *Staphylococcus aureus* colonization. *Ann Intern Med.* 2006;144(5):318–325.

33. Huang SS, Platt R. Risk of methicillin-resistant *Staphylococcus aureus* infection after previous infection or colonization. *Clin Infect Dis.* 2003 Feb 1;36(3):281–285. Epub 2003 Jan 17.

34. Shurland S, Zhan M, Bradham DD, Roghmann MC. Comparison of mortality risk associated with bacteremia due to methicillin-resistant and methicillin-susceptible *Staphylococcus aureus*. *Infect Control Hosp Epidemiol.* 2007 Mar;28(3):273–279. Epub 2007 Feb 15.

35. Selvey LA, Whitby M, Johnson B. Nosocomial methicillin-resistant *Staphylococcus aureus* bacteremia: is it any worse than nosocomial methicillin-sensitive *Staphylococcus aureus* bacteremia? *Infect Control Hosp Epidemiol.* 2000;21(10):645–648.

36. Kuehnert MJ, Hill HA, Kupronis BA, Tokars JI, Solomon SL, Jernigan DB. Methicillin-resistant-*Staphylococcus aureus* hospitalizations, United States [published correction appears in *Emerg Infect Dis.* 2006;12(9):1472]. *Emerg Infect Dis.* 2005;11(6):868–872.

37. Association for Professionals in Infection Control and Epidemiology, Inc (APIC). Guide to the elimination of methicillin-resistant *Staphylococcus aureus* (MRSA) transmission in hospital settings, March 2007. Available at: www.apic.org/Content/NavigationMenu/GovernmentAdvocacy/ MethicillinResistantStaphylococcusAureusMRSA/Resources/ MRSAguide.pdf. Accessed November 8, 2007.

38. Huang SS, Datta R, Platt R. Risk of acquiring antibiotic-resistant bacteria from prior room occupants. *Arch Intern Med.* 2006;166(18):1945–1951.

39. Siegel JD, Rhinehart E, Jackson M, Chiarello L, Healthcare Infection Control Practices Advisory Committee. Guideline for isolation precautions: preventing transmission of infectious agents in healthcare settings 2007. Available at: www.cdc.gov/ ncidod/dhqp/gl_isolation.html. Accessed November 8, 2007.

40. Siegel JD, Rhinehart E, Jackson M, Chiarello L, Healthcare Infection Control Practices Advisory Committee. Management of multidrug-resistant organisms in healthcare settings, 2006. Available at: http://0-www.cdc.gov.mill1.sjlibrary.org/ncidod/dhqp/ pdf/ar/mdroGuideline2006.pdf. Accessed November 8, 2007.

41. Van Trijp MJ, Melies DC, Hendriks WD, Parlevliet GA, Gommans M, Ott A. Successful control of widespread methicillin-resistant *Staphylococcus aureus* colonization and infection in a large teaching hospital in the Netherlands. *Infect Control Hosp Epidemiol.* 2007 Aug;28(8):970–975. Epub 2007 Jun 19.

42. Vos MC, Ott A, Verbrugh HA. Successful search-and-destroy policy for methicillin-resistant *Staphylococcus aureus* in The Netherlands [letter]. *J Clin Microbiol.* 2005;43(4):2034.

43. Jones RN. Microbiological features of vancomycin in the 21st century: minimum inhibitory concentration creep, bactericidal/static activity, and applied breakpoints to predict clinical outcomes or detect resistant strains. *Clin Infect Dis.* 2006;42(suppl 1):S13–S24.

44. Wang G, Hindler JF, Ward KW, Bruckner DA. Increased vancomycin MICs for *Staphylococcus aureus* clinical isolates from a university hospital during a 5-year period. *J Clin Microbiol.* 2006 Nov;44(11):3883–3886. Epub 2006 Sep 6.

Address correspondence to Priya Sampathkumar, MD, Division of Infectious Diseases, Mayo Clinic, 200 First St SW, Rochester, MN 55905 (sampathkumar.priya@mayo.edu).

From *Mayo Clinic Proceedings,* December 2007. Copyright © 2007 by Dowden Health Media. Reprinted by permission.

The Noisy Epidemic
Physical and Mental Stress in a High-Decibel World

Elizabeth Svoboda

After physician Louis Hagler retired, he set himself a single goal: to learn to play the piano. He bought himself a wooden upright and vowed to crank out scales and chord progressions every day at his home in Richmond, California.

But as Doctor Hagler embarked on his self-teaching regimen, he encountered an unexpected obstacle. "I lived close to a railway crossing, and slow-moving freight trains would constantly be coming through," he says. The blast of train horns was so deafening that he could scarcely concentrate or hear the notes his fingers were striking. "And it wasn't just train horns," he says. "There were boom cars on the streets that were noisy beyond belief."

Doctor Hagler's frustration set him thinking about the impact of excessive noise on the world around him. If train noise stopped him from learning to play piano, a relative luxury, what about children trying to learn in schools next to fire stations, or singles trying to converse with future spouses in bars blaring heavy metal music?

When Doctor Hagler began his in-depth research on noise (published last spring in the *Southern Medical Journal*), he found that study after study confirmed his worst suspicions: Excessive noise made people more violent and aggressive, increased their risk of heart problems and sleep deficits, decimated their productivity, and impaired their ability to learn. In short, unwanted noise degraded almost every aspect of their lives.

But if noise is a blight on society, it's largely an ignored one, and Doctor Hagler realizes this can make the political will for change elusive. Most people don't think of loud sounds as harmful. Rock concerts and demolition derbies are embraced as exciting; noise is viewed as a backdrop of life with no consequences for mental or physical health. It is an awareness gap that Doctor Hagler and other anti-noise crusaders are now trying to close. "In 1964, the Surgeon General came out and said smoking was bad, but it took years for people to do anything about it," he says. "Now we know secondhand noise is as bad for us as secondhand smoke."

Noise and Violence

Two years ago, Nashid Muhammad shot Ronnie Rose in the parking lot of a Cincinnati, Ohio, gas station after a dispute involving loud music from Muhammad's car stereo. When Rose asked Muhammad to turn down the stereo, the two began arguing. Rose shut the car door on Muhammad's leg, and Muhammad responded by shooting him twice in the chest. Rose died almost immediately.

Would the confrontation ever have escalated if Muhammad had kept his music turned down? It's impossible to say for sure, but studies linking noise and aggression suggest skirmishes like this are far from coincidental. Russell G. Geen and Eugene McCown, psychologists at the University of Missouri, exposed male subjects to loud and unpleasant noises, then allowed them to give other subjects electrical shocks. The participants exposed to uncontrollable noise gave their partners shocks that were unusually long in duration. This indicated that the noise had raised their aggressive hackles, making them more prone to lash out at others.

Reactions like these don't surprise Ron Czapala, head of Kentucky's chapter of Noise Free America. "Having to put up with boom cars and loud mufflers every day can make you a little crazy," Czapala says. "There's an increasing number of people becoming violent as a result of excessive noise." New reports of noise-induced foul play hit Czapala's inbox almost every day. Stuart Holt of Lancashire, England, was recently stabbed after leaving the volume on his stereo system cranked up for hours on end. Prince Ernst-August of Hanover, husband of Monaco's Princess Caroline, beat the owner of a nightclub in Kenya because he was so enraged by the loud music blaring from inside.

Our evolutionary roots may make us prone to respond violently to excessive noise. Whenever we're presented with an impulse we see as threatening, our immediate instinct is to retaliate. "The body reacts to noise with a 'fight or flight' response," Doctor Hagler says. In other words, we're genetically primed to react to weed whackers and backyard boom boxes the same way we would to robbers or wild animal intruders.

Noise and Well-Being

Anger is just one facet of the noise-induced "fight or flight" response. When a glass unexpectedly shatters or a Vespa screeches by, our bodies respond with an array of hormonal, nervous, and vascular changes. Blood pressure and heart rate peak, arteries and veins constrict, and levels of stress-related hormones like epinephrine and cortisol spike.

When we experience these physiological changes repeatedly over long periods, our health can suffer. Stefan Willich, an epidemiologist at Berlin's Charite University Medical Center, found that people exposed to chronic noise were more likely to have heart attacks. He interviewed more than 2,000 heart attack survivors from thirty-two Berlin hospitals and asked them to rate their exposure to noise over the course of recent years, then compared their histories with those of non-heart attack sufferers. Male patients exposed to excessive environmental noise had a 50 percent increased risk of heart attack, and female patients who fit the same description had a 300 percent increased risk. The risk was greatest for people who regularly experienced noise above the sixty-decibel threshold—about the level of background noise in a busy mid-sized office.

Some researchers believe that noise can produce social and behavioral consequences, a fact they are still trying to test and quantify. No direct association between noise and mental illness has yet been found; because psychiatric conditions are the result of genetic and environmental factors operating in concert, analyzing each case to determine what role noise might have played is a tall order. Still, a number of population studies have shown that people living in noisy areas tend to report lower levels of well-being, take more psychoactive drugs, and experience more sleep disturbances. All of these factors could put them at risk of developing mental disorders.

Excessive noise made people more violent and aggressive, increased their risk of heart problems and sleep deficits, decimated their productivity, and impaired their ability to learn.

Excessive noise can adversely affect happiness and productivity even if listeners don't end up in mental hospitals. A steady background thrum—like the drone of riveters at a construction site or the thunder of planes overhead—can put those experiencing the racket on edge and distract them from their daily responsibilities. Arline Bronzaft, a professor emeritus of psychology at Lehman College, helps field 350,000 noise-related complaints per year as chair of the noise committee of New York City's Council on the Environment. "When I take calls, I often have to calm people down because they're so distressed and angry about what's going on," she says. Gary Evans, an environmental psychologist at Cornell University, found that workers in noisy surroundings made forty-four percent fewer attempts to solve difficult puzzles than their counterparts in quiet offices. This may be because ever-present noise generates psychological stress that dampens motivation and scuttles the focus needed to finish a task.

Noise and Learning

Whenever she watched her grandson play, Bronzaft grew more certain that neighborhood noise was nipping his learning and concentration skills in the bud. "The family lived near La Guardia airport, and every time a plane came by, he'd hold his ears," she says. "Every plane stopped him from what he was doing." When the perceived threat had passed, he'd go back to his toys and books. But he remained ultra-sensitive to outside stimuli, as though decibel bombardment had made him overly vigilant.

Bronzaft established a broader correlation between noise and learning problems when she and colleague Dennis McCarthy tested the reading ability of two groups of children at New York's Public School 88. One group of students was assigned to classrooms on the "quiet side" of the building, and the other group was on the "noisy side," where elevated trains whizzed by every four minutes. "By the sixth grade, kids on the noisy side of the school were about a year behind in reading," Bronzaft says. "When the trains went by, they were so loud that the teachers actually had to stop teaching." Like Bronzaft's grandson, the students would take several minutes to regain their focus after such an intrusion, resulting in thousands of lost minutes of instructional time each year.

Dozens of studies in classrooms all over the world have since confirmed Bronzaft's theory that noise intrudes on children's learning. Gary Evans, a professor of design and human development at Cornell University, recently uncovered one possible explanation for these detrimental effects. He found that children in noisy classrooms typically responded to the racket by tuning out speech in addition to other, less relevant, sources of sound. When children become used to noise, Evans explains, they don't just tune out the sound of cars and airplanes—they tune out everything else as well, which affects their reading and language development.

Bronzaft's story had a happy ending. She was able to persuade New York transit authorities to install rubber pads on train tracks near the school to cushion some of the noise, and school officials also approved the construction of acoustical ceilings in the noisiest classrooms. "The classrooms were six to eight decibels quieter after that," she says. "Eventually, both sides of the school had the same reading scores." But she worries about all the schools nationwide that aren't taking precautions to protect students from noise. "Children need to learn to sit back, think, and reflect in order to have new ideas. To get that result, you have to foster quiet."

What Are the Solutions?

Doctor Hagler describes noise as an "unwanted airborne pollutant," and though that description would strike many Americans as too strident, officials in many European Union countries agree with his assessment. The EU has seized the initiative in developing a governmental plan to combat noise, mandating that all European cities with populations over 250,000 assemble digital maps spotlighting where environmental noise is worst. After these hot spots are identified, local authorities will be better able to implement anti-noise measures like diverting train and automobile traffic away from schools and residential areas.

The U.S. government has shown no signs of following suit. Though the U.S. Environmental Protection Agency boasted an Office of Noise Abatement and Control back in the 1970s, it was shut down two decades ago for lack of funding. Though EPA spokesman John Millet admits it's hard to argue with research

Getting an 'Earful'

Decibels measure sound intensity, while "loudness" is subjective for different individuals. Federal rules urge that workdays inflict no more than an average of 85 decibels on workers.

	Decibels	Range
Sound Studio, Rustling Leaves	20	20–40 Very Quiet
Library, Soft Whisper	30	
Living Room, Quiet Office	40	40–60 Moderate Quiet
Light Traffic, Average Home	50	
Air Conditioner, Conversation	60	60–80 Moderate Loud
Noisy Café, Office, or Street Traffic	70	
Vacuum, Alarm Clock, Shouting, Fast Automobile	80	80–100 Very Loud
Heavy Truck, City Traffic, Noisy Bar	90	
Firecracker, Subway, Power Lawnmover, Walkman	100	100–120 Uncomfortable
Rock Concert, Discotheque	110	
Jet Takeoff	120	120–140 Deafening
Thunderclap	130	130 Pain Threshold
Rocket Launch	160	160 Perferation of Ear Drum

that demonstrates noise's impact on physical and mental health, he fears funding for national noise-control measures will not be forthcoming unless the public demands them.

That's the crux of the problem, according to Doctor Hagler. Most people aren't aware of noise's detrimental effects, so they're not inclined to demand change—they'd rather see government funds going to solve other problems that are seen as more pressing. "We have a history in this country of being slow to recognize health effects, and once we recognize them, we are slow to respond," he says. "The lightbulbs will go on slowly. There's not going to be a quick fix." And it's a mistake to expect boombox and motorcycle owners to have an innate sense of civic responsibility, he adds. "We no longer live in a society where good manners count, where being thoughtful is automatic—it's an I-Me-Mine-Now way of looking at life. But we all own the air, and none of us has the right to ruin it for anyone else."

Since the federal government isn't likely to budge on the noise issue anytime soon, anti-noise crusaders may end up tallying their most significant victories at the local level for the foreseeable future. After New York City received a record number of noise complaints in 2006, for instance, mayor Michael Bloomberg passed a new noise code that placed specific restrictions on noisy stereos, air conditioners, and car alarms.

Doctor Hagler's battle against excessive noise in Richmond was successful from a legislative point of view. He and other concerned citizens persuaded the town government to pass an ordinance stating that train horns would not be used in the area if other safety precautions were taken. But it was a Pyrrhic victory. Long before the law was passed, Doctor Hagler got so fed up with the constant noisy blasts that he and his wife moved to a quieter neighborhood in the Oakland Hills. "You still hear the kids coming out of school, and occasionally, you get motorcycles screaming down the road with after-market pipes," he says. "But things are much better." He's even starting to regain his enthusiasm for learning to play the piano.

ELIZABETH SVOBODA is a writer living in San Jose, California.

From *Science & Spirit*, January/February 2008. Copyright © 2008 by Heldref Publications. Reprinted by permission.

Test-Your-Knowledge Form

We encourage you to photocopy and use this page as a tool to assess how the articles in *Annual Editions* expand on the information in your textbook. By reflecting on the articles you will gain enhanced text information. You can also access this useful form on a product's book support website at *http://www.mhcls.com*.

NAME: DATE:

TITLE AND NUMBER OF ARTICLE:

BRIEFLY STATE THE MAIN IDEA OF THIS ARTICLE:

LIST THREE IMPORTANT FACTS THAT THE AUTHOR USES TO SUPPORT THE MAIN IDEA:

WHAT INFORMATION OR IDEAS DISCUSSED IN THIS ARTICLE ARE ALSO DISCUSSED IN YOUR TEXTBOOK OR OTHER READINGS THAT YOU HAVE DONE? LIST THE TEXTBOOK CHAPTERS AND PAGE NUMBERS:

LIST ANY EXAMPLES OF BIAS OR FAULTY REASONING THAT YOU FOUND IN THE ARTICLE:

LIST ANY NEW TERMS/CONCEPTS THAT WERE DISCUSSED IN THE ARTICLE, AND WRITE A SHORT DEFINITION:

We Want Your Advice

ANNUAL EDITIONS revisions depend on two major opinion sources: one is our Advisory Board, listed in the front of this volume, which works with us in scanning the thousands of articles published in the public press each year; the other is you—the person actually using the book. Please help us and the users of the next edition by completing the prepaid article rating form on this page and returning it to us. Thank you for your help!

ANNUAL EDITIONS: Health 10/11

ARTICLE RATING FORM

Here is an opportunity for you to have direct input into the next revision of this volume.
We would like you to rate each of the articles listed below, using the following scale:

1. **Excellent: should definitely be retained**
2. **Above average: should probably be retained**
3. **Below average: should probably be deleted**
4. **Poor: should definitely be deleted**

Your ratings will play a vital part in the next revision.
Please mail this prepaid form to us as soon as possible.
Thanks for your help!

RATING	ARTICLE	RATING	ARTICLE
	1. Are Bad Times Healthy?		26. Is Pornography Adultery?
	2. The Perils of Higher Education		27. 'Diabesity,' a Crisis in an Expanding Country
	3. We Can Do Better—Improving the Health of the American People		28. Sex, Drugs, Prisons, and HIV
			29. The Battle Within: Our Anti-Inflammation Diet
	4. On the Road to Wellness		30. Who Still Dies of AIDS and Why
	5. Redefining Depression as Mere Sadness		31. A Mandate in Texas
	6. Stressed out Nation		32. Pharmacist Refusals: A Threat to Women's Health
	7. Seasonal Affective Disorder		33. Curbing Medical Costs
	8. Dealing with the Stressed		34. Thanks, but No Thanks
	9. Fat City		35. The Silent Epidemic—The Health Effects of Illiteracy
	10. Eating Well on a Downsized Food Budget		36. Incapacitated, Alone and Treated to Death
	11. Suck on This		37. Dentists Frown at Overuse of Whiteners
	12. An Oldie Vies for Nutrient of the Decade		38. Medical Tourism: What You Should Know
	13. What Good Is Breakfast?		39. Caution: Killing Germs May Be Hazardous to Your Health
	14. A Big-Time Injury Striking Little Players' Knees		40. Tattoos: Leaving Their Mark
	15. The Skinny Sweepstakes		41. Hazardous Health Plans
	16. Dieting on a Budget		42. When Government Makes Us Sick
	17. "Fat Chance"		43. From Smoking Boom, A Major Killer of Women
	18. Great Drug, but Does It Prolong Life?		44. Sound the Alarm? A Swine Flu Bind
	19. Some Cold Medicines Moved Behind Counter		45. Chemical in Plastic Bottles Fuels Science, Concern—and Litigation
	20. Drinking Too Much, Too Young		46. HIV Apathy
	21. The Changing Face of Teenage Drug Abuse— The Trend toward Prescription Drugs		47. Methicillin-Resistant *Staphylococcus aureus*: The Latest Health Scare
	22. Helping Workers Kick the Habit		48. The Noisy Epidemic: Physical and Mental Stress in a High-Decibel World
	23. Scents and Sensibility		
	24. Love at the Margins		
	25. Girl or Boy? As Fertility Technology Advances, So Does an Ethical Debate		

NO POSTAGE
NECESSARY
IF MAILED
IN THE
UNITED STATES

BUSINESS REPLY MAIL
FIRST CLASS MAIL PERMIT NO. 551 DUBUQUE IA

POSTAGE WILL BE PAID BY ADDRESSEE

McGraw-Hill Contemporary Learning Series
501 BELL STREET
DUBUQUE, IA 52001

ABOUT YOU

Name   Date
_____

Are you a teacher? ❏ A student? ❏
Your school's name
_____

Department
_____

Address   City   State   Zip
_____

School telephone #
_____

YOUR COMMENTS ARE IMPORTANT TO US!

Please fill in the following information:
For which course did you use this book?
_____

Did you use a text with this ANNUAL EDITION? ❏ yes ❏ no
What was the title of the text?
_____

What are your general reactions to the Annual Editions concept?
_____

Have you read any pertinent articles recently that you think should be included in the next edition? Explain.
_____

Are there any articles that you feel should be replaced in the next edition? Why?
_____

Are there any World Wide Websites that you feel should be included in the next edition? Please annotate.
_____

May we contact you for editorial input? ❏ yes ❏ no
May we quote your comments? ❏ yes ❏ no

NOTES

NOTES

NOTES

NOTES

NOTES

NOTES

NOTES

NOTES

NOTES